W9-AJU-905

Dear
PLAYBOY
ADVISOR

Dear PLAYBOY ADVISOR

Questions *from* Men *and* Women *to* *the* Advice Column *of* Playboy Magazine

CHIP ROWE

PLAYBOY PRESS

NEW YORK, NEW YORK • HANOVER, NEW HAMPSHIRE

SPECIAL THANKS TO MICHAEL OSTROWSKI AND LYNN STROM
FOR THEIR ABLE ASSISTANCE, AND TO JAMES R. PETERSEN FOR SETTING THE STANDARD.

For information about permission to reproduce
selections from this book, write to:
Playboy Press / Steerforth Press
25 Lebanon Street
Hanover, New Hampshire 03755

Library of Congress Cataloging-in-Publication Data

Rowe, Chip.
  Dear Playboy advisor : questions from men and women to the advice column
of Playboy magazine / Chip Rowe. — 1st ed.
    p. cm.
  ISBN-13: 978-1-58642-118-2 (alk. paper)
  ISBN-10: 1-58642-118-2 (alk. paper)
  1. Sex customs — United States. I. Title.
HQ18.U5R69 2006
306.70973—dc22

                                2006013064

Alternative Cataloging-in-Publication Data

Rowe, Chip.
Dear Playboy advisor : questions from men and women to the advice column of
Playboy magazine.

Includes material on men-women relations, affairs, anal sex, cars, cigars, contraception, etiquette, "getting hitched," kinky sex, "the married life," masturbation,
oral sex, orgasm, the penis, prostitution, pornography, semen, sex toys, "the
single life," and STDs.

1. Man-woman relationships. 2. Advice columns — Excerpts. 3. Questions
and answers. 4. Sex instruction. 5. Sex customs. 6. Adultery. 7. Anal sex.
8. Contraception. 9. Etiquette. 10. Married people — Sexuality. 11. Single people
— Sexuality. 12. Oral sex. 13. Masturbation. 14. Orgasm. 15. Penis.
16. Pornography. 17. Semen. 18. Sex toys. 19. Adultery. 20. Sexually-transmitted
diseases. I. Title: Playboy Advisor. II. Playboy
(Chicago, Ill.).
HQ18.U5R69 2006
306.7—dc22

FIRST EDITION

CONTENTS

INTRODUCTION

In 1997 the *New York Times* asked me to share the most memorable question I had received in my role as the Playboy Advisor. Here it is:

> Each summer, I drag a recliner into the woods near my house. When I feel horny, I sit in the chair in the nude and spray insect repellent everywhere on my body except my genitals. Is this normal?—*G.B., Fort Lauderdale, Florida*

My response was simple. I asked G.B., "Have you seen any other chairs out there?" If only every letter were so offbeat. Instead, I feel a tinge of anxiety each month as I read through the new batch of reader mail. Will we receive enough questions that we haven't already answered? There's reason to feel insecure. Since the Advisor debuted in September 1960, *Playboy* has published more than 6,500 questions, of nearly 400,000 received. And yet, month after month, the magazine's readers surprise me. This book contains the most interesting, enlightening and entertaining letters of the past decade. I hope my responses can be described the same way, although when I am too flippant, or cross that line between being honest and brutal, I am sure to hear about it. The readers keep me honest, and informed.

To prepare the first column, the editors solicited questions from friends, including whether to wear a tie with tweed, whether the salad is served before or after the entrée and whether one should answer the phone during sex. Sixty-three readers wrote in before the next issue—a rousing response. (The number of letters has been carefully tallied ever since. Today we receive 100 letters and 500 e-mails each month, nearly all of which receive a personal reply.) The wide range of subjects covered in the column—we have promised for 45 years to answer "all reasonable questions, from fashion, food and drink, stereo and sports cars to dating dilemmas, taste and etiquette"—reflects the magazine's belief that a person interested only in sex isn't very interesting. But that policy also leads to ribbing. Jay Leno, for example, once asked on *The Tonight Show*, "Did you ever notice the Playboy Advisor tells you about your love life and your car problems? Do you generally go to the garage and say, 'Clem, I'm bothered by sexual dysfunction'?"

The most interesting part of writing the column is the dialogue that some topics provoke, such as whether masturbation is cheating on your spouse with your hand. About 30 percent of the letters we receive are from women, many of whom pick up their husband's or boyfriend's issues but many of whom subscribe on their own. Their contributions are invaluable. The most common question, without a doubt, is a simple one: Am I normal? Inevitably the answer is yes. Or, at least, you're as normal as you need to be.

Some readers wonder what makes me qualified to be the Playboy Advisor. When I appeared as a guest on *Politically Incorrect* a few years ago, comedian Paul Rodriguez asked this question directly, saying, "Who died and made you Sex God?" No one had to die. Because I am a journalist and not a doctor or academic, I don't presume to know anything. Instead, my skill is that of a perverted reference librarian. I can find someone qualified to answer even the most offbeat question, and I'm not shy about asking. That is what *Playboy* makes me say, anyway. The reality is that I do know everything, and that I am the world's greatest lover.

Thank you to the thousands of readers who have shared their knowledge, experiences and questions over the past four decades, including Barry Manilow, who wrote in 1965 to ask if he should leave his day job to pursue his musical wild oats. (We told him to go for it.) Keep the letters coming.

Another batch of mail has arrived, so it's time to sit in my chair in the woods. You pick up some strange habits at this job.

Chip Rowe
New York City

AFFAIRS

Is it cheating? Ask your spouse.

What is this guy thinking?

I had an affair with a guy for two months, but a girlfriend told me afterward that I did some dumb things when going about it: (1) Since he's married (so am I), he didn't want anyone to see him sign into the motel. So he had me do it. (2) He paid for the room the first time, but thereafter let me do it. (3) He always said he had to hurry home because he felt guilty. He wouldn't even walk out of the room with me. I always checked out by myself. (4) We never went anywhere because he was afraid someone would see us. We would only meet every two weeks, even though we live near each other. (5) After I got home I would e-mail him sweet things but would not hear back from him for days. I know the problems are glaring. But can you tell me, from a man's perspective, what he was thinking?—K.C., Cleveland, Ohio

You wanted romance, he wanted sex, and he got what he wanted. Plus, you picked up the tab. Throw in a massage and an order of wings and you're every man's fantasy. You might do better telling your husband what you want, and asking what he wants, and figuring out together how you can provide for each other, than looking for answers in a motel with a guy who treats you like a prostitute. FYI: He didn't feel guilty, and he had done it before.

She fantasizes about cheating

After we'd fought, I invited my girlfriend over so I could apologize. We ended up having great make-up sex. The thing is, we fell into this weird cheating fantasy. She kept saying things like, "I hope your girlfriend won't mind me sucking your cock right now" and "I can't wait until the next time my boyfriend and I fight, so you can fuck me." It spooked me. If she gets off on the idea of cheating, maybe she has already cheated, or she will. I was hoping that you could give me your take.—M.E., Shelton, Connecticut

If your girlfriend were cheating on you, she wouldn't need to fantasize about it. Encourage her to tell you more of her bad-girl fantasies, then make them happen. Try this: Call her at work at noon and give her a room number at a

nearby motel. Be waiting for her there in a suit. After your quickie, hide her panties. Back at work, she'll think about you every time she shifts in her seat.

Is a cheating employee bad for business?

A woman who has worked for me for 12 years is having an affair with a service technician who visits my shop. Her husband also works for me. I am concerned that if or when she is caught, she and her husband will both quit, which will be bad for my business. I've become involved to the point where I schedule the husband's business trips to coincide with when his wife is over her period so she and the tech can more easily have sex. My questions are: (1) Do you have any statistics that report the outcomes of these situations? (2) Should I be this involved? I am a married man who several years ago also had an affair with this woman, but it ended without anyone knowing.—C.F., Seattle, Washington

Not only did you step in it, you jumped up and down. Unless the woman or the tech calls it quits, this is going to end badly. Do your best to distance yourself; if she wants to cheat, make her work at it like everyone else. When it all goes to hell, hire the technician to replace the husband. Or is he married, too?

Maid to order

I came home early from work and found our new maid on the couch masturbating. When I asked her to explain herself, she walked over, unzipped my pants and gave me a blow job. The next week I faked being sick for three days and went home early on the other two to have sex with the maid. I would fuck her in the afternoon and then fuck my wife at night. But two days ago, out of the blue, my wife fired her. I asked why, but she didn't give me a straight answer. Does she know? I love my wife but miss the maid.—R.B., Phoenix, Arizona

Of course she knows. Didn't you notice the house was a mess?

Is my husband cheating with my sister?

My husband and I hang out with my sister and brother-in-law quite a bit. They have a "nude-only" hot tub. My husband hurt his back and used the tub one afternoon. My sister also was home. When my husband returned he was acting funny. He said, "Nothing happened with your sister." I asked what he was talking about. He said, "Nothing happened, and nothing ever will." I am assuming that something almost happened and he was embarrassed. My sister is constantly talking about my husband. She craves attention, so maybe this is her way of getting it. What do you think is going on here?—J.A., San Diego, California

Here's what we think happened: Your husband arrived at the house, removed his clothes and lowered himself into the tub. Your sister, who has been gauging his reaction to the possibility of an affair, also removed her clothes and climbed into the tub. Your husband felt uncomfortable. Your sister propositioned him and said that if he declined, she would tell you that the two of them had sex. He declined, came home and, as a preemptive strike, assured you that nothing had happened. Your sister needs to be convinced that nothing ever will.

Should I have sex to prevent an affair?

I'm 21 and have been married for a year. I love my husband, but he's the only person I've slept with. There's this hunk at work who wants to fuck me. I don't want to cheat, but I don't know if I'll be able to help myself. Should I have sex with this guy so I can stop thinking about him all the time? And did I make a mistake in getting married so young?—J.M., Wausau, Wisconsin

You think it's tough to resist this guy now? Sleep with him and see how bad it gets. Lusting for people besides your spouse is okay. The marriage changes only how you respond to that lust. Ideally, you'd be able to go home, tell your husband about this hot guy (since he's felt the same way about other women and since he trusts you) then ride that energy into the bedroom. Perhaps he's mature enough to do that, but we doubt your relationship is. In that sense, you married too young.

How many people cheat?

A *Playboy* survey of 1,432 adults found that 75 percent of men and 82 percent of women had never cheated on their partners. Have other surveys found similar numbers? If you watch TV, you'd think only one in five doesn't cheat.—K.I., Sarasota, Florida

Researchers from the University of Chicago interviewed 3,342 adults and found that more than 80 percent of women and 65 percent to 85 percent of men said they had slept with only their spouse while married. The researchers concluded, "No matter how sexually active people are before or between marriages, no matter whether they lived with their partners before marriage or whether they are virgins on their wedding day, marriage is such a powerful social institution that, essentially, married people are nearly all faithful." This is reflected in the finding that half of all adult Americans have three or fewer lovers in their lifetime and in the fact that cheating is usually not what leads couples to divorce. They have bigger problems.

A cheating dream

I am 28 years old and engaged. I have never considered straying and never intend to. However, my fiancée recently told me that she overheard me talking in my sleep. She said it sounded like I was on the phone. I was trying to get someone to come to our apartment because "she doesn't get off work until five." This obviously bothered my fiancée. How can I explain to her that it was just a dream when it seems I subconsciously want to cheat?—B.A., Nashville, Tennessee

Your fiancée isn't sure what to make of this—even if you aren't cheating, what sort of man dreams about it? Every sort of man, of course. That's biology. There's no way to explain this in a way that will satisfy her, but the prospect of committing to sex with one woman for the rest of your life can cause anxiety that seeps out in guilty fantasies. Many women would be relieved to have boyfriends, fiancés and husbands who only dreamed of taking lovers.

Of all the things dreams might be, unconscious yearning doesn't make the list anymore. Dreams are about data mining, pattern recognition, image respooling and verbal reassembly, current feedback, broken snippets of conversation, TV commercials—hell, he might have been repeating something from a radio commercial that he heard on the way to work. Omens and lusts are stuff of romance novels but not dream processes. Next you'll be suggesting that dreams predict the future.—A.K., Fort Myers Beach, Florida

His dream may have been all that and more, but it doesn't resolve the larger dilemma, which is that his fiancée heard him talking in his sleep as if he were cheating. We still believe there's no way to explain this in a way that will satisfy her, regardless of whether he offers your scientific explanation or our Freudian one.

"When are you going to fuck me?"

I am a retired Marine Corps officer now on my second career. An attractive co-worker has made it clear that she would like to have an affair with me. If

I were single, I'd take her out in a second. But I've never cheated on my wife, and I'm not about to start after 25 years of marriage. This woman and her husband have become friends of my wife's as well. The four of us socialize frequently. I want to keep her and her husband as friends. I told her this, but she acted like she hadn't heard me. She just said, "So, when are you going to fuck me? It's inevitable that we'll end up in bed, so why prolong the agony?" I asked my father for advice and he told me to treat her as a professional colleague and stop socializing. But I don't want to piss her off, either. Hell hath no fury. . . . What do you think?—J.C., Tampa, Florida

Father knows best. This woman is no friend. Be polite but firm in your dealings with her. If she propositions you again, follow her lead and act as if you didn't hear. It's a tough cross to bear, being so desirable to women.

Their lying eyes

Can you tell just by looking at someone if he or she is lying?—R.T., Philadelphia, Pennsylvania

Most people aren't accomplished enough liars to conceal their guilt. Former FBI profiler Jack Trimarco says you should be suspicious of any person who: (1) changes his usual speech patterns—a person may also pause as he invents a lie or repeat the question to buy time; (2) subconsciously lowers his voice because he's ashamed of the lie he's about to deliver; (3) denies specifics, such as insisting she didn't cheat with the neighbor because the guy actually lives three doors down; (4) remains calm while working hard to convince you that you're mistaken—an innocent person is more likely to grow angry, and his denials to grow stronger; (5) changes the subject; (6) displays conflicting verbal and nonverbal behaviors, such as saying no while nodding yes; (7) changes her story over time ("A lie is hard to remember, while the truth is easy," Trimarco says); (8) avoids eye contact. Someday you may not need intuition to ferret out untruths. A few British insurance companies use voice-analysis software to identify people who call in with false claims (about 10 percent are identified as suspicious), and scientists are scanning the brains of volunteers to see if they can identify which areas light up when a lie is told.

Pool party

I have been dating the same woman for 10 years. We live in different states but see each other as often as we can. The other night I called her at 12:15 A.M., but she didn't answer. The next morning she told me she had gone to a neighbor's pool party and gotten home at midnight. I investigated and heard from one of her female neighbors that my girlfriend had sex with the host and his brother next to the pool. In fact, this neighbor had filmed the whole thing from her window and sent me the tape. When I confronted my girlfriend, she played dumb, saying she remembered the neighbor hitting on her but nothing else. We even went to a hypnotist, but he couldn't help. Should I believe her?—*G.A., Warren, Michigan*

It hardly matters. The relationship is over. And where was it going anyway?

Falling for my boss

I'm a 43-year-old secretary who's falling in love with her married boss. Until a few months ago he had been all business. But one afternoon he called me "darling" and asked if I was "planning to stick with him." I felt dizzy—a schoolgirl realizing her crush. Since that day, we have engaged in a flirtation that is alternately thrilling and excruciating. We haven't gotten physical, but he has informed me, in a roundabout way, that he's well hung, told me to "plug him in there tight" when I offered to update his planner, let me know that he "loves to give me a hard time" and intimated that he suspects that I have to resort to masturbation after working with him all day. When he drove me home from work, I became wet sitting so close to him. Another time I was taking dictation when I looked up at him and we smiled and stared at each other for half a minute. Is there anything more thrilling than falling in love? I suffered from depression for many years and my only intimate contact with a man was more than 25 years ago, when I was date-raped as a teenager. How can I curtail my randiness before this situation gets out of hand?—L.P., Houston, Texas

Your background reveals more about this situation than anything else. You don't have much more sexual experience than a nun. We both know what your boss is up to, but if his flirtation leads to an affair, it won't end well. The best thing for your emotional well-being is to extract yourself, even if that means finding another job. You deserve a partner who doesn't need to make wisecracks to conceal his lust or betray someone to be with you. It's time you make a serious effort to find a relationship that will move your life forward.

Is it cheating to masturbate together?

A married man whose wife is out of town visits a bar with friends. He strikes up a conversation with an attractive woman. She too is married and her husband is away. They decide to have a nightcap at her place. Although the conversation is somewhat sexual, there is no physical contact. As the evening is winding down, the woman tells the man that she plans to masturbate after he leaves, and that she assumes he will do the same when he arrives home. She suggests they masturbate together. They disrobe and masturbate within sight of each other, but they never touch beyond a chaste kiss as he gathers his clothes to leave. Is this considered cheating?—E.A., The Woodlands, Texas

You bet. The couple shared sexual intimacy, and that meets the definition of adultery even if the participants can't see each other, such as during phone sex or while online. If the guy had returned home to masturbate, he might have escaped on a technicality. But his judgment would still be suspect—married guys generally don't have nightcaps with women they meet in bars.

Seducing married women

I am a single, average-looking businessman in my mid-40s. During the past three years, I have slept with every married woman I have desired. I meet them in supermarkets, bookstores and record shops. I invite them in for coffee and the rest is easy. From these encounters I have observed the following: (1) I have not met a woman whose husband has made love to her properly in the past six months. (2) Many of these women had never had a multiple orgasm. Two had never had orgasms until we went to bed. (3) None of these women experience any major guilt from these encounters. Most feel they are neglected and view our time as luxurious sin. In the meantime, I have collected a casual harem. I am never pushy—they call me. Can you explain why so many married men are such neglectful lovers?—T.G., Los Angeles, California

Because they don't read the Advisor. Your letter sounds like a challenge, and we've just become your worst enemy by publishing it.

You pointed T.G. in the right direction, but let an old stud put it more plainly. He needs serious advice before his swelling head, or something else, bursts. Every woman tells every man that he is the best—that's good manners. What T.G. is hearing is the modern version of "Be gentle, I'm a virgin." After he has each of the women in his "harem" 200 or 300 times and nurses them through a couple of hangovers and some PMS, he will see the situation differently. In the meantime, he asks, "Where are these women's husbands?" Well, son, their husbands are out doing and hearing the same things you are.—D.P., Honolulu, Hawaii

We're sure T.G. isn't listening.

Can my husband be friends with an ex-mistress?

My husband fell in love with another woman and left me and my children. A week later he said that he shouldn't have left and moved back into the house. The woman has moved to another town, but I know they talk on the phone. He argues that they were friends before the affair so they can be friends after. What should I do?—R.R., Cambridge, Massachusetts

Your husband is confused. A mistress is not a college girlfriend. If he's serious about saving your marriage, then he'll hang up the phone and talk to you instead. Your husband can't just move back to the house. He has to move in.

Desperately seeking permission

While drunk, my girlfriend admitted to her best female friend and me that she had a dream in which her friend and I were having sex and she didn't care. After she sobered up I asked her if she actually would care. She said, "Not really." I think her friend may like me. Would it be okay to have sex with her?—M.T., Shippensburg, Pennsylvania

Sorry, but that wasn't enough of a yes—and we have pretty low standards. But you have a good line on a threesome.

Meet me after class

I'm a dance student and part-time instructor. Whenever I dance I get incredibly horny. After class I always end up staying an extra hour to fuck the teacher while my boyfriend waits outside. Even when I teach, my student ends up in me somehow. Is this called something? Is there anything I can do to hold out?—C.T., Bayside, New York

It's called a lack of self-control. Try dancing with your boyfriend. At the very least tell him to pick you up an hour later so you're not wasting any more of his time.

Brotherly love

My husband put an ad on the Internet without my knowledge. It has all his data—height, weight, profession, favorite quotes—but a photo of his brother. He swears it's an ad for his brother, who is in prison, but I didn't know they were even in touch. My husband says he meets women through the ad and gives them money. He says they are interventions but won't explain what that means. He went to Vegas to meet one of these women after telling me he was going to a different city on business. I found out only after he totaled our car. I am convinced he is cheating. He refuses to discuss it and says he is working on getting someone else in the family to take over his brother's ad. What do you think?—K.C., Walnut, California

Not only is your husband cheating on you, he's doing it badly, which is no tribute. You can probably do better for yourself without walking more than 50 feet in any direction.

My dad is cheating with a hooker

I've learned that my father is cheating on my mother with a hooker who meets him at his office. This could ruin not only my parents' marriage but my reputation ("There's the guy whose father cheated on his wife"). What's the best way to end this before my mother finds out?—P.R., New Orleans, Louisiana

Could you pay the hooker more than your father does? Confront him, then mind your own business. (Your concern about your reputation is overblown.) Your father may be scared straight, but it's more likely he'll become more discreet, to the point that you'll no longer know whether he's cheating, which is the way it should be. One of the unfortunate side effects of adultery is that it draws others into the lie.

Wife wants to visit her "best friend"

My wife's best friend is a man. They grew up together and had a couple of intimate moments but never dated. He lives in California. When she e-mails him she begins with a "Hey, baby" and ends with "Love, your girl." This makes me uncomfortable. We call each other baby and I thought she was my girl, legally and emotionally. I haven't asked her to stop because I don't know if I'm blowing this out of proportion. She wants to fly to California to spend a week with the guy, whom she hasn't seen in 10 years. Please help.—C.G., Atlanta, Georgia

You're right to be suspicious. It's okay for your wife's best friend to be a guy, as long as that guy is you. You can't stop her from going to California, or flirting with her old buddy, but you can let her know it's damaging her marriage. Then she'll decide.

Advisor, your response was too harsh. I've had several strictly platonic relationships with women. In each case, once the boyfriend or husband found out, every one of them became jealous, and the woman and I had to break off the friendship even if we'd known each other for years. If the reader can't trust his wife, the trouble is on his end, not hers.—G.M., San Jose, California

Fair enough. But how many of your married female friends write you e-mails signed "Love, your girl" and visit you for a week without hubby?

ANAL

It's the new oral.

Anal 101

I'd like to try anal sex with my wife, but she says it would be too painful. If it's painful, why does anyone do it?—L.J., St. Louis, Missouri

With the right preparation and care, anal sex can provide immense pleasure for a woman. The anus and vulva share major nerves, and penetration may provide enough indirect pressure to stimulate her G-spot. "Anal sex shouldn't hurt even a little bit," says Tristan Taormino, author of The Ultimate Guide to Anal Sex for Women. *"Start with your pinkie and a lot of lube. Then work up slowly. Try a finger, then two, then a slim butt plug. This progression doesn't have to happen in one night." Plus, she says, "Anal sex can also build intimacy. The woman might find herself thinking, We worked up to this and I trust this guy. As for men, it's in their best interest to make sure their lovers experience only pleasure from anal sex. A woman's butt will remember pain for a long time."*

Emotional breakdown

I've been with my boyfriend for eight months. The relationship is wonderful and the sex is awesome. The other night we engaged in anal sex, which we have both done before, but this time I had a total emotional breakdown. My orgasm was accompanied by a crying episode so intense it took us both by surprise. Everything was great and I didn't experience pain, but the tears came in buckets. Can you tell me if this is a normal reaction or why it happened?—T.G., Memphis, Tennessee

It's nothing to worry about. We carry more stress than we realize in our sphincters. Penetration requires the muscles to relax, and the tension can dissipate in ways that surprise us. Annie Sprinkle calls this emotional release a crygasm. "I've talked to so many women who tell me that when making love or having an orgasm they have a little cry at the same time," she says. "It feels so good." There was a time when lovers were expected to cry. "Eighteenth century novels are full of scenes that suggest or, in a few cases, represent orgasm with tears as the most sublime experience possible," notes historian Tom Lutz, author of Crying: The

Natural and Cultural History of Tears. *"Weeping in love was considered the norm, and a lover who couldn't weep wasn't worth having."*

Adventures in butt-kissing

I've been licking women's asses for more than 30 years. It started with my wife. We were in a 69 and I found her cute ass inches from my nose. Later we became swingers, and I tongued dozens of women. (A buddy once persuaded an uptight librarian he was dating to let him try anilingus; before long she was showing up at all hours saying, "Get on your knees, you disgusting pervert, and lick my ass like a good boy.") When licking a woman's ass, it is important to be as hygienic as possible. Use an antibacterial soap to prepare, and never lick her ass and then move to her pussy. After you've finished, wash your mouth with antibacterial soap, then gargle with mouthwash and warm water. For best results, put a bit of Vaseline and a mild skin rub that contains menthol on your tongue (but again, don't go near her pussy). If you want to see something erotic, watch women lick each other. We were at an orgy once when one woman bet another that she couldn't lick her own pussy. She lost the bet and, as a result, had to lick the woman's asshole. They put on quite a show. The other females oohed and aahed. The men were mostly silent.—W.R., Lehigh Valley, Pennsylvania

You know you're at a hot party when anilingus is the icebreaker.

Shit doesn't happen

I haven't been able to nuzzle up to a butthole since my undergraduate studies in microbiology (I'm now in med school), when I learned that one gram of feces contains 100 million bacteria and that fecal matter is 60 percent bacteria. In addition, hepatitis A and other nasties are commonly transmitted via oral-fecal contact (which doesn't necessarily mean ass licking but rather eating contaminated food, such as from a salad bar, but I suppose with anilingus one bypasses the salad). To the old coot who wrote to boast that he had given his old lady anilingus for 25 years: Think about all this the next time you kiss your grandchildren.— B.N., Lincoln, Nebraska

Rimming does have risks. When you lick an anus, even an enema-clean anus, you may ingest trace amounts of feces. That's the reason God created barriers such as dental dams, plastic wrap, unlubed condoms cut lengthwise and the fingers of

latex gloves—*she wants us to stay safe while enjoying the amusement park of nerves around the butthole. "With rimming you're not going that far into the rectum, so sticking a soapy finger up there before your anal date is going to take care of most of the fecal matter and bacteria," says Tristan Taormino. "Lots of people have been licking lots of buttholes for lots of years, yet we haven't seen widespread E. coli outbreaks. This student is joining rimming and fecal matter when the two don't necessarily happen at the same time." We'd add that your comment about the "old coot" is too judgmental for us or for the medical profession in general. By your reasoning, you shouldn't offer your hand to shake if you've ever wiped your ass with it.*

Does anal sex make you gay?

My wife and I were in a 69 when she began to lick my asshole. I was a little surprised, but it felt great. She told me to position myself on all fours while she retrieved her vibrating dildo. What could I say? After teasing my balls and anus, she pushed it slowly into my ass. As she pushed it in and out, she began giving me head. She asked me what I thought of being butt-fucked; I had to admit I loved it. Does this mean I might be gay?—E.C., Sacramento, California

Sliding a finger, sex toy, corncob or any other object into your butt doesn't make you gay. Being gay makes you gay. Write again if you start fantasizing that Tom Cruise is holding the dildo. When we receive letters like this, we recommend the instructional video Bend Over, Boyfriend *(goodvibes.com, or 800-289-8423). Its producer and star, Carol Queen, points out that anal play is a great way for a man "to explore the various ways he can be sexual and climax without his cock being touched." During one of the film's demonstrations, she tells her antsy partner, "Wait a minute. I want to fuck you, and then you can fuck me back."*

Does anal sex make you loose?

My husband's anal techniques are beyond wonderful; the sensations he provides me are becoming an addiction. There's one problem: I think my sphincter is getting loose. After intercourse it feels relaxed for about an hour. This never happened in my early anal days (I can't believe I just wrote that). Can you help?—N.A., Tucson, Arizona

No need. What you're feeling is normal. You've had enough experience with anal sex that you've learned to release the tension we carry around in our butts. An hour sounds about right for your anus to return to its naturally puckered state.

The male G-spot

I received an e-mail that promised to reveal the location of the male G-spot for $25. My husband is chomping at the bit. Is there such a spot and how do we find it?—M.E., San Ramon, California

Save your money. The male G-spot, better known as the prostate gland, is a mystical place beneath your husband's balls. To find it, insert your index finger about 1.5 inches into his anus and make a come-hither motion against the front wall of his rectum. He may have had a doctor do this during an exam, but it's quite a different sensation when you're highly aroused, the finger belongs to your wife and insurance companies aren't involved. Suzi Godson, in The Sex Book, *offers further instruction. Have your husband lie on his back. While stroking his cock, press gently but firmly on the area between his balls and anus to stimulate the prostate from the outside. As you slide your latex-gloved, lubed finger into his anus, his sphincter will twitch. This may feel uncomfortable for your husband, but after about 30 seconds the spasms will stop. Caress his prostate gently. He may feel the urge to urinate (but won't). If he can speak, ask him what motions feel best. As he approaches orgasm, his sphincter will tighten and the gland will swell. Because it supplies part of the fluid that makes up his come, the gland will contract as he ejaculates. When you remove your finger, your husband will deflate.*

Anal surprise

While making love with my girlfriend, she inserted a finger into my rectum and rotated it. I had the most intense orgasm I've ever experienced. Is there a reason for this, or did the shock of feeling her finger in my ass just catch me by surprise?—B.T., Leeds, England

It's always refreshing to meet an anal-inventive woman. Your lover has learned somewhere (probably from being on the receiving end) that the anus is filled with nerve endings and becomes engorged and aroused during intercourse just as genitals do. We suggest using a water-based lubricant if you plan to return the favor, and make sure to trim your fingernails, as the interior of the rectum is delicate. Cathy Winks and Anne Semans, authors of The Good Vibrations Guide to Sex, *offer this guidance: After applying a lubricant, "circle your finger around the soft folds of anal tissue. Many people find that gentle stroking of the anal opening is all the anal stimulation they desire. If your partner becomes sufficiently relaxed, she or he may bear down and slide right onto your finger. Your fingertip should reach toward the front of the body rather than crook up toward the tailbone. The sphincter muscles may tense up automatically as soon as you enter, so hold your finger still at first until the anus relaxes around it. Then feel free to insert your finger deeper, exploring the outer rectum. You can circle your finger, tap and stroke the walls of the rectum or move your finger gently in and out."* If your partner has never experienced anal penetration, don't be surprised if she or he finds the sensation unsettling when you first slide in. By the way, Winks and Semans also advise that you *"take the time to look at your partner's anus. You may be surprised at how sweet and innocent it looks—not like an 'ass-hole' at all."* That changes everything: What are we supposed to yell at bad drivers?

Should I bleach my anus?

The skin around my asshole is sort of brown. My boyfriend says it's normal, but he's just trying to make me feel better. I am a very clean person. Is there a way to make my anus go back to its natural pink? I've heard you can bleach it.—L.T., Houston, Texas

We never imagined we'd write these words in the Advisor, but here they are: Do not bleach your anus. Despite rumors that asshole brightening is the latest Hollywood craze, it's a stunt that belongs in the next Jackass *movie, not in your bedroom. Your boyfriend is right. Brown is your natural color, although your anus may appear more pink when you're aroused.*

Bleaching is crazy. Instead, leave some petroleum jelly down there. After three days your anus will look and feel much lighter and cleaner.—L.L., San Jose, California

And you'll be prepared should any spontaneous butt fucking break out.

Honey, have you seen my vibrator?

My girlfriend wants to experiment with anal penetration, but I've heard stories about embarrassing trips to the emergency room because of "misplaced" sex toys. How can we be sure things don't get stuck?—J.H., Los Angeles, California

Be very, very careful. If that vibrator or butt plug doesn't have a flange, or rim, think long and hard before sticking it in anyone's bum, no matter how good you think it might feel. If there is an accident, don't hesitate to visit the emergency room, and be honest when you get there. The doctors on duty have seen it all, evidenced by their habit of sharing outrageous pelvic X rays with medical journals. Besides dildos and vibrators, physicians have removed screwdrivers, artillery shells, curling irons, spatulas, baseballs, flashlights, candles, vegetables, a polyethylene waste trap from the U-bend of a sink, sewing needles, salami and shampoo bottles. For God's sake, people, there's no shame in buying and using toys designed for anal pleasure. It's certainly safer than grabbing whatever's handy.

AURAL
Stop, look, listen.

How can I make my boyfriend scream?

I'd like to make my boyfriend scream during sex. I get low growls and the occasional "Oh, yeah," but I want him to yell stuff like "Yeah, baby!" or "Faster!" What can I do better?—J.L., Seattle, Washington

It's not you. Few people outside porn are screamers, though they always seem to live next door. The only reliable way to make a guy yell in bed is to grab his balls and pull. The best you can do otherwise is provide pleasant surprises—finger his ass while you blow him, lick his ass while you stroke him, do your Kegel exercises and squeeze his erection like a pump. He'll probably just moan louder, but he'll owe us a big favor.

I like to hear about his ex-girlfriends

My boyfriend is 37, and I'm 23. When we're in bed, I like for him to pretend I'm someone from his past. I ask him first to give me details, such as how one of his ex-girlfriends liked to be fucked or who had the tightest pussy or the biggest tits. Then I pretend I'm her. While the sex is great, he is sometimes reluctant to do this, saying he just wants me to be me. I want him to do it every time we have sex, and I'm worried he'll get bored with it. He says he's never had any lover who wanted to play this game, but I am much younger and full of curiosity. Is this normal?—E.P., Carpentersville, Illinois

He's already bored. Your curiosity is understandable, but there is something to be said for being yourself. Role-playing once in a while is fun, but you're not learning anything about yourself or him by constantly revisiting old ground. The question you should be asking is, What did each of your exes do that turned you on? Gather some intelligence, then mix their best moves with your own and give him something to remember you by.

What does he mean, "talk to me"?

My girlfriends and I were discussing this during a girls' night out: When you are having sex with a guy and he says "talk to me," what is it he wants to hear?—N.C., Des Moines, Iowa

That's an easy one. He wants a pause in the lovemaking to analyze the strengths and weaknesses of your relationship, dissect a scandalous conversation you overheard at work and confirm that one of your girlfriends is indeed making a mistake by not inviting her mother's cousin's wife to her baby shower. Please. A guy who makes that request wants you to talk dirty. He wants to know he's turning you on. He wants you to tell him what feels good, why it feels good, how he can continue to make you feel good and what you're thinking about doing to make him feel good. He wants you to make demands—"Fuck me, now." He wants you to be overcome with desire: "Oh my God, that feels so good!" Turn off the sound during a porn movie and notice how quickly it goes from erotic to uninspired. That's because the female performers are accomplished actors—at least during the sex scenes. They moan, groan, coax, reassure, respond, plead and command. Some pretend to be aroused, some are aroused, some become aroused by talking as if they're aroused. There's a lesson in that. There are many formulas to talking dirty, and not all of them involve explicit language. In her guide to erotic talk, Exhibitionism for the Shy, *Carol Queen suggests an exercise: Describe what's happening. It may start simply—"You're kissing my neck, you're tugging at my nipples . . ."—but it always becomes more heated as you progress.*

Love noises

My girlfriend and I often stay with friends on weekend trips. This past weekend the walls were so thin I could hear the clock ticking one floor down. In this situation is it rude to make "fun noises"? Keep in mind that there is no way for us to be quiet. We have a good time and like to hear it. The bed will rock, the floor will creak, the windows will rattle.—R.W., Chicago, Illinois

You obviously don't have kids. If you tend to fuck with volume, why not explore a new sexual frontier by hitting the mute button? First, place a private wager: If either partner makes a noise louder than the ticking of that clock, he or she will pay a fine to be decided by the other. It can be as simple as having to wash the dishes for a week. Then communicate only with facial expressions and by guiding each other's hands. You'll find that fucking in silence slows everything down—it's hard to thrust like a madman when you can't make squishing noises. You'll also look into each other's eyes longer and pay closer attention to breathing and body language. Each moan that escapes will sound like a trumpet. Trust us, concentrated silence will make you feel like teenagers again, and no one will suspect a thing.

Did I ruin the mood?

My girlfriend is turned off by dirty words. Once I told her, in the heat of passion, that I loved her beautiful ass. Another time I blurted out, "Fuck me!" In both instances she said I had ruined the moment. Can you suggest words we could use in bed that aren't too clinical or crude?—J.S., Manhattan, Kansas

Perhaps you should learn a foreign language. Carol Queen recounts how one of her lovers enjoyed the sound of the French tongue. "I once impelled her to tear my clothes off in the middle of the afternoon by reading aloud to her from a Sabatier kitchen knife brochure." Queen suggests that couples who have a problem with slang—or who prefer English—invent their own bedroom language. She recommends Nicholson Baker's The Fermata *for inspiration and provides an entertaining appendix of erotic words and phrases to expand your vocabulary. As Queen points out, it's not what you say but how you say it. "If your arousal is reflected in your voice, cries of 'Oh, yeah, do that!' or 'Please put your mouth on me now!' can be devastatingly hot, even though you haven't used a single 'dirty' word." Still, there's no substitute for a good "Fuck me!" once in a while (we always add "please"). When you're so turned on you need that pussy, that ass, that mouth or those tits more than your lungs need air, you don't want to fuss with Shakespeare.*

Give me a moan

Why do I get so turned on by listening to my wife as she becomes aroused and then climaxes? My moans and groans don't seem to have the same effect on her.—R.G., Atlanta, Georgia

She's reining you in. Evolutionary biologists suggest a woman's moans are designed to help her control your arousal, increasing her chances of capturing your sperm while minimizing the time she is vulnerable (i.e., that you're on top of her). What little research there is on vocalized sounds made during sex has found that men rate them as more arousing than women do and that women tend to make more of them. The topic screams for more study. For example, does a woman make less noise after her partner has ejaculated? Do the sounds of climax correspond with genital contractions? Scientists have found that people open their mouth more often during sex than during masturbation, which may be a response to the hyperventilation that occurs as they get aroused. Is moaning designed to increase this hyperventilation and improve the high? Perhaps the woman's moans dictate the rhythm of the man's thrusts. Are moans during clitoral stimulation different from those produced by touching the G-spot? Do women make different noises during masturbation? Do they moan less after menopause, when they can no longer become pregnant? Scientists can't rely on anecdotal evidence to answer these questions, but we sure as hell can.

AUTOMOTIVE
The need for speed, and oil changes.

The best car for a ride

Which is the best car for sex?—D.B., Cleveland, Ohio

Short of a limo, a van or a vintage Nash Airflyte (in which the interior seats can be folded down into a bed), having sex in an automobile isn't the most comfortable experience. And yet almost everyone you ask has fond memories. That's because car sex is risky and typically rushed, which makes it exciting. It also forces you to be creative. The British sex columnist Grub Smith once made the keen observation that "the sexier a car appears, the harder it will be to actually have sex in it." He also made note of an exercise known in the U.K. as the hot bonnet, in which the woman leans back or forward over the warm, vibrating hood. Parking brakes on, everyone.

Wife says I have to ask to use 'vette

For her 40th birthday, I bought my wife a 1982 Corvette. We are Corvette nuts—for more than 20 years I've been buying, restoring, selling and maintaining them. I own a 1972 convertible that is my treasure. It's a little tricky to drive, so she had always asked me before she took it. Now the tables have turned. She says I must ask to take her car—the one I bought, maintain, fix, clean, polish and wax. She checks the mileage and last night threw a fit because I had used her car to go to lunch. I sold my Camaro Z-28, my motorcycle and my kid's four-wheeler to get this car for her. I consider myself the leader of the household and I'm not inclined to ask her to drive the car. I recognize that it's hers—her name is on the title—but who's out of line here? I think she's being ungrateful. Frankly, I'm sorry I bought her the car. I am not so sure I don't want her to pack her shit in it and take off.—J.C., Memphis, Tennessee

Didn't we see you on Jerry Springer? *You have a lot of control in the relationship, and your wife sees the car as a way to claim some for herself. So, leader of the household, share the power. Tell your wife you'll ask. Accept her decisions graciously (once she sees you respect her wishes, she may not turn you down often). In the meantime, put aside the idea that you earned chits by cleaning the car, waxing it, etc. You're not doing that for her benefit. Don't make us come down there to straighten this out, because we'll take both cars away.*

How to avoid a ticket

What is the best way to get out of a speeding ticket?—P.L., Spokane, Washington

Let's start with the strategies that don't work. We asked Robert Snow, a police captain who has stopped thousands of motorists in and around Indianapolis, to run through his list: (1) Giving the officer a lame excuse you concocted in the 30 seconds it took him to reach your vehicle's door. "I've heard them all," Snow says. "The brakes failed, though they work now; you were racing home before your tire went flat; a foot spasm made you hit the gas; you were going too fast to stop. The problem with excuses is that they all fall apart with the slightest investigation." (2) Feigning bewilderment. "A stop sign? Where?" Any driver that inattentive or careless deserves a ticket. (3) Blustering about your connections. "Just wait until the mayor/chief/governor hears about this!" A driver with real clout would accept the ticket politely, then get it fixed. (4) Denying the charge, which implies that you consider the officer to be corrupt, blind or stupid. It may not always work, but the best strategy to avoid a ticket is to admit your error. "Only two drivers have ever done that to me," Snow says. "I was so flabbergasted, I sent them on their way."

Standard procedure requires officers to write down relevant comments made during stops, so admitting your guilt may not be wise if you later decide to fight. *Beat Your Ticket*, a guide written by a California lawyer, advises drivers who are stopped to be pleasant but never to admit guilt. You also should be as forgettable as possible—if the officer is honest and can't remember you in court, you win. Furthermore, many officers and prosecutors are as confused by traffic laws as drivers are. Here in Columbus, a posted speed limit of 35 mph is presumed safe. But if an overzealous officer gives you a ticket for going 43 in light traffic on a wide roadway with no pedestrians and clear weather, a judge may decide that your speed wasn't unsafe. (This happened to me.) The law you are accused of violating will be noted on the ticket, so make sure you did what the officer accuses you of doing. You may save yourself money on the fine, insurance and work-related problems if you drive for work.—T.D., Columbus, Ohio

I am a lawyer who used to be a highway patrol officer and traffic-court marshal. Arguing that your speed wasn't unsafe only works in states that have presumed speed limits. Some states have absolute limits—one mile per hour over and you're guilty. Others have absolute limits on freeways but presumed limits elsewhere. As for avoiding a ticket, you should never attempt to manipulate an officer, because it creates resentment. This includes women who shift their clothing to reveal their assets and drivers who threaten to waste the cop's time by calling him to court. He'll just earn overtime for being there.—H.F., Richmond, California

I received a ticket in North Carolina for driving 15 mph over the limit. What would have happened had I not mailed in the $111 fine?—T.C., Royal Oak, Michigan

If you ignore a ticket for a moving violation, it's sent to a judge, who could revoke your license and issue a bench warrant for your arrest, making you a fugitive from traffic justice. If you pay the fine, you're pleading guilty. In either case, the DMV notifies your home state under a reciprocal agreement called the Driver License Compact. If your state also is a member of the Non-Resident Violator Compact, it's obligated to suspend your license until the fine is paid. The last time we checked, only two states (Michigan and Wisconsin) didn't belong to one or the other.

Renting Luxery Cars

Is it possible to rent a Lamborghini? How about a Ferrari?—L.K., San Diego, California

This is America—you can rent anything. Hertz offers Jaguars and Lincolns in 50 cities; Avis has Cadillacs. Beverly Hills Rent-a-Car (bhrentacar.com or 800-479-5996), which supplies the movie industry, will rent you a Rolls Royce convertible or Ferrari Modena 360 Spyder for $3,500, a Lamborghini Diablo VT or Bentley Azure for $2,800, a 1966 Cadillac DeVille for $550, Maserati Spyder GT for $950, or, if you're on a budget, a Hummer H2 for $350, a Jaguar XK8 for $400 or a Porsche Boxster for $300. What it won't do is sell you insurance, meaning you'll need your own coverage (this isn't a good way to practice for your stunt-driver career) and the Beverly Hills agency requires that you have $20,000 free on your credit card to take the priciest cars. Many cities have agencies that specialize in high-end vehicles; search online for "exotic car rental." If you're ready for a *long-term relationship, Exoticcarshare.com (847-358-7522), sells shares in fancy wheels. You can own one-fifth of a Lamborghini Murcielago, for example, for $25,000 plus an annual fee of $15,000, which covers maintenance, insurance, storage and the cost of delivery and pick-up anywhere in the continental U.S. (The company is based near Chicago.) Your share gives you seven weeks alone with the Lamborghini each year—two in the spring, three in the summer and two in the fall. Or pay $60,000 plus the annual fee to own an equity share, which allows you to receive at least $25,000 back when the car is sold after three years.*

How often should I change the oil?

Oil companies, automakers and mechanics say to change your oil every 3,000 miles or three months. I've always thought that was just a ploy to get more business. Am I right?— C.O., San Mateo, California

There's no grand conspiracy; 3,000 miles is considered the minimum for vehicles subjected to "severe driving." That's the industry term for stop-and-go traffic, idling for prolonged periods and short trips. There are other factors to consider, such as climate. If you live in Miami, which has high heat and humidity, or endure the extremes of Chicago, it's wise to have the oil changed by the book. If you live in a milder spot such as southern California, you may be able to go 5,000. If you're using a synthetic oil, you can wait 6,000 to 7,500 miles.

What about the car's other fluids?—A.H., Dallas, Texas

Providing hard and fast rules is difficult because so much depends on the make of your vehicle and how often and how far you drive. MotorWatch.com tried to establish guidelines by creating a chart that outlines intervals for severe and normal driving. It immediately drew criticism from the site's 48-member technical committee, with advisors representing automakers who say the intervals should be longer and mechanics who insist they should be shorter. The guidelines state that drivers who generally make trips of 10 miles or less in each direction should have their coolant/antifreeze changed every two years or 24,000 miles (whichever comes first) with conventional coolant and every three years or 36,000 miles with long-life. Brake fluid should be changed every two years or 24,000 miles on cars with antilock brakes and every three years or 36,000 miles on vehicles without them. Power-steering fluid should be changed every three years or 36,000 miles. Transmission fluid should be changed on automatics every three years or 36,000 miles and every 10 years or 100,000 miles on manuals. If most of your trips are longer, you can wait three years instead of two (or 36,000 miles instead of 24,000), or five years instead of three (60,000 miles instead of 36,000) for fluid changes. If you're driving a mix of short and long distances, the intervals are somewhere in between.

Breaking a lease

Is there any way to get out of an auto lease early?—G.J., Detroit, Michigan

Just ask the dealer nicely. No go? You can post an ad online and hope someone will assume the payments. The two major sites for unloading leases are Swapalease.com, founded in 1999 by a chain of Cincinnati dealerships hoping to turn lessees into buyers, and LeaseTrader.com, created in 1998 by a Miami businessman who didn't want to forfeit $14,000 to dump his Beemer. The services charge $40 to $50 for a basic listing, plus $95 to $150 if you make a transfer. It may help to offer an additional cash incentive or to be unloading a sports car—the five most traded vehicles on LeaseTrader are the BMW 325i, the Audi A4, the Mercedes C230, the Porsche Boxster and the BMW X5. The finance company must approve the deal, but that's usually a rubber stamp. If you're lucky, your freedom will cost only a couple hundred dollars.

How to become a stunt driver

Car commercials on TV always include a disclaimer that reads, "Professional driver. Closed course." How do you become one of these drivers, what is the pay, and is it necessary to become a professional to drive a car for a commercial? —Z.C., Albuquerque, New Mexico

It's harder than it looks. First you'll need a Screen Actors Guild card and a reputation with directors. The former is easier to get than the latter. For the past 20 years Georgia Durante has operated Performance Two, which specializes in providing drivers for TV ads. She says wannabes need to be trained in precision driving at schools such as those run by Bobby Ore, Rick Seaman and Skip Barber. "A big part of the job is keeping pace with the camera car," Durante says. "You see a car traveling down the road and it's serene, but the driver may have been behind a truck holding a camera boom inches over his hood. I had one driver who ducked just as the boom ripped the top off the car." Durante says her drivers all make six figures, with one earning more than $500,000 during a particularly good year. That's in part because they receive residuals each time a commercial airs. To qualify, a driver has to perform a stunt. That can involve executing a controlled

27

skid or jump; having his or her vision impaired by the camera, fog or smoke; or being asked to drive too fast for the conditions. Before you get any bright ideas about instant riches, Wally Crowder, editor of the Stunt Players Directory, *points out that there are already 1,200 professional drivers hungry for work.*

Is it faster to change lanes?

My wife and I commute together and always get stuck in freeway traffic. If a lane adjacent to us is moving faster than the one we're in, I'll switch. My wife says I should sit tight, because everyone is switching and making the fast-moving lanes more congested. Who's right?—T.W., Los Angeles, California

Changing lanes in a traffic jam might save you a few minutes, but most of the time it only increases your risk of being involved in an accident. That causes a big delay for you and everyone behind you. According to researchers armed with computer simulations and videotape evidence, most lane changes in a traffic jam are pointless because the average speed of each lane is the same. But because the speed of each lane isn't constant, and because drivers gauge the speed of adjacent lanes only when they are stopped (i.e., every time you check, you're in the slow lane), one or another lane always appears to be moving faster. We also tend to ignore cars we're passing or have passed (since they leave our vision) and concentrate on those that move ahead of us, creating the illusion that we're falling behind.

How to store your baby

I would like to store my 1971 Chevy Nova for the winter. What should I do before parking it for six months?—B.D., Lakewood, Ohio

We always cry a little. If you're storing the car outside, park it on cement covered with plastic to prevent moisture from reaching the undercarriage. Leave the windows open a quarter inch. Change the filter, oil (use a synthetic), brake fluid and antifreeze. Top off the tank and add a gas stabilizer, then run the engine long enough for the stabilizer to reach the carburetor. Remove the battery (store it on plywood) and use a trickle or solar battery charger. To keep varmints out, close the vents, cover the tailpipe and place mothballs or camphor crystals in and around the vehicle. Inflate the tires to 35 pounds and put the car on jacks. Some people suggest starting it periodically, but that's a bad idea because it leaves moisture in the crankcase and exhaust. Before you revive the car, give it a thorough visual inspection. Then crank the engine with the coil disconnected until the oil light goes off.

Pumping up the gas

Do fuel additives do any good?—M.M., Santa Barbara, California

Sure. Although today's cars are better at keeping the fuel injectors clean, the detergents added by law to gas still help. In fact, these additives are the only thing that distinguish one brand of gas from another. Lately, some oil companies have drastically reduced the amount of detergents in their products, both to save money and supposedly because modern fuel injectors can handle it. That may be true, but some mechanics report increased carbon build-up in other parts of the engine, which affects gas mileage and power. (Carbon problems are often misidentified as a slipped timing belt or bent valve.) Our mechanic suggests using an additive such as Redline SI-1 with each fill-up.

Do radar jammers work?

I have a device in my car that supposedly jams police radar. I've heard that I could be charged with obstruction of justice. Is that true?—S.A., El Paso, Texas

Yes, but in most states that will happen only if a state trooper makes a federal case of it. Jamming or attempting to jam a police speed gun has been a federal crime since 1997, but the feds don't enforce the law. State troopers in Florida and Ohio are the most aggressive about initiating obstruction charges, and California, Colorado, Minnesota, Nebraska, North Carolina, Oklahoma, Utah, Virginia and Washington, D.C., have jammer bans of their own. The larger problem might be finding a jammer that actually works—you can buy legal defusers that foil some laser guns, but any product that claims to block radar is probably bogus. Carl Fors of Speed Measurement Laboratories, which tests products for police agencies, says the latest police laser guns have such short bursts that they're invisible to jammers or detectors.

Restoring a rare Porsche

Do you remember that 1989 Porsche Speedster owned by Nicolas Cage that was stolen and dumped into the Lake of the Ozarks? It had only 100 miles on it. I read the other day that the thief got five years in prison. He ripped out the stereo before pushing the $100,000 black beauty into the drink. The windshield was crushed and the convertible roof was torn half off. Can a Porsche in that condition be restored? Five years wasn't long enough for that punk.—H.T., New York, New York

We tracked the Speedster, one of only 802 made, to Jerry Hawken of Hawken Paint and Body in Osage Beach, Missouri, who bought it from Cage's insurance company. Hawken won't reveal what he paid but says salvage jobs typically run 15 percent to 25 percent of retail. He cleaned off the mud, drained the fluids ("The transmission fluid was like honey") and repaired the suspension. He had the gauges rebuilt, replaced the computer, electrical components and headlights and next plans to straighten the damaged panels and replace the $4,000 windshield. "People see the car and say, 'What a shame,'" he says, "but I'm optimistic. And I have a clean title signed by Nicolas Cage."

How is fuel efficiency determined?

How do automakers determine fuel efficiency? The numbers seem precise, but I've found a lot of variance with my car.—J.K., Chicago, Illinois

As they say, your mileage may vary. Automakers test preproduction models and submit results to the Environmental Protection Agency, which retests about 10 percent for accuracy. The vehicles are driven in a lab on a treadmill-like machine. The city test is an 11-mile, cold-start, stop-and-go trip with an average speed of 20 mph and a high speed of 56 mph. The trip takes 31 minutes, with 23 stops and about six minutes of idling. The highway test is a warm-start, 10-mile trip and averages 48 mph with a high of 60 mph and no stops. The EPA reduces the results by 10 percent for city and 22 percent for highway to reflect real-world conditions. In early 2006 the EPA proposed that, beginning with model year 2008, the calculations also account for high-speed/rapid acceleration driving, use of air conditioning and cold-temperature operation. Visit fueleconomy.gov to check your vehicle's projected miles per gallon. The average car or truck manages 20 mpg—about the same as in 1980.

Going to the source

I've heard that if you buy a BMW you can arrange to pick it up at the factory in Germany and test-drive it on the autobahn before you bring it home. Is that true?—N.M., Denver, Colorado

Yes, although you're setting yourself up for disappointment when you get the vehicle back to 55 mph land. Five European automakers offer factory packages— BMW (Munich), Mercedes (Sindelfingen) and Porsche (Stuttgart or Leipzig) in Germany, and Volvo (Göteborg) and Saab (Trollhattan) in Sweden. With the exception of Porsche, which charges at least $1,150 for the privilege, the companies *discount seven to nine percent off U.S. sticker prices. At a minimum the packages include duties and shipping costs; some also offer perks such as airline tickets, hotel stays and short-term insurance. You can tour Europe with your purchase for up to six months before a hefty sales tax kicks in (it's 16 percent in Germany). Each year about 6,000 people buy cars this way. Everything is arranged months in advance through stateside dealers because each vehicle must be built to meet U.S. pollution-control and safety standards. That's the catch if you attempt to buy and ship a car on your own. Making it street legal here can cost thousands of dollars. A few models aren't available for pickup; BMW's Z4 and X5, for example, are made in South Carolina.*

Your car's little black box

I've read that some newer cars have a factory-installed black box like one you'd find on an airplane. What sort of data do they store? Can it verify your speed? Which vehicles have these boxes, and can they be removed or disabled?—D.N., Sioux Falls, South Dakota

The latest boxes record your speed during the few seconds before impact, as well as whether you accelerated or braked and whether your seat belt was fastened. They can be useful to police in reconstructing accidents. In one case in Florida the data helped convict a man charged with manslaughter. He had been driving his 2002 Trans Am on a residential street when he collided with a car pulling out of a driveway; two teenagers were killed. He admitted to going 60 mph. The accident investigator calculated his speed at 98 mph. The black box recorded it as high as 114 mph. He got 30 years. As many as 40 million vehicles, including every GM since 2000 and every Ford since 2002, have electronic data recorders. Safety researchers, insurers and prosecutors love EDRs; opponents see them as a potential violation of your right against self-incrimination. (One defense attorney compared the technology to having a government agent in the backseat.) Automakers take the position that the data belongs to the vehicle's owner—GM collects it for safety studies only with permission—but that doesn't stop a judge from issuing a court order. In 2003, California became the first state to require automakers to inform buyers if their new cars have EDRs. The technology is difficult to remove because it's integrated with the system that controls the air bags.

How much safer is the backseat?

How much safer are you in the backseat without a belt than in the front?—M.L., Springfield, Ohio

You're safer in a head-on, but not by much. Researchers at the University of Buffalo who analyzed 300,000 fatal crashes found that the force of an unbelted adult slamming against the driver's seat nearly triples the chance the passenger will die and doubles the chance that the driver will. We don't mean to sound like safety nerds, but we prefer that our readers die while having sex.

How to read an oil can

What does it mean when an oil is 5W-30 or 10W-30? Which is best?—K.M., Kansas City, Missouri

The two numbers indicate how the oil performs when the engine is cold and hot. The 10W-30, for instance, contains polymers that allow it to act like a thinner 10-weight oil as the car is started and a thicker 30-weight oil while it's operating. This is important because when you first start the engine the oil is thinner and pumps more quickly. As the engine gets hotter the oil thickens, which provides better protection for its moving parts. (This innovation—adding polymers to oil that make it thicken as it gets hotter when it naturally would become thinner—is one reason engines today can last well beyond 100,000 miles.) In Maine the temperature goes below zero often enough that many people use 10W-30. In the Midwest 5W-30 is sufficient.

Customize your ride

Why don't the customizers you see on the Discovery Channel have to build their motorcycles in accordance with state and federal safety regulations? That is, how do they get around requirements such as blinkers or a horn?—D.W., Miami, Florida

Every bike taken onto a public road is supposed to comply with safety and pollution-control laws. Custom bikes are required to have, among other things, headlights, a rearview mirror and approved tires, rims and brakes. State laws may require side mirrors, a speedometer, muffler and brakes on both wheels. There are illegal cycles (and cars and trucks) out there, but the people who can afford to have them built can also afford the tickets. In fact, what makes a bike unsafe has been a point of contention since the days when the feds went after choppers for their extended front ends. The custom shows on cable have been great for the industry but also draw attention to its extremes, and regulators have taken notice. In December 2004 the National Highway Traffic Safety Administration, in what many saw as a preemptive strike, fined a custom shop that does work for MTV's Pimp My Ride *$16,000 for removing a driver's-side air bag to install a video screen in the steering wheel. As of 2006, the Environmental Protection Agency allows customizers to build 24 motorcycles that don't meet emissions standards (allowing for shorter and more attractive exposed exhausts and better performance). The catch is that they can be ridden only to and from bike shows. The agency will also allow individuals to build one exempt cycle with no travel restrictions. However, the exemption applies only once per lifetime, so if you wreck or sell your dream bike, you can't replace it.*

CIGARS
Sometimes it's just a cigar.

Storing cigars without a humidor

I don't own a humidor, so I've kept the boxes in my bedroom closet. The cigars are in the boxes, in metal tubes, with a leaf in each tube. When I went to smoke one the other day I noticed what looked like mold on some of them. What can I do about this? Should I keep them in the basement? Please help me prevent a good thing from going to waste.—C.C., Trenton, New Jersey

First, make sure it's mold and not bloom, which is a grayish white powder caused by oils that the tobacco exudes as it ages. Mold is bluish green and stains the wrapper; bloom is harmless—the equivalent of dust on a bottle of wine. A closet is a good place for your stash because it's dark and remains at a relatively constant temperature close to the ideal of 70 degrees. But it still might have heat spikes, which can lead to trouble. That's why you should invest in a small humidor or cedar cigar box or, at the very least, use an airtight container that you've lined with cedar strips, which are the "leaves" wrapped around your cigars now. Cigars will dry out if you don't add moisture (the goal is 65 to 70 percent humidity), so include a paper towel or small sponge soaked in distilled water or use a product such as Evermoist. Don't let water come in contact with the wrappers. Dry cigars can be rehumidified as long as their oils haven't evaporated.

Are Cubans that great?

Are Cuban cigars all they are said to be? I have found a place that sells Cubans and I wonder if I should switch from my current brand.—G.G., Atlanta, Georgia

The quality of Cubans has declined in recent years, and some smokers say they were never that great. Joel Sherman, author of Nat Sherman's Passion for Cigars, *notes that Cuban cigars are usually rushed to market because they're in such demand. "When you take a puff on most Cubans, you feel a burning sensation in your chest—testimony to the high ammonia content due to lack of proper aging," he writes. "Back in the 1950s, like a lot of smokers, I clenched my teeth and grinned through the experience of smoking a Havana. They had to be good, right? It took* *an almost macho disregard for comfort to smoke one all the way down." Expect to pay $25 to $50 each for handrolled Cubans, which have been contraband in the U.S. since a trade embargo was enacted in 1963. Cohibas are the Cubans of choice, but it's often difficult to tell if you're holding the real thing. A third to a fourth of so-called Cubans are phonies. How can you spot a fake? Sherman suggests checking each cigar because "boxes of Cubans are notoriously inconsistent in color." And if you don't feel that burn, you're probably not smoking what you paid for.*

What is the penalty if you're caught sneaking Cubans into the U.S.?—H.B., Akron, Ohio

If you are smuggling a box or two, a friendly U.S. agent will seize them. (Customs says it incinerates about 240,000 Cubans each year.) If you're a serious smuggler with a suitcase, you'll face jail time and/or a hefty fine. Keep in mind that you don't have to visit Cuba to lose your stash—the ban applies to Cubans purchased anywhere in the world. You can challenge a seizure, but don't expect much. A Philadelphia man who lost 100 cigars purchased in Havana took the government to court, arguing that because he had purchased the cigars on the black market, he hadn't enriched the Castro government and thus didn't violate the embargo. A federal judge congratulated the cigar lover for his "quite attractive" argument, then ruled in favor of the government. In 2004 the Treasury Department Office of Foreign Assets Control tightened its regulations of Cuban cigars, ruling that it's illegal for Americans to buy or smoke them anywhere in the world.

Should you remove the band?

Should you remove the band before smoking a cigar?—A.H., Pittsburgh, Pennsylvania

Keep the band on, for several reasons. First and foremost, removing it can damage the wrapper. Richard Carleton Hacker, author of the Ultimate Cigar Book, *finds that the band also is a good reference point for where to hold the cigar (in Victorian times, the band kept the fingers of a gentleman's glove from becoming stained with tobacco, or with the powder used to give cheaper cigars a uniform color). The band is also a way to announce your allegiance. As Hacker says, you wouldn't buy a sports car and rip the emblem off, so why do it with your fine cigars? That attitude doesn't play well overseas (where the band is always removed), but Hacker observes that European cigar smokers, especially the French and English, are hypocrites. "They claim that leaving the band on a cigar is ostentatious," he says. "So what they do is carefully place the band face-up in the ashtray, where everyone can see it."*

The proper cut

Is there any way to open a cigar if you don't have a cutter handy?—H.T., Peoria, Illinois

Many smokers in the Caribbean and Central America have never used a cutter. Instead they incise with their thumbnail around the head of the cigar, then remove the cap. If you don't have experience with this technique, it's best to save it for emergencies because it's easy to muck up. We prefer cutters: they contribute to the ritual and showmanship of lighting cigars, and that's half the reason we smoke them. We also aren't keen on sticking a thumbnail into the same leaf that's about to go into our mouth.

You write that you like cutters because they "contribute to the ritual and showmanship of lighting cigars." What a crock of elitist crap. Over the years I have used various cutters (V-cut, guillotine, bore, etc.) but have never found anything better than the one used by millions of smokers: their teeth.—F.U., San Francisco, California

You can bait us, but we're not biting.

Best way to beat a runner

What's the best way to get rid of the runner in a cigar?—P.R., Philadelphia, Pennsylvania

When a cigar burns faster on one side than the other, it's generally a lost cause. Tunneling occurs because of poor fermentation of the leaf, a natural flaw in the cigar or improper rolling. You can try to recut above the run, but a cigar that has already been lit never tastes as good the second time around.

Thanks to a technique I learned from the good people at De La Concha Tobacconist in New York City, a tunnel can be recovered. Lick your thumb and wet the length of the cigar several times from the tip of the run to the end of the cigar. In many cases, this will slow down the rate of burn behind the tunnel, and allow the opposite side to "catch up." It doesn't work on every run, but it's worth a try.—P.L., New York, New York

Several readers asked why you can't repair a runner by holding your lighter under the slower-burning side. The technique sounds simple but never works because typically the flaw continues for the entire length of the cigar. That explains why the De La Concha method gets the job done—sometimes.

How far should you go?

I was at a party when the host invited us to smoke cigars on the porch. Everyone had a different opinion about how long a cigar should be smoked. That is, do you continue until you hit the band, or until you can't hold it any longer? Also, how much of the tip should be cut off?—S.H., Allen, Texas

If you're smoking a great cigar, you can continue until your facial hair bursts into flames. So says Richard Carleton Hacker: "Some people stop when they hit the band," he notes. "Others take the band off, which I don't recommend because it provides a good place to hold the cigar and lets others know what you're smoking. Every cigar burns differently and has a characteristic taste, but they all tend to get a little more rank as you get closer to the end and have less tobacco to filter the smoke. It's not unusual for many cigars to begin smoking poorly halfway through." As for the head, slice it from the top, just as the tip starts to curve outward.

COLLEGE LIFE

Let's party.

Reach out and touch someone

A college friend invited me to come along on a weekend boat trip. I grabbed my bikini and we drove to a lake in a van with four guys she knew. When we arrived, there were about 30 boats tied together on the water. After about two hours, a guy grabbed a bullhorn and announced it was time for Raise the Flag. Everyone climbed over the boats to a stage that was built from two pontoons. Four guys volunteered to have strings tied around their waists with flags that draped down over their crotches. They also had their hands tied behind their backs. Four girls then climbed onstage and paired off with the guys. The women yanked down the guys' swim trunks and were handed bottles of oil to rub on themselves and anywhere on their partners except their cocks and balls. Prizes were awarded each time a flag was raised. Two guys also won $100 when they allowed the women to measure their erections. The game continued on various boats. My girlfriend had a tape measure, so we both got our hands on a few penises. At one point I watched the guys bring my friend to orgasm with their hands, and I found myself getting very turned on. I touched only one guy, and he was the only guy who touched me. We've talked on the phone a few times since, and now I'm torn between going on the next trip and wanting to be with him. Any suggestions?—A.R., Oklahoma City, Oklahoma

God bless America—after all that, you ask the Advisor a relationship question? We need a moment to calm ourselves. Ask this guy out, already. Getting to know him better is the only way to determine if you should pledge your allegiance, or if he wants it. At the very least, you'll have a chance to raise his flag in a sovereign state—your bedroom.

The stray hair

One afternoon my roommate's girlfriend came into our dorm room when my roommate wasn't around. She started paging through one of our copies of *Playboy*. She commented on how beautiful the Playmate was and then unfolded the centerfold. That's when it happened. A strand of pubic hair fell out. She looked at me and said, "I see you like her too!" I turned beet red and didn't know what to say. Now when we see each other, she teases me about it. Thankfully, she has a heart and never says anything when others are around. Should I try to discuss it with her? I haven't mentioned the *M* word, but she knows what's going on.—L.A., Los Angeles, California

A strand of hair proves nothing. Demand a DNA test! It looked like a chest hair to us! You were framed! Okay, the situation doesn't look good, but here's some news: Your roommate's girlfriend masturbates. Your roommate masturbates. Everyone in your dorm masturbates. It's normal. Being aroused by the image of a beautiful, nude woman is normal too. So your friend is ribbing you for being normal. She's playing with you and that's cool—we like her sense of humor and discretion.

My room is a sex hut

Last semester I transferred to a new college. I have yet to find my niche, so I spend a lot of time in my room. At least five times a week my roommate's girlfriend comes over and they fool around. I sit outside until they're finished. Other times she shows up in the middle of the night and they wake me up with their love vibrations. I don't feel comfortable saying anything because my roommate doesn't say anything when I smoke pot in the room. What should I do?—A.S., Oneonta, New York

Your roommate is not going to curtail his sex life on the suspicion that it bugs you. Make it official. Tell him you don't want to be a cockblocker but that your grades and sleep are suffering. Ask if he'd be willing to limit his girlfriend's visits to two weeknights and one on the weekend, during which time you'll make yourself scarce (you're doing that anyway, so it's a good negotiating position). If he hesitates, offer to keep your reefer unlit when he's around. While compromise is grand, the more important point is that you need to get off your ass. Find a few girlfriends so you can kick your roommate out once in a while.

So many girls, so little time

A buddy and I live in a coed dorm and both have girlfriends. About three weeks ago two girls who live upstairs came down to visit. Soon the talk turned dirty enough for us to joke about getting naked, and weird enough that these girls did. They must have planned the encounter because they took turns on us. Afterward nothing was said except that it was great and they shouldn't tell our girlfriends. Now our upstairs friends are visiting three or four times a week, always late at night. We can't keep this up because there's too much pressure to perform well for them and our girlfriends. Also, we're not getting enough sleep and our grades are suffering. I'm afraid if we tell the girls to stop coming they'll rat on us. What should we do?—T.S., East Lansing, Michigan

Isn't this half the reason you went to college? If you're tired, lock your door twice a week, and don't answer.

Analyze this

I'm a 28-year-old graduate student who most people would judge to be hand-some. Earlier this year, I began noticing a gorgeous student from another department. We seemed to keep similar schedules, and I would often see her in the library or the cafeteria. We have never met, but for a long time we exchanged semiflirtatious smiles and glances. Often, I would look up and catch her staring at me, and then she would quickly look away. Many times she caught me doing the same. A few times we passed on campus and said hello. After several months of this, I waited for the right moment to intro-duce myself. Then something strange happened: For no reason that I can dis-cern, the smiles and glances stopped. I have a clear vibe about this: If she's aware of my presence, or if she spots me on the street, she makes an effort not to look my way. Naturally, I take this as a bad sign, but some of my friends think her new body language might be good news. Perhaps she feels rejected because I didn't talk to her when I had a window of opportunity. Or maybe she's interested but just nervous. Obviously, she's aware of my pres-ence. Then again, maybe she just thinks I'm a creep and hopes I'll get lost. Is there any way to tell these things before I walk up to her and risk making a fool of myself?—J.M., Boston, Massachusetts

Yikes. The energy you've wasted analyzing this situation could power every street lamp on the eastern seaboard. Quit waiting for the perfect moment, because it will never arrive. Make eye contact, smile, say hello and tell her, "I've seen you around for months and thought it was time to introduce myself. I'm sorry I didn't do it sooner." C'mon, man, this is a gimme. Ask her out for coffee. We can't imagine she'll turn you down, but if she does, a quick sting is better than smol-dering regret.

Two girls at once

A few of my fraternity brothers like nothing better than to double-team a girl. It's gotten to the point where they would rather tag-team someone than have sex with her alone. I prefer one-on-one or maybe two girls at once. The last thing I want to see while having sex is my buddy's erection. Am I being too uptight?—J.W., Kansas City, Kansas

It's not unusual to want sex with a woman only when she's not fucking another guy. It sounds like your buddies have been watching too much porn, or perhaps they feel they are performing a public service for women who fantasize about pulling a train. Whatever the case, don't fret about this; take advantage. In their absence you have more old-fashioned girls to choose from.

Meeting women in class

Can the Advisor provide any tips on how to meet women in the classroom?—J.M., Shreveport, Louisiana

You've come to the right place. Back in the day, we put the stud in studious. College classrooms are ideal places to meet women—you have a common interest (passing the course), plus you see each other a few times each week. That gives her time to size you up, and it gives you repeated chances to chat. Here are two lines that worked for us: "Hi" and "Is this seat taken?" Introduce yourself, ask if she enjoys the class, find out where's she from—you know the drill. If she's friendly (or, hell, even if she's not), ask if she'd like to make a study date or have a cup of coffee. If she declines, express disappointment, but don't give up. Continue to say hello. You may grow on her—and if she misses a class, you can offer a copy of your notes with your number at the top.

Why can't college guys get it up?

Why do college guys have a hard time getting it up? Seventy percent of the guys I've slept with could not get an erection. Isn't it enough to have a naked woman saying "Fuck me now"? What am I doing wrong? I'm not ugly, and I don't smell.—S.E., South Bend, Indiana

We'll take a wild guess here, but have 70 percent of your partners been intoxicated? That would explain a lot. Yet even if they were sober, many college guys have never encountered a girl like you. They're used to being in charge, and now they have a partner saying "Gimme!" If a guy loses his erection, don't make a big deal of it. He's not a machine. But he does have a tongue. As you meet guys with more experience and who use other methods besides booze to get you into bed, this will be less of a problem.

Roommates who touch themselves

I'm an 18-year-old female high school senior who will soon be living in a dorm room with three women I've never met. The problem is, I love to masturbate. One afternoon after sex ed class I came home and "found myself." I haven't gotten into or out of bed since without masturbating. And I'm not shy about it with my close friends or family. (I have 10 siblings and share a room with three sisters.) My parents bought me my first vibrator. I love toys, but some of my best orgasms have been with my fingers while pulling on my nipples. My dad says to do it only when I'm alone; my mom says to be open with my roommates about it. I'm not a screamer, but my sisters know I usually thrash around. What happens if one of my roommates freaks and tries to ruin me? Can you give me any stats to show that this is normal?—J.S., Los Angeles, California

Throwing statistics around won't help. Rest assured that most women masturbate, although perhaps not as frequently or openly as you. You're ahead of your time. This isn't about masturbation as much as the compromise required for any sort of group living. To avoid friction you may need to make minor adjustments to your routine, such as holding your hands behind your back until you get to the shower. But don't be surprised if at least two of your roomies also routinely masturbate and have their own concerns about privacy. Why do we think we'll see you on The Real World?

CONTRACEPTION

Don't forget your rubbers.

My girlfriend wants to go "natural"

My girlfriend planned to save herself for marriage but has changed her mind. The problem is, she insists that her first time be "completely natural." Can you tell me what the chances are she'll become pregnant from one instance of unprotected sex?—D.J., Toronto, Ontario

How good are you? If you have the self-control, you might slide inside her a few times before you slip on the condom; that may satisfy her curiosity. But given your girlfriend's inexperience, your first time together won't be as magical as she imagines, and contraception isn't going to make or break the encounter. We recommend that you play it safe. If she wants all natural, have sex outdoors with a lambskin condom and water-based lube. And appeal to her romantic side: Tell her she isn't going to write in her diary that her first time was special because you didn't wear a condom, but because she was with you.

Risky business

I have been using the withdrawal method to keep from getting my girlfriend pregnant. That is, I come on her stomach. She takes a shower after sex, and I'm wondering if the water can carry the sperm into her vagina. Have you ever heard of that happening?—V.T., Lansing, Michigan

No. Even with the best of intentions, it's much more likely you'll get her pregnant before she hits the shower. Coitus interruptus is better than nothing, but that's about the only good thing we can say about it. The technique's failure rate is estimated to be about four percent with perfect use, meaning that over a year's time, four of 100 women using it will get pregnant. However, given that highly aroused men are involved, a 19 percent failure rate is thought to be more realistic. About the only birth-control methods more risky are the rhythm method and crossing your fingers. For many years researchers thought the high failure rate could be attributed to pre-come, which is produced by the Cowper's gland and emerges during foreplay in quantities ranging from a few drops to a teaspoon, probably to lubricate the urethra and head of the penis. However, several small studies have found no sperm or only immobile sperm in the fluid, so human error remains the chief culprit. If you don't want to see something else being pulled from your girlfriend's vagina, we suggest using a more reliable contraceptive, such as the pill or a condom.

Who's your daddy?

My wife and I are swingers. We want to have a child, but I'm concerned. Is there a time frame during which a fertilized egg would be in danger from another man's sperm in the event that a condom broke?—R.T., Orlando, Florida

Once the egg is fertilized, there's no risk of anyone else's becoming the father. Before that happens, it's a simple race, and the sperm of the second (or third) man to ejaculate inside a woman often scores a come-from-behind victory. In extreme cases, a woman might have fraternal twins (i.e., from two eggs), each by a separate father. This is most apparent when the children are of different races. Studies indicate that 10 percent of children worldwide are not sired by the men who believe they're the father—and that some additional percentage are conceived this way but miscarried or aborted. There's another important risk to consider: Anything that alters the delicate balance of bacteria in the vagina, including genital-tract infections and STDs, can contribute to early labor. That, in turn, can lead to serious lifelong problems for the child, including cerebral palsy, mental retardation, blindness, deafness and respiratory problems. The risk of infection increases when the mother and/or father have sexual partners besides each other.

Finding a condom that fits

Whenever I use a condom I have a hard time keeping it from slipping off. Is there anything I can do?—R.Z., Pittsburgh, Pennsylvania

For health and liability reasons, most condoms are longer than most guys—that is, standard condoms are seven inches, while standard guys are between five and six. The idea is that it's better to have too much protection than not enough. The problem is that the typical guy ends up with an inch of latex rolled up at the base of his penis. Besides being uncomfortable, this makes the condom more prone to unroll or catch inside his partner. That inspired Adam Glickman, founder of Condomania.com, to introduce custom-fit condoms. Download, or request by phone (800-926-6366), a "fit kit"—two paper rulers to measure the length and girth of your erection. With that info you can select the best fit from 55 sizes. A 12-

pack is $12. "We've sold every size, but it's trending toward narrower and longer," Glickman says. "That makes sense, since the early adopters are guys who are the most unhappy with one-size-fits-all." While the company expects to have one of the more interesting databases out there—hundreds of thousands of penile measurements—Glickman says customers need not worry about their personal data being shared with anyone.

Super-thin condoms

To me, wearing a condom is like kissing through a screen door. It deadens sensation to the point that I'm nearly incapable of achieving orgasm and quite often lose my erection. The only condoms I can live with are superthin lambskins, but they're not effective in protecting against sexually transmitted diseases. Short of suggesting a vasectomy, can you give me any guidance?—D.K., Atlanta, Georgia

Don't give up yet. Condoms are essential, but they're also no fun. That's why condom manufacturers are always tinkering with them. There are superthin condoms that protect against STDs, but they aren't always available in drugstores. Condomania.com (800-926-6366) offers several brands, including latex condoms from Crown of Japan. You might also try X-tra Pleasure by Lifestyles, which features a baggy tip to allow more friction against the head of the penis. Finally, take heart in news from Quebec City's University Laval. A team led by Dr. Michel Bergeron is developing what he calls an "invisible condom." The product is a non-toxic liquid at room temperature that thickens to a water-soluble gel after being injected with an applicator into the vagina or rectum. It remains effective as a barrier for at least 48 hours. Early studies have shown that the gel can stop the transmission of HIV and herpes. It may also prevent pregnancy, especially if bolstered with spermicides.

When discussing superthin condoms, you didn't mention polyurethane. Why is that?—W.D., Las Vegas, Nevada

We're careful about recommending polyurethane condoms to anyone who isn't allergic to latex, which is the only FDA-approved use for them. The agency has yet to okay the product (made by Durex under the brand name Avanti) as a contraceptive or barrier against sexually transmitted diseases. That's largely because of concerns about its durability. In a 1997 study involving 800 couples, 8.5 percent of the Avanti condoms broke or slipped off during intercourse or withdrawal, compared with 1.6 percent of latex condoms. About 30 percent of the men said plastic condoms were difficult to put on. Still, polyurethane has its fans. It's twice as thin as latex and allows more heat transfer. It's also odorless and safe with oil-based lubricants.

Sexual sandwich

My fuck buddy and I were getting ready to go at it when I realized I didn't have a condom. She's not on the pill, and I don't trust where she's been, so instead of going to bed with blue balls I put a sandwich bag on my penis and held it in place with a rubber band. The sex felt great! Is there anything wrong with this kind of contraception?—S.S., Winfield, Kansas

Good grief. What did you use for lube, peanut butter and jelly? A sandwich bag is better than nothing, but not by much.

Reversing a vasectomy

Three years ago I was in a relationship with a woman who did not want children. She told me that in order to show my commitment to the relationship I should get a vasectomy. Two years later she left me. Do I have any legal recourse?—A.B., Sterling, Colorado

No. But you may have medical recourse. Vasectomies have been reversed as long as 30 years after the procedure. About 60 percent of men who have microsurgery to reconnect the vas deferens produce children.

The condom ripped

The condom ripped as my girlfriend and I were having sex last night. What are the chances that she's now pregnant? This is the third condom we've ripped in the past three weeks.—H.N., Trenton, New Jersey

Chance has nothing to do with it. By now, either she's pregnant or she isn't. It's extremely rare for condoms to break because of structural defects. Our guess is that you're pulling them on too tight. Once you've unrolled the condom over your erection, gently pinch at least a half inch of airless space at the tip. This allows a place for the semen to be deposited, and it provides room for the condom to move as you thrust.

When is she most fertile?

When is a woman most fertile? My girlfriend makes me wear a condom when we have sex, but she can't possibly be able to get pregnant every day of the month.—T.R., Los Angeles, California

According to a study published in the New England Journal of Medicine, *a woman has a window of about six days during her monthly menstrual cycle when she can be impregnated. Her hot zone is the day of ovulation, during which one of her ovaries releases an egg into one of her fallopian tubes to hook up with any available sperm. Your girlfriend's remaining fertile days occur during the week or so before ovulation, and in some cases a day after. Researchers calculate that fertile women who have unprotected sex once a week over the course of their menstrual cycle have about a 15 percent chance of pregnancy; those who have sex every other day, a 33 percent chance; and those who have sex daily, a 37 percent chance. Those are good odds only if you're trying to have a kid. Keep your condom on and leave the body temperature charts, hormone tests and guesswork to couples who are ready for the miracle of life.*

The male pill

Can you give me an update on a contraceptive pill for men?—T.A., Detroit, Michigan

Researchers have been searching for years for a pill that could shut off the sperm factory as relatively easily as the female pill shuts down a woman's reproductive cycle. There have been many false starts. One problem is that hormonal methods can lower sperm counts to zero but usually have serious side effects, such as reduced libido, loss of muscle mass or liver damage. However, progress is being made, and there's talk of a male patch or implant on the market in Europe by as early as 2009, followed by a U.S. debut. One promising technique is a progestin implant that reduces the hormones in the male brain that control sperm production, supplemented by a testosterone injection every 90 days to keep everything in balance. Other scientists are working on ways to make sperm too tired to swim very far, or to keep them from attaching to the egg. Keep your vasa deferentia crossed.

Hot, hot, hot

I saw some Brits on the Discovery Channel who soaked their testicles in hot water for a few hours a day, with the idea that your testicles must be cooler than your body temperature to make sperm. That's why your scrotum hangs away from your body. It took a few weeks, but eventually the guys shot blanks. It struck me—why not create a discrete pouch to keep guys' balls overheated? People have laughed when I explain my idea, but I think it could change the world, and make me rich.—W.S., Madison, Wisconsin

We're sorry to disappoint you, but you're 80 years behind the curve. Scientists have been studying the effects of heat on sperm production since at least the 1930s, and several inventors have attempted to market testicle pouches and insulated underwear without success. Heating your balls does seem to work, but it takes discipline. One widely cited 1946 study with nine volunteers found that men who soaked their balls in 116-degree water for 45 minutes a day for three weeks become sterile for about six months. Other research has found that holding the balls extremely close to the body raises the temperature enough to impede production. But that too is a tough sell, and we wouldn't trust either method. We've been writing about research into male contraception for years, and there is always something revolutionary just over the horizon. The latest technique that doesn't involve hormones is Reversible Inhibition of Sperm Under Guidance, which is currently being tested in India. Doctors inject a gel into the vas deferens that causes the heads of passing sperm to explode. RISUG appears to be reversible when the gel is flushed, although removal requires a combination of vibration, electric current and rectal massage. Elaine Lissner of the Male Contraception Information Project (newmalecontraception.org) notes that there have been 25 years of research on RISUG but it's still a long way from being approved in the U.S. or Europe. "This is the most promising method because we know it works," she says. "Several dozen men in India have been using it for a decade without problems and 140 others for three or four years."

My girlfriend is horny on the pill

Ever since my girlfriend went on the pill, she's gotten really horny. Is it me, or could it be the drug?—T.S., Trenton, New Jersey

It's you—maybe. Your girlfriend may be more interested in sex because a big risk (pregnancy) has been all but eliminated. Her interest might also depend on what type of pill she's taking. While past research has shown that the pill lowers the hormones thought to affect sexual desire, a recent study of 364 women suggests that certain types of pills may inhibit them less than others. Writing in the

Archives of Sexual Behavior, *researchers at San Francisco State University found that users of triphasic pills, which vary the level of progestin released during the pill's 21-day cycle, reported more sexual thoughts, fantasies and arousal than those taking monophasic pills, which maintain a consistent level of the hormone. Surprisingly, women taking triphasics also reported more sexual thoughts and interest than women who weren't using oral contraceptives, but pill users may be hornier to begin with. Another interesting finding: Women not taking the pill reported more and better anal sex.*

What are the odds?

My wife says birth control pills fail about three percent of the time, while I've read that condoms fail about 12 percent of the time. So what would the failure rate be if a couple used both the pill and a condom—0.36 percent?— J.T., College Station, Texas

Your calculations are on target, but they're based on the worst-case scenario, i.e., the woman forgets to take her pill, the guy is a klutz with the condom and they don't use spermicide. In the best-case scenario, in which both people know what they're doing and do it well, the probability of simultaneous failure is one in a million. About the only way to get better odds is not to have sex.

Morning-after pills

I've heard there's birth control that can be taken after sex. Is that true? My girlfriend and I had a scare after a condom broke, so we're curious about any safety valves out there.—R.W., Oakland, California

Given our culture's reliance on pills to battle everything from tension headaches to lackluster personalities, it's surprising that we haven't embraced more drugs that combat the serious social problem of unwanted pregnancies. There are two methods. The first is to take a specific dose of common birth control pills within up to five days after unprotected intercourse (it's most effective within 120 hours). There are two types, both of which work by preventing the fertilized egg from implanting in the uterus. The first contains estrogen and progestin and can reduce a woman's chance of getting pregnant by at least 75 percent. The other, known as Plan B, has just progestin. The latter is preferred by many women because there is less chance of nausea and vomiting and it reduces the risk of pregnancy by 89 percent. The second method is a copper-T intrauterine device inserted by a doctor within seven days after intercourse. You can get more information, including a list of birth-control pill brands and a list of health-care providers at a site maintained by the Office of Population Control at Princeton University and the Association of Reproductive Health Professionals. It's located at not-2-late.com.

COOKING

Hey, good looking . . .

Do certain foods cause sex dreams?

Have any studies found a connection between the foods we eat and the dreams we have? If so, what foods create the sexiest dreams?—T.G., Seattle, Washington

There's no surefire way to determine if a person is having an erotic dream other than waking him to ask, and no sleep scientist has felt the need to do that and also record what the subject had for dinner. Even an erection isn't a reliable gauge, since they occur whenever a healthy male is dreaming about anything. Many people believe that heavy or spicy meals induce vivid dreams, but it may be that certain foods simply cause more frequent awakenings, which increase recall. In an earlier time, authorities speculated on diets that could prevent "pollutions," or wet dreams. Our dusty copy of The Illustrated Encyclopedia of Sex, *published in 1950, asserts that "erotic dreams mainly come to persons who during the day too frequently nurse erotic desires." To prevent sexual intrusions, the authors recommend an anti-erotic vegetarian diet rich in vitamins and salts. "Whole wheat bread, potatoes, vegetables, salads, fruit, etc., also prevent constipation," they noted, while "stimulating foods" such as game, fish, eggs, cheese, mushrooms and alcohol only cause trouble. Whatever your diet, you're more likely to have pleasant dreams when you're relaxed. Anxiety can produce landscapes you may not want to visit: running into your mother at an orgy, discovering strange plants growing from your genitals or realizing at a crucial moment that you left your penis in your other pants—but that your girlfriend brought hers.*

Sexy recipes

I would love to have some sexy recipes to impress my girlfriend. Any suggestions?—L.W., Phoenix, Arizona

We recently came across a tantalizing work in progress, Simple Recipes That Will Help Get You Laid, *by a photographer who goes by the online nickname Short2000 (short2000.com/simple). She uses color, fruit and scotch to get the job done. Examples: (1) Place fresh pineapple chunks and maraschinos on skewers, then throw them on the grill for a few minutes until the pineapples are slightly caramelized. For extra impact, serve with coconut ice cream. (2) Blend two cups of frozen mango chunks, or two large, soft but not mushy mangoes, with a cup of yogurt and a cup of vanilla rice milk until thick and smooth. Serve in a frosted wine glass, and top with fruit. (3) Mix salad greens, pomegranate seeds and balsamic vinaigrette for a "sweet, crunchy, juicy, tangy, leafy" salad. (4) Pour single malt scotch into a colored glass and call it a butterfly wing. "The name alone will get you some action, and its color will cast spells. Just don't use a glass that says SeaWorld or anything like that." If any of this gets you laid, drop Short2000 a line to thank her.*

Serving caviar

What is the best way to serve caviar?—D.S., Cleveland, Ohio

Place the open container in a small glass or porcelain bowl, surrounded by crushed ice. Don't use a metal or stainless steel serving spoon, which can spoil the taste. Some caviar lovers insist the roe should be served only with lightly toasted bread points, or with a squirt of lemon juice if you're serving a lesser-quality grade. You don't want to serve chopped eggs, onion, sour cream, crème fraiche or anything that overpowers the roe. The drinks of choice are dry champagne or frozen vodka. Adventurous hosts use caviar to top dishes such as omelettes, pasta, salads or fish. In preparing caviar, never freeze or cook the eggs, and finish eating the roe within a week of opening the tin. Store fresh caviar in the coldest part of the refrigerator, or in a bowl of crushed ice; unopened tins will remain fresh a few weeks at best. Traditionally, the best roe (beluga, oestra and Sevruga) comes from the Caspian Sea, but because of concerns about overfishing, the U.N. has banned the international trade of wild sturgeon caviar. Fortunately, some American caviar is also excellent.

How to sharpen a blade

My set of cooking knives includes a metal rod with a wooden handle. I assume this is to sharpen the blades, but I have no idea how to use it. How do you hold it?—K.L., Atlanta, Georgia

The steel isn't designed to sharpen a dull blade; instead it maintains the edge of an already sharp knife. A chef or butcher will use the steel every few minutes; for cooking at home, it's sufficient to steel after each use. Many people simply flail the steel and edge together, but craftsman Keith De'Grau, who runs HandAmerican.com, a site devoted to cutting tools, says control is the key. "My preference is to hold the steel vertically and then tip it 10 to 20 degrees one way or the other, depending on the angle of the edge," he says. "Run the blade straight down the steel, from bolster to tip, drawing it toward you. Repeat for each side." (His site has photos.) Regardless of your technique, most steels are heavily grooved, which means that each time you run an expensive knife over them, the blade is serrated. This creates the illusion of sharpness but damages the knife. De'Grau suggests running 400-grit silicone-carbide paper over your steel for five minutes to make it less aggressive. If you aren't comfortable using a whetstone to sharpen your trusted knives, have a professional do it for you every 12 to 18 months.

Grilling tips

My neighbor moved and gave me his gas grill. I'm new to the art. Can you run down a few basics?—P.S., Mesa, Arizona

Let's talk steak. (1) Trim fat edges to a quarter inch to reduce flare-ups and heart attacks. (2) Sprinkle both sides of each steak with kosher salt and pepper, then drizzle with oil. Start with high heat, char both sides, then move the meat to a cooler area. Keep your steaks about an inch apart. (3) Use tongs rather than a fork so you don't pierce the meat and let juices escape. (4) Cook with the cover closed. Let the steak sit for five minutes after you take it off the grill so the juices have time to settle back to the center.

That's good advice, but what's the best way to know when a grilled steak is medium rare?—R.R., Boston, Massachusetts

Most grillers press on the steak with tongs to measure its resistance; beef becomes less springy as it cooks. To get an idea of how it should feel, press the fleshy part of your hand between the index finger and thumb. That's rare. For medium rare spread your fingers out and poke the same spot. For medium make a fist. Or spend five bucks on a meat thermometer. The FDA recommends cooking beef to at least 145 degrees for medium rare, 160 for medium and 170 for well-done. Whole poultry should be cooked to at least 180 degrees, measured at the thigh. Chicken breasts should be cooked to 170 degrees, pork and ground beef to 160.

Sushi bar etiquette

What is the protocol while eating at a sushi bar?—G.G., Citrus Heights, California

Never dip your sushi rice-side, and don't soak it—the sauce should complement the fish, not kill its flavor. The ginger is there to cleanse your palate. The green stuff *(wasabi) is hot; mix bits of it with your soy sauce to taste. It's best to eat each piece in one bite, but in the West that's not always practical because sushi tends to be larger. Never pass food with your chopsticks; in Japan, this resembles a Buddhist ritual in which bone fragments from a cremated body are passed at a funeral. Instead, offer the plate. It's okay to pick up sushi with your fingers, but always use chopsticks for sashimi. When you are not using your sticks, place them on the small, decorative hashi oki. If you take food from a shared plate, turn the sticks around so you're not using the ends that you put in your mouth. It's bad form to smoke. And while you should leave a tip on the bar for the chef, keep in mind that the people who handle the food never touch the money.*

Charcoal vs. gas

A friend has been giving me a hard time about my new gas grill. He's convinced it's my plebeian attempt to be a griller. To hear him talk of charcoal you'd think he was indulging in foreplay. "The longer, the sweeter," he says. But I grill almost daily, at times for breakfast, lunch and dinner. (Pancakes, eggs and pizza are some of my favorite meals.) I enjoy it as much as he does, but I do it more quickly and more often. In the end I think a juicy, satisfying sirloin is more a matter of technique. What does the Advisor say?—S.P., Kirchenthumbach, Germany

The Advisor says, "Will you two shut up and flip our steak?" You each have what you need. Although there is no question that meat grilled over charcoal tastes better, you can't beat the convenience of gas. Don't give up on charcoal; a chimney starter cuts down on the prep time considerably while eliminating the need for lighter fluid. And we prefer hardwood charcoal, which burns faster and with greater intensity. For some reason it's a great comfort to tend that dancing flame.

Who says meat grilled over charcoal tastes better? Charcoal, like gas, is just fuel. The grilled flavor comes from the smoke that rises when the juices and marinade drip onto the briquettes. Gas grills approximate this with bars or rocks. I am an experienced griller and can taste no difference. However, the convenience of gas can't be beat. It also allows you to grill in the winter.—R.G., Lake in the Hills, Illinois

In 2000 a research firm hired by Kingsford charcoal gave a blind taste test to 796 adults in four cities and found that around 65 percent preferred chicken and

hamburgers cooked over charcoal—by someone else, notably. But Weber, which makes both types of grill, says it has conducted repeated surveys in which people report they can't tell the difference. As one griller puts it, a lot depends on whether you're into the journey or the destination. Some people compromise—gas during the week, charcoal on weekends.

I am a propane cooker myself and challenge any briquette lover to serve a better meal. My secret is wood chips. Soak two cups of them in water for half an hour, drain and place in a foil pouch. Punch a few holes to vent and place as close to the flame as possible. You can buy smoking pellets, but they last only 15 minutes. Real wood chips smoke for up to 45. They also come in different flavors: hickory, mesquite, apple wood.—C.T., South Lyon, Michigan

You're looking for trouble with that throw-down.

Propane toasting is not barbecue. Barbecue is cooking large cuts of meat for long periods of time at lower temperatures. Stop buying grills because they are shiny. Stop trying to cook a cheap hunk of meat at 600 degrees in two minutes. Stop using Italian salad dressing as a marinade. Then we can talk about a grill-off.—R.K., Los Angeles, California

As we have discovered, it's dangerous to stand between two men wielding tongs.

Preparing truffles

A friend gave me a jar of black truffles from Italy as a gift. These things have such mythical status that I'm not sure how to use them to their best effect. I'm an adventurous cook within striking distance of a gourmet grocery, so anything is possible.—C.O., San Carlos, California

You don't need adventure or gourmet groceries. In fact it's best to keep it simple. "The traditional truffle dish is eggs," says chef Peter Urbani, whose family runs Urbani Truffles (urbani.com). "Add a quarter teaspoon of truffle butter or oil, and shave your black truffle over them." Urbani says your gift is either summer truffles (Tuber aestivum Vitt.) or winter ones (Tuber melanosporum Vitt.). "Look for tuber on the jar," he says. "If you don't see it, it's not a European truffle and you probably paid too much for it." With any luck you have winter truffles, which are more flavorful. "It's like the difference between catfish and sea bass," Urbani says. He recommends using a microplane to shave your truffles onto a risotto or pasta with cream sauce. Unlike white truffles, the black variety can also be added to the dish near the end of the cooking process.

Choosing the best cheese

How do you select interesting cheeses to serve at a party? I always get safe bets such as Swiss or Gouda, and I have no idea which of the hundreds of cheeses at the local deli might be good.—J.N., Chicago, Illinois

The proprietor of any good cheese shop can lead the way. That's why we called chef Terrance Brennan, proprietor of the 10,000-square-foot Artisanal Cheese Center in New York City (artisanalcheese.com). He suggests serving three to five cheeses arranged on a plate from mild to strong, with the mildest at six o'clock. Present as much variety as you can, considering the regions where the cheeses originated, the type of milk used to make them and their textures, flavors and shapes. To get started Brennan suggests Uplands Pleasant Ridge from Wisconsin for a cow's-milk cheese, Montenebro from Spain for a goat's-milk selection and Spenwood, a sheep's-milk cheese made in a small English village. Always include a blue cheese, because it's a crowd-pleaser and a great finisher. Brennan recommends Colston Bassett Stilton from England; we also like Cashel Blue from Ireland. Plan on two to three ounces per person. Artisanalcheese.com has more information on pairing wines. (The Uplands is great with merlot.) In general, if you're serving a red, keep it young, light and fruity. White wines are easier to match; you can't go wrong with a sauvignon blanc.

Aging beef at home

How do restaurants age beef? Can it be done at home?—A.K., Dallas, Texas

They store it for three or four weeks in the walk-in cooler, typically at between 32 and 34 degrees Fahrenheit with 85 percent relative humidity. This allows the muscle fibers to slowly decompose, making the meat more tender. At the same time, it loses water, making it firmer and more flavorful. Most meat is wet-aged, meaning it is vacuum packed in its own juices and stored only until it's sold and served. The meat becomes more tender, but its flavor doesn't change. Merle Ellis, who has been a butcher for 50 years, offers this recipe to dry-age a loin at home: Pat the meat dry with paper towels, then store it for a week with the fat side down on the refrigerator shelf that has the best air circulation—usually the bottom one, which is also often the coldest. The surface will darken and dry, but that's okay.

Check often to wipe away any moisture, or wrap the meat in clean white cotton dish towels and change them daily. After 10 to 14 days, cut steaks from each end and allow the rest of the loin to continue to age. "I'd be willing to bet that after dry-aging even under less than the best of conditions, the beef will be better than it was the week before," Ellis says.

DESIRE

Feast or famine.

My spouse has no interest in sex

In the beginning of our marriage, my wife was very passionate. Now, 10 years later, she says she has no interest in sex. She treats it like a chore. She makes me feel like it's something I do to her rather than with her. I've tried to talk to her about the situation, but she gets angry at me for bringing it up. Everything in the marriage is fine except for the intimacy. Any advice?—D.M., Baltimore, Maryland

Without the intimacy, it's not much of a marriage. The typical advice you'll get from self-help books is to be more attentive to your wife's emotional needs and the sex will follow. We wonder why the equation can't be turned around: If your wife fucked you more often, she'd have her emotional and every other need met—and then some. That's why we like what we hear from Michele Weiner Davis, author of The Sex-Starved Marriage. *She stands up for guys, noting that it's not fair for a wife to refuse to fulfill her husband's desires while demanding monogamy. "A lot of women need an emotional connection to feel aroused," she says. "They can't fathom how to have sex if there's tension in the air, or the kids are home, or there are clothes to be folded. Desire is a decision. I tell women to succumb to their husbands no matter their mood, and see what happens." One group was amazed at the response—their husbands suddenly read to the kids, set aside time to talk, fixed things. And women who think they aren't in the mood often end up enjoying themselves immensely. "Men tell me that sex with their wives is about more than just getting off. It makes them feel wanted, loved, appreciated, masculine. If the wife shuts the husband out, he has one of two reactions: (1) He becomes highly critical because he's so angry, or (2) he withdraws. Neither response will get you laid. My advice for guys is to explain how they feel when they're refused. A husband told his wife in a session with me, 'When I reach for you and you reject me, there's no lonelier feeling.' His wife responded, 'When you touch me the only thing I can think about is whether I'm in the mood.' That was a start."*

The reader who wrote because his wife never wants sex can take comfort in the fact that other aspects of his marriage are fine. My husband's excuse is either "I'm tired" or "My back hurts." I've gone from being hurt to angry to indifferent. Now I take what I can get, and I rely on my vibrator. It's sad, but many of us need more than our spouses are willing to give.—J.D., New York, New York

Indifference is a sign of real trouble. An angry spouse is at least motivated to take action. In his book Great Sex, *Michael Castleman observes that, over time, sex in any relationship becomes less like the Fourth of July and more like Thanksgiving. He summarizes the attitude of the spouse who wants more sex as "You used to want sex five times a week. If I'd known you'd eventually want it only twice a month, I'm not sure I would have stuck around. But now we're married and have kids and a mortgage. I love you, and to me love means sex. I feel that you don't love me. I also feel that you tricked me. Now I feel stuck." The other partner thinks, "If I'd known you were such a sex fiend, I'm not sure I would have stuck around. I love you, but there are big differences between love and sex. You're insatiable. I feel stuck." Couples in this situation often slip into one of two modes: bickering or silence. The higher-desire person will often stop initiating sex to see how long it takes for the partner to ask for it—the long wait often makes him or her even angrier. The couple stops hugging, kissing, holding hands or cuddling because the partner who wants sex sees these activities as foreplay. Castleman notes that couples have three choices: Break up, live in misery, or compromise. Therapists find that both partners typically desire the same thing: more nonsexual affection and more attention from their spouse in general. Good sex comes out of a good marriage, not the other way around.*

Burdensome fantasies

My boyfriend informs me that he sees women all the time who he wants to have sex with. That made me feel insecure and paranoid. It's not that I don't fantasize about other guys, but I keep my thoughts private and I don't harbor the images for longer than that person is in my sight. I asked my boyfriend how often these fantasies happen; he said he couldn't say. When do these thoughts become too much for a relationship to bear? And is it normal to envision others when you are being intimate with the one you allegedly love? Am I asking too much for my lover to focus on me when we are having sex?—A.H., New York, New York

Your boyfriend is normal; his mistake, apparently, was to be honest with you about his erotic daydreams. Many women would interpret that sort of honesty as a sign of trust, but you scolded him for it. That's too bad. If you accept that every person is a sexual being, and that most men are stimulated visually more than women are, it's easier not to get worked up about fantasies—even those that occur in bed. (As Johnny Carson once said, when turkeys mate, they think of swans.) The important thing isn't whether your boyfriend is dreaming about fucking other women but whether he's doing it. There is a point where your boyfriend may be pushing it—he should not be turning his head when he's with you—but that's a matter of etiquette.

Sexual addiction

How can you tell if you're a sex addict? I think about sex constantly. I download porn. I have a large collection of adult videos. I masturbate an average of three times a day. The littlest thing about a woman turns me on. I get agitated if I don't get sex. I can't always tell if I love someone or if I just want the sex. I've had women say that I'm a different man after sex. Beforehand I'm crabby; afterward I'm happy and glowing and ready to party. I have to have sex before I go out! It's always sex, sex, sex.—B.L., St. Louis, Missouri

Welcome to the club. The behavior you describe doesn't make you an addict. It makes you a guy. The idea of sexual addiction has become a cottage industry—its roots lie in the idea that yielding too often to masturbation, pornography, homosexuality and other "sins" will make you mentally ill. It was popularized by a 1989 book called Contrary to Love, *which includes a ridiculous "screening test" with such questions as: Have you ever subscribed to sexually explicit magazines such as* Playboy? *(Yes.) Do you often find yourself preoccupied with sexual thoughts? (Yes.) Do you feel that your sexual behavior is not normal? (Yes.) Are any of your sexual activities against the law? (Yes, in many states, until recently.) Have you ever felt degraded by your sexual behavior? (Yes.) Has sex been a way for you to escape your problems? (Yes.) When you have sex, do you feel depressed afterward? (Yes.) Do you feel controlled by your desire? (Yes.) Sign us up! We're not dismissing the idea that sex can be a destructive force, but as one of our favorite vixens, Annie Sprinkle, has written, "compulsion," "problem" and "challenge" may be better words than "addiction" to describe the situation. It's sex, not heroin.*

As the director of the Minnesota Institute of Psychiatry and author of the first psychiatric textbook on sexual addiction, I agree that the behavior the reader described does not make him an addict. I also agree that the concept of sexual addiction has been misused by hucksters and charlatans. However, discussing whether sexual addiction is a valid concept makes sense only in the context of a meaningful definition. I like this one: It's a condition in which some form of sexual behavior is employed in a pattern characterized by (1) a recurrent failure to control the behavior, and (2) continuation of the behavior despite significant harmful consequences. In other words, whether a pattern of sexual behavior qualifies as addiction is determined not by the behavior, its object, its frequency or its social acceptability but by how the behavior affects a person's life. You suggest that compulsion may be a better term. But by definition, compulsive behavior does not produce pleasure or gratification.—Dr. Aviel Goodman, St. Paul, Minnesota

We appreciate the letter, but we'll stick with our deeply cynical view of this "affliction." It seems to us that a person cannot be diagnosed as having a problem with sex unless he gets no pleasure or gratification from it, and that would qualify as a compulsion.

Peggy Kleinplatz of the University of Ottawa and I have written about how psychiatry deals with sexual concerns in general and have particular concerns about flaws in the idea of "sexual addiction." The criteria presented by Dr. Goldman, which include recurrent failure to control sexual behavior and continuation of the behavior despite harmful consequences, are quite problematic. By those criteria, many teenagers would be classified as sex addicts by virtue of their masturbation habits and their suffering from socially imposed guilt. The problem occurs when people believe that sex in general—the wrong type of sex or the wrong amount, however they define it—is sick and then look for rationalizations for their values.—Dr. Charles Moser, Institute for Advanced Study of Human Sexuality, San Francisco, California

Why are some people beautiful?

Has there ever been any research on why some people are considered beautiful and others are not? I've been attracted to many types of women—slim, tall, short, with long faces, round faces, etc.—but find it curious that nearly everyone agrees that supermodels such as Carol Alt or Cindy Crawford are gorgeous.—D.R., New Orleans, Louisiana

Researchers have found that even across different races and cultures, men generally prefer women with large pupils, widely spaced eyes, high cheekbones, a small chin and upper lip, a generous mouth and shiny, smooth skin. A psychologist at the University of Louisville took the measurements further after asking 150 male students to rate 50 women's faces. Among the faces deemed pretty, each eye was one-fourteenth as high and three-tenths as wide as the face, the nose took up no more than five-percent of the face, the distance from the bottom lip to the chin was one-fifth the facial height and the distance from the middle of the eye to the eyebrow was one-tenth the facial height. Surprisingly, when the faces of models are superimposed on that image, they don't match up. Instead, the composite resembles someone's mom. Women, meanwhile, consider a man's maturity and dominance with cues such as thick eyebrows, a strong jawline, prominent chin and cheekbones and a small nose. If your features don't match that scientific standard, don't despair: You probably have a great personality.

She doesn't like sex

I am a 24-year-old woman in my second relationship. The problem is that I hate sex. I feel no desire to be sexual with anyone, male or female. I don't like foreplay. I don't like trying new positions. I like it one way, with my boyfriend on top, and quick. I don't like giving or receiving oral sex. I don't masturbate and don't think I've ever had an orgasm, nor do I want one. Between relationships I didn't miss sex in the least. In fact, I was relieved that it wasn't part of my life. I haven't been molested or raped, if that's what you're thinking. I just think sex is overrated and a nuisance. Any idea what might be wrong?—M.A., Fitchburg, Massachusetts

We'll give your boyfriends the benefit of the doubt and suggest that you have a low libido or perhaps none at all. The question is whether you suffer from a physical or mental condition that can be treated (psychiatrists call it hypoactive sexual desire disorder) or whether you are naturally asexual, which is a controversial diagnosis. Brain chemistry plays a huge role in our feelings of falling in love and in lust and long-term attachment—perhaps some people lack the chemicals for lust. It may be helpful to read posts from other people who feel as you do. There's a forum at asexuality.org and even a dating service at asexualpals.com. The online definition of asexual *is inclusive: It applies to people who say they masturbate but can't feel romantic love and those who say they have never been horny but feel romantic passion. Before we accept the existence of amoeba man, we'd like to see a few proclaimed asexuals in the lab. If scientists ever document a human being with no measurable libido, we'll let you know.*

I am so easily turned on

I'm writing to you because I'm not sure who else to ask. I am easily turned on. I mean, very easily turned on. If I am washing the dishes and touch my clit against the sink, I can have an orgasm. Once I was wearing tight pants and driving, and I had to park and fuck my pants until I came. I've been with the same guy for three years. I sometimes make him park and fuck me. Once, a guy who was walking his dog spotted us. I refused to stop, and the guy got an eyeful. I can't wait for the first big snowfall so my boyfriend can eat me out in the snow. (He says it'll be too cold, but I'm going to drag him out there by his jacket collar.) Last week at a dinner party I was walking toward him, but before I could say anything he smiled and said sweetly, "No." Later he said he thought I was going to ask him to fuck me under the dinner table. (So I was—is that a crime?) Is there something wrong with me? My sister says I'm sick and need help, but it's not like I'm fucking every Tom, Dick and Harry in town.—M.D., Philadelphia, Pennsylvania

You sound fine to us. Horny, but fine. Your sister sounds as if she suffers from what we call the Helms syndrome: She believes that anyone who has more and better sex than she does is a pervert. You should be concerned only if your desires interfere with your life. That is, pulling over to fuck your pants is an impulse. Pulling over every mile to fuck your pants is a compulsion. And it makes you late for work.

Turned on by his clothes

While my husband and I were window-shopping at a mall, he whispered to me that he had an erection. He said, "My silk boxers are rubbing me the right way." He put his hand in his pocket to disguise his excitement, but I quickly slipped my hand in his other pocket and began rubbing his balls as we walked. I was so aroused I didn't care if other people noticed our antics. Thank God we had driven the minivan so we could lie down in the back, where I sucked him off. Is it natural for a man to get an erection from the way his clothes rub him?—T.S., Jackson, Michigan

You bet. If only it were natural to have a woman stick her hand into his pants every time it happened.

Scentsational sex

Nothing in the world smells so good as my girlfriend's body. I love to close my eyes and put my nose against her hair and skin. If my cock gets lazy during sex, I put my nose into her pussy and it never fails to arouse me. She no longer wears perfume. She knows it doesn't turn me on. Why am I so affected by her scent?—G.E., Martinez, California

You're attracted to your girlfriend's scent because it was designed to attract you. Every person has a unique odor. Scientists believe its purpose is to help us determine if a potential mate has a sufficiently different genetic makeup. Body odor is created when hormones secreted from glands concentrated in the armpit and groin interact with bacteria on the skin and are dispersed by body hair. Because as a culture we wash daily with scented soaps, these natural pheromones often are removed or overpowered. Women also typically shave their underarms and sometimes their genitals, removing hair that might otherwise distribute what Baudelaire called their "scent of fur." The poet shared your love of eau de femme (he found great meaning in erotic sweat), as did Napoleon, who famously wrote Josephine, "I will be arriving in Paris tomorrow evening. Don't wash." Resourceful French prostitutes once dabbed vaginal fluid behind their ears. In Shakespeare's time, a love-stricken woman would place a peeled apple under her arm, saturate it with sweat, then offer the "love apple" to her paramour to inhale. (Try that the next time your girlfriend packs your lunch.) Today, scientists wonder if our habitual cleanliness creates a subconscious hunger for pheromones, and if that has led to more exposed flesh and more oral sex. If you and your girlfriend want to experiment with your natural attraction, you'll find fragrance-free soaps and shampoos at stores such as mothernature.com. You'll find apples at the supermarket.

My friends and I split the cost of a pheromone-based cologne additive that claimed it would boost our sexual attractiveness. After using the product carefully and religiously, we concluded that it made no difference. Do pheromones work? The manufacturer claims its product is extracted from the armpit sweat of healthy young men. Should that have tipped us off that we were getting ripped off?—F.B., New York, New York

Not necessarily. If humans secrete sex pheromones, a sweaty armpit is a likely place to find them. In this case, however, you purchased a drop of science distilled in a barrel of marketing. Human pheromones can influence people in subtle ways, but they aren't powerful enough to convince a woman you're sexually desirable if she doesn't already believe that. Elsewhere in the animal kingdom, of course, pheromones are an essential part of the mating ritual. If a sow in heat gets a whiff of androsterone, a steroid found in boar saliva, she'll stop in her tracks, arch her back and present her genitals. How easy is that? Male underarm sweat contains a similar steroid, but if you lift your arm over a woman's nose, the only thing you'll see is the door. That's not to dismiss the idea of subliminal scents entirely. One study found that undetectable steroids produced by the body do elevate a woman's mood—as long as you dab them right beneath her nose. Distilled in a cologne or additive, these steroids are diluted enough that a woman would have to be close enough to kiss you to inhale them. If she is, you don't need help.

Recovering her libido

I have no desire for sex, which frustrates my wonderful husband of 10 years. I began losing my libido after the birth of our son. My husband deserves better. Can you help?—T.G., Dallas, Texas

We'll try. Let's run through the most common reasons women suffer a loss of libido. Perhaps one or more will strike a nerve: (1) A diminishing sex drive isn't unusual during pregnancy and after childbirth, especially among women who breast-feed. Children can be exhausting in general. A British study of 1,000 women ages 30 to 55 found that one in three reported being too tired for sex and attributed it to working full-time while also running a household. (2) Health problems such as diabetes or thyroid disease can make sex uncomfortable, and many women suffer from dyspareunia (pain during intercourse). Depression may be the most common libido killer. (3) Medications such as birth control pills, antibiotics, antihistamines and antidepressants may hamper desire. At the same time, some studies suggest that the antidepressant Wellbutrin can help restore lust in some women. (4) Relationship problems can spill into the bed-room, as can body image issues—with your own body or that of your partner. (5) Hormonal changes in a woman's late 30s, 40s or early 50s may play a role. About a third of women report a loss of libido in the years before menopause, and about 40 percent in menopause. What treatments are available? Estrogen or testosterone may help. Regular exercise is often overlooked as an aphrodisiac. Some therapists recommend a steady diet of literary erotica. Artificial lube is a great salve. As we've mentioned in the past, a classic treatment is sensual massage. It not only relieves stress but also redefines sex as more than intercourse that leads to orgasm.

Unleashing the wild woman

Last summer, my shy music-teacher wife shed every extra pound and got a boob job. Yet she still didn't feel confident about how she looked. I suggested that she submit her photos to *Playboy*, but she had another idea. A friend of mine planned to visit us for the weekend. She asked what I would think if at some time during my friend's stay, she allowed him to see her nude. I said I had no problem with this; the idea turned me on. When I brought my friend home from the airport, my wife was in the pool in a teeny, nearly transparent bikini I hadn't known about. My friend appeared to be in shock. The show continued the next day when she allowed him to catch glimpses of her naked breasts as she sunbathed. That night we all climbed into the hot tub and soon began talking about my wife's new body. There didn't seem to be any problems with her modesty: She scooted up on the edge of the hot tub and removed her bikini top. She and I began to make out and invited my friend to join in. The three of us wound up on the living room floor. My wife had never allowed me to come in her mouth but now swallowed from both of us. Later she asked to be "double fucked" with me in her vagina and my friend in her ass. She kept screaming, "Fuck me!" I was blown away; I had never seen this side of her. The next morning she asked if she could take my friend to catch his plane home. She returned horny as hell and we had a fantastic day of sex. She later told me she had given my friend "the blow job of his life" in the airport parking lot. This may sound stupid, but I'm wondering if I should feel jealous. Also, my wife was vocal and frantic during our threesome. I want that every night, but it hasn't happened since. She says the situation was a total loss of control on her part, and that she would be embarrassed otherwise. How can I unleash the wild woman again?—R.T., Seattle, Washington

You're overlooking the larger problem: How are you going to keep her? If you listen closely, you'll hear what she's saying: "I'm the new me, but you're the old you." She lost weight, felt the stares of other men and realized how bored she had become.

That puts you at a disadvantage, but the situation is not hopeless. First, recognize that you could tell her 50 times a day that she's irresistible and it wouldn't have the same effect as one stranger winking at her. She's ready to explore, and standard sex from hubby isn't going to hack it, especially as her confidence grows. You have to show her it's worthwhile to stick around. Get wild yourself: Introduce fun sex toys, blindfold her, eat dessert off her body, massage her, make love to her on the hood of the car. Love her like she's not yours. If you don't, your wife may again blow another guy at the airport—then get on the plane with him.

Is sex necessary?

Do people need sex? My friend says he doesn't, yet he masturbates. Isn't that a need for sex?—F.J., Albany, New York

People do need sex. Your friend's masturbation involves fantasy, which reflects his need for intimacy. We can survive without that, but it's a life less lived. Some people will argue that we need sex only to reproduce, but that can now be done in a lab. Fucking for no biological reason is what makes us human. In that sense, we need it bad.

"Fucking for no biological reason" isn't an exclusively human trait. Dolphins are said to have sex for pleasure, for example. And my dog tries to have sex with everything. Is he not seeking pleasure?—G.K., Madison, Wisconsin

Sure, but that's not why he's horny. He doesn't think about what he's doing; he knows only that he must have sex. By contrast, human males are driven by . . . wait a minute. That doesn't work. What makes us human is that we can choose not to have sex. No other animal has that luxury, regardless of the consequences. When a male honeybee ejaculates, for instance, his genitals fall off and he explodes (we've all been there). Evolutionary biologist Olivia Judson, author of Dr. Tatiana's Sex Advice to All Creation, *says that many animals besides dolphins and humans have been observed having sex even when reproduction isn't possible. Some species of duck have sex in winter, when the male's testes are regressed and the female isn't producing eggs. Indian-crested porcupines do it when the female is already pregnant. One type of wood roach fucks constantly. The list goes on. The most notorious swingers in the animal kingdom are bonobo chimps, who are unusual in that they have intercourse face-to-face. They also masturbate and enjoy oral sex and orgies.*

Horny women

A friend's recently divorced sister-in-law, whom I've never met, is apparently open to the idea of us being fuck buddies. Is this weird? I'd be going on a blind date with the expectation of sex.—M.D., Chicago, Illinois

You know how women are—it's always sex, sex, sex. See how it goes, but don't put out until you know her better.

I know you were being facetious, but you may want to give women more credit for their general horniness. I read recently about a study done at Ohio State, where researchers asked 201 students to record their sexual histories. The women reported an average of 2.6 partners, the men an average of 3.7. Then the researchers hooked the students up to a (fake) lie detector. The men's responses stayed virtually the same, but the women's average jumped to 4.4. The women also reported masturbating and watching porn twice as often as they had on the surveys. So it looks like women do love sex as much as guys—they just don't like to admit it.—T.R., Oberlin, Ohio

Can women get blue balls?

Guys get blue balls. What do girls get?—R.B., Wheeling, West Virginia

They get laid.

Your response is too flippant. A woman's genitals become engorged with blood during arousal. If that blood isn't released back into the body by orgasm, the woman feels the same swelling, pressure and discomfort that a man would.— D.S., Pullman, Washington

You're right, of course. Women can get frustrated to the point of painful vaso-congestion, but it's reported far less often. That's why it doesn't have its own slang. When a woman has the equivalent of blue balls, her inner labia may double in size and burn bright or deep red, depending on whether she's given birth.

My human sexuality professor at Arizona State calls the female equivalent of blue balls "violet vulva." It's actually known as *protracted resolution*, because the genitals return to their unaroused state without orgasm prior to the resolution stage.—D.S., Chandler, Arizona

Most guys live in a state of protracted resolution.

I'm a 28-year-old married bisexual woman. I laughed at your blue balls remark because it assumes that women can get sex whenever they want. As any woman can tell you, that isn't true—especially if you're dating another woman.—S.J., San Francisco, California

You're married, bisexual and female and still frustrated? What does it take?

Morning wood

My boyfriend almost always wakes up with an erection. When I ask him why, he says he's been dreaming about me. I'm not that gullible. Is there a medical reason for morning erections?—M.B., Birmingham, Alabama

Of course he's dreaming about you. Or he may be dreaming about red pickup trucks, fresh artichokes, being chased by Roseanne or going to class in his underwear. Regardless of what's on his mind, every healthy male experiences spontaneous, involuntary erections as he dreams. They occur every 90 minutes or so during the dream stage of sleep. Scientists aren't certain why sleep erections occur, but one prevailing theory is that they are a natural systems check or some kind of exercise program to keep the penis in shape. A woman might interpret morning wood as an invitation for sex. That's a good instinct. But the guy's immediate thought is probably, How am I going to pee with this thing?

Do women have similar patterns? And why do scientists measure sleep arousal?—E.R., Tulsa, Oklahoma

Women apparently do experience similar sleep arousal. But while blood flow to the penis can be monitored by attaching an expandable ring, measuring blood flow to a woman's genitals is more of a challenge. Sleep erections are typically monitored to determine if erectile dysfunction is a physical or a mental problem.

ETIQUETTE

Do the right thing.

Can I keep copies of her dirty photos?

When my girlfriend and I were together, she let me take nude snapshots of her, including a few where she's giving me head. Now that we're breaking up, she wants the prints and negatives. I don't want to be a bastard, but I also wouldn't mind having the photos for reference. At one point, I scanned a bunch into my computer and burned a CD. Does that count as something that I have to give her?—A.L., Huntsville, Alabama

In other words, can you return the prints and negatives, but keep copies? Sure. The photos were taken during private moments in your ex-girlfriend's life, but those moments also happen to be part of your life. The courts call it joint custody. That said, only a real shit would share these images with anyone, for any reason, be it carelessness or revenge. One reader attempted to solve this problem by offering nude images of himself to his ex. She didn't consider it a fair trade.

Tipping tips

I found myself in an uncomfortable situation on a business trip to Los Angeles. When the limo driver dropped me at the airport, I realized I had only two singles. I wasn't sure what to do. Should I have offered him the two bucks with an apology? Instead, I shook his hand and thanked him. Now I feel like a schmuck.—K.T., Chicago, Illinois

If you find yourself short of cash, apologize and ask for his card. Then send a thank-you note with a tip. Copy his boss. That way you're a schmuck only if you don't follow through.

Last month a reader asked about a friend who would not tip on the alcohol portion of a restaurant meal. You didn't address the larger issue, which is why we're expected to tip on meals at all. We need to stop looking down on people who are willing to pay only the price on the menu.—J.S., Vermillion, South Dakota

You can pay the price on the menu, but who's going to bring you the food? Skipping out on a tip might have worked in the Middle Ages, when leaving extra

was done solely in gratitude. But like it or not, tipping is now a form of compensation. Early Americans considered it undemocratic, but that changed in the late 19th century after wealthy Americans saw that it was done in Europe. Hotel and restaurant owners encouraged the practice because it allowed them to reduce wages and supervision of their staff. So many workers became dependent on tips that customers who held out paid for their insolence: Bellmen made chalk marks on the bags of nontippers so they would remember which ones to drop; in Chicago in 1918 police arrested 100 waiters for spoiling the meals of repeat customers who refused to tip. Tipping can be confusing. Our advice is to trust your instincts. If it feels as if you should tip, make sure you do. If it feels as if you should give a little more, then do that, too.

When traveling, I've noticed that people in some countries expect a tip in advance of a service. Isn't this a bribe?—R.S., Honolulu, Hawaii

A tip is given in appreciation; a bribe is given in anticipation. When traveling in many parts of the world, it's a good idea to recognize both. In the Middle East and Indonesia, a small bribe (pretip?) for services to be rendered is known as baksheesh; *in Mexico it's* la mordida *(little bite); in Kenya it's* chai. Grease *is the term we grew up with. Any good travel guide will provide the going rates and customs. No matter where you are, it's best to be discreet and not to offer cash until absolutely necessary. If you don't offer at least minimal resistance, you'll be marked as a rube. Government officials in some countries can spot a mark at ten paces, and it's not beneath them to take your bribe and then "fine" you for bribery. Relative to what you're spending on the trip,* baksheesh *won't add up to much, but it will make your journey a great deal smoother.*

Returning the favor
How do you ask a friend to return a favor without holding it over his head?—R.T., Denver, Colorado

You don't. A favor doesn't create debt. You can, however, cash in a favor to assist a third party, such as another friend. If you need a favor yourself, describe the situation in general terms and hope your previously favored friend takes the hint. If he doesn't, don't push it. While reporting on the favor economy for Chicago *magazine, writer Marc Spiegler articulated the rules power brokers seem to follow: (1) Never give a favor expecting a specific reward, or demand repayment—you shouldn't know or care if you're paid up or paid back. (2) The value of a favor can rise or fall (e.g., securing Bulls tickets is no longer any great* shakes). (3) *Personal and professional favors are interchangeable. (4) Favors are often better than money, and generally tax-free. (5) Always offer a favor before it is requested. (6) Don't abuse the system, or you'll be frozen out.*

The limits of PDA

Where does the Advisor draw the line on public displays of affection?—T.R., Des Moines, Iowa

No tongues. We also prohibit baby talk and sliding a hand into your lover's back pocket. Frantic groping in the bushes is okay.

The lady in red

A few months ago the CEO of my company died. He had worked his way from the mail room to the top. In the process, he stepped on plenty of toes. One woman lost her job when the executive promoted her boss but wouldn't allow her a transfer. At the funeral she wore a red dress louder than any fire engine. Some people thought it was tacky, but I thought it was great. I didn't like the guy, either. Should she have worn a traditional dress and not expressed her feelings? And what should a man wear to a funeral to express his loathing?—D.G., New York, New York

Tacky, tacky. We don't approve of making a spectacle of anyone's grief. A simple man who loathed the dead would skip the memorial. A gentleman would attend, dressed appropriately, and keep his mouth shut out of respect for the widow and family who had to live with the deceased.

How should I handle the office party?

I just landed my first job. The office holiday party is approaching and I'm nervous about it because I'm afraid I'll do something stupid. Any advice?— T.H., Philadelphia, Pennsylvania

If nobody did anything stupid at holiday parties, who would go? The best advice is to limit your alcohol intake to that warm, friendly point just before you can't legally drive, and never get drunker than your boss. Consider it an opportunity to get to know co-workers who might become friends and perhaps help you advance (or keep you out of trouble). There's another benefit to attending: A British newspaper surveyed 1,000 people and found that about 10 percent had started a relationship at a company holiday party. In addition, five percent said they had removed some of their clothes. We'd guess many in the second group also belong to the first.

Turf wars

I'm in a bar with a date and excuse myself to use the rest room. When I return, a guy is hovering over my chair, talking to my date. I linger, play the jukebox, etc. I didn't want to dive in like a possessive boyfriend. Later, my date said I should have come right back because the guy was a loser and she was dying to get rid of him. A week later, I'm on a date with another woman. This time when I come out of the john and see a guy talking to her, I head straight for the table, excuse myself and take my seat. My date later tells me that I acted like a jealous he-man claiming his turf and should have given her time to take care of the situation. I guess the only solution is to ask my dates before I take a leak, "If there's a guy with you when I come back, how would you like me to handle it?" How does the Advisor deal with the man-in-my-chair situation?—C.T., Santa Barbara, California

We put our hand on the back of the chair and say hello. It's a bar, after all—lots of friendly people. But we're confused by the women you're dating. How hard is it to tell a chummy guy that you're with someone? It's okay to expect your date to save your seat.

The revolving door

What is the protocol for walking women through rotating doors? Ladies first and make them push, or gentleman first in order to do the pushing?—A.F., New Orleans, Louisiana

We think ladies first, for the same reason it's always ladies first—so you can check out her ass. Did we say that aloud?

Best time to break up

When is the best time to break up with someone?—K.J., Chicago, Illinois

Right after they've won the lottery, so they know you're serious. There's no good time for the person getting dumped.

A friendly squeeze

My best friend went to the Caribbean for his honeymoon. One day he got a massage. He told me that the masseuse "hooted" him—that is, she squeezed his penis. Embarrassed, he ignored the gesture. The masseuse continued the massage as if nothing had happened. Was she sending a signal that she'd be willing to give him some X-rated attention? If so, what's the proper response?—M.K., Somerville, Massachusetts

Have you already booked your flight? Before we hear from any outraged masseuses, let's say first that you should never expect or request a happy ending. We've enjoyed hundreds of massages over the years and have never been hooted. Then again, we don't find our masseuses in the sports section of the newspaper. There is no secret meaning to a woman grabbing your cock, in any context. It means what you think it means. The best response, if that sort of thing interests you, is, "That felt nice."

Nipple patrol

While at the beach my sister-in-law and I were talking after she had come out of the cold surf. I noticed that her nipple was exposed. She left to get a soda, then marched back and asked why I hadn't told her about her nipple. I hemmed and hawed and finally said, "I hoped it would slip back on its own." Later, after a few drinks, we all had a good laugh about it. But what should I say next time it happens? With her breasts I'm sure it will.—D.T., Miami, Florida

Do they call you Mr. Smooth? No need to be coy. If her nipple escapes again, tell her to watch her top.

Follow-up visit

Is it ethical for a patient to ask out his nurse?—B.S., Pittsburgh, Pennsylvania

Sure. She's already seen your penis. But it's not ethical for her to accept.

Caller I.D.

What is the etiquette for answering a phone that has caller ID, specifically at work? Should you greet the person by name or use a more generic hello?—D.Y., Phoenix, Arizona

Answer with your name instead of theirs. Someday that caller ID is going to be useful, so keep it close to your vest.

Are those real?

I have become friends with an attractive woman at work. She speaks freely with me about her new breast implants. How can I ask her to show them to me without destroying the friendship?—N.B., Bedford, Texas

You won't ask her that, especially not at work. Given the boob jobs we've seen in test shots, her tits probably look better in her shirt. Enjoy the fantasy.

Everyone hates his wife

My best friend has married a woman who is such a bitch that no one in our circle of friends, including my girlfriend, wants to be around her. How do I tell him that everyone hates his wife?—J.P., Chicago, Illinois

He already knows—or he should, since he's probably seeing a lot more of his wife's friends than his own. Good friends are often the first victims of bad marriages.

Sending flowers

Is it customary for a gentleman to send flowers after the first time he has sex with a lady, or is chivalry dead?—N.P., Rushmore, Minnesota

If you were chivalrous you'd marry her. Once you've been intimate you can't go wrong sending flowers.

Calling her by the wrong name

What should a guy say when he calls his partner by another name while making love?—B.F., Van Nuys, California

There's not much to say. This is why early man invented the word "baby."

Susan Sarandon delivered a great line in *Bull Durham* regarding this. She asked, "Would you rather I were making love to him using your name, or making love to you using his name?"—M.S., Portland, Oregon

FASHION

Looking good.

Making an impression

The other day my boss commented on the fact that the pants of my suit did not have cuffs. He said that because I am tall (6'3"), it is considered a faux pas. He said my cuffs should be 1¹/8 inches wide. He also commented on my tie, saying it should have a dimple (he has a full Windsor knot). Finally, he didn't like the monochromatic look of my tie against my shirt. Should I consider any of his comments?—T.M., Beverly Hills, California

It depends. What is the nature of the business? If you're meeting regularly with clients, your boss sets the standard. Traditional pleated trousers should have cuffs, but a width of 1³/4 inches is more appropriate for your height. If you're wearing slender, fitted pants, cuffs aren't necessary. Your tie should have a dimple, but stick with the common four-in-hand knot; the Windsor isn't practical unless your shirts have spread collars. "Most well-dressed men don't use Windsors because the knot looks much too self-conscious," says Alan Flusser, author of Dressing the Man. *"A four-in-hand is infinitely more stylish." Monochromatic also works, for now. However, it may not work for your boss.*

Fighting yellow pits

My deodorant creates yellow stains on the armpits of my white dress shirts. Is there any way to prevent this?—K.R., Los Angeles, California

The stains aren't caused by deodorant but by secretions from your apocrine glands, which are found in your pits and near your genitals and produce those funky pheromones designed to turn the ladies to mush. The more stressed you are, the more secretions. Although the secretions should decrease as you get older, your cleaner is right—there's not much you can do to prevent stains except to wear undershirts, throw each shirt into the wash instead of the hamper or retire to a beach resort. One fashion maven we saw on Howard Stern's TV show demonstrated how she puts maxipads in the armpits of her jackets to protect them. You could try that, but don't get caught.

White vinegar can get rid of those stains. Sponge it on or soak the stains for 30 minutes, then launder the shirts in the hottest water safe for the fabric.—B.M., Cedar Hills, Texas

Thanks for the tip. Another reader suggested pouring an equal mixture of laundry soap, bleach and dishwasher detergent (granules) into a hot-water wash, letting it dissolve and adding the shirts. After about three washes, she says, your whites will be white again. Or try a prewash scrubbing with a baking soda paste or a shampoo designed for oily hair.

Match game

When you wear dress shoes and trousers, should your socks match the shoes or your pants?—R.H., Ormond Beach, Florida

Your socks should match your trousers. For example, if you choose a dark gray suit and brown shoes, wear charcoal gray socks. And make sure your socks extend well above your ankles. The most serious hosiery faux pas is allowing a patch of skin to show when you sit down.

I've been told that your shirt-pants-shoes color combination should alternate—that is, light-dark-light or dark-light-dark. What do you think?—S.C., San Antonio, Texas

That's not the place to start. The goal of dressing well is to draw attention to your face. The first thing to consider is the contrast between your skin and your shirt, and your jacket and tie if you wear them. Selecting colors is trickier, but if you stand in front of the mirror and hold up enough colors to your face, some will stand out (you don't want to look pasty or pink). Eye color and suntan are also factors. "If you have blue eyes, you definitely want to wear blue shirts or ties with some strong blue in them," says Alan Flusser. "A dark tan tends to mean you should wear more contrast. That's why men tend to dress more colorfully in the spring and summer." If you play with contrast, be careful. Too much and you'll look like a Creamsicle. Still confused? Stick with the classics: black jacket with gray pants, blue jacket with khakis.

Can you wear a striped tie with a striped shirt or suit?—A.A., New York, New York

You want tough? Throw in a striped suit. "I've seen a photo of Fred Astaire wearing three stripes, and it looks wonderful," says Flusser. "It requires a delicate

touch. The more sophisticated the dresser, the more likely he'll attempt patterns together." Most guys can handle mixing three solids (one color should stand out) or two solids and a pattern. Fewer can find their way with two patterns. Ideally, one should be stripes, both should share a color and each should have a different scale. "If you're wearing a suit with stripes that have an inch of space between them, choose a shirt that's more of a pinstripe," Flusser says. "If you have a striped tie, make sure it's closer to the scale of your suit than to that of your shirt. You want to avoid wearing small stripes next to small stripes."

David Letterman often wears white or cream socks with a dark gray or navy double-breasted suit. My late father, who sold clothes for 50 years, would have had a fit. Is this something that only Letterman does, or is it a trend?—W.D., Memphis, Tennessee

It's a trend among late-night hosts who make $14 million a year and have no one left to impress. After all, style is just shorthand for "What can I get away with?" White socks work for Letterman because he's a comedian. They wouldn't work so well if he were handling people's money.

The proper length of pants

I've been dressing myself for 40 years with no complaints. I recently took up residence with a much younger woman who gripes about the length of my pants. My girlfriend insists that I buy pants so long I walk on them after slipping off my shoes. I tend to wear them only long enough to cover the tops of my shoes. What is the proper length for a pair of pants? Is it different for dress slacks and jeans?—P.W., Helper, Utah

Your pants should have a single break in the front and hang about a quarter inch above the top of your heel in the back. In the front, they should be long enough that the cuffs cover one-half to two-thirds of the length of your shoes. The weight of your cuffs keeps them in contact with your shoes. "You see a lot of athletes and rap stars with their suit pants bunching up by the ankles," says Playboy's *fashion director, Joseph De Acetis. "Don't do that." The quarter-inch rule also applies to jeans, although the trend lately is to wear them dragging below the heel, giving the edges a ragged look. You can get away with that, De Acetis says, but you'll still be considered fashionable if the denim stops before it hits the asphalt. Propose a compromise: Your dress slacks will remain at, or be adjusted slightly to, their proper length, and your girlfriend can buy you a new pair of jeans that are long enough to walk on.*

Business casual

Some time ago I took a job with a company that has a business casual dress code. For that reason, my wool suit jackets have begun to lose their shape. Do you have any storage tips for suits that are in the closet more than they're on me?— W.K., Omaha, Nebraska

You need stronger hangers. Thin hangers (especially those made of wire) allow the shoulder pads to shift, giving your suits that wilted look even when they're not in the closet for a season. For those that have already sagged, ask your tailor or retailer to replace or press the pads. Have your suits cleaned before putting them away, and don't leave them inside the retailer's garment bag, which can trap moisture and create wrinkles. Instead, cut the bag so that only the shoulders are covered. Also, make certain the suit is stored with a solid front; that is, the panels should overlap slightly so that the button holes line up with the buttons.

Is my tie like a penis?

When my wife and I go to parties, she constantly fiddles with my tie. I mentioned this to a colleague. He said not to worry about it because my tie represents my penis, and therefore my wife must adore it. He was joking, but it made me wonder if there's any truth to his theory.—R.T., Atlanta, Georgia

We like everything about the analogy except the knotting and tugging part. Believe it or not, the Guild of British Tie Makers has studied the interaction between women and men's ties. "The tie is a very psychological garment," a guild spokesman told a London newspaper. "Very simply, it protects the jugular. It's a man's warrior shield. So a woman touching a man's tie in public is a clear sign that she is laying claim to him." According to the guild, women enjoy a variety of necktie nuances, including a simple touch (to gauge a man's response), the brush (to show she's interested), straightening (a sign of desire for intimacy), adjusting (a power move), loosening (to lower a man's defenses, possibly to say she's ready for sex), untying (staking her claim) and tying (possession, especially if she bought the tie). Let's be careful out there.

The lines of the tie

I was complimented on my tie by a friend, who then flipped it over to take a closer look. He said tie quality is determined by horizontal lines enmeshed in the fabric. Is that true?—G.B., Orlando, Florida

That scene says more about your boorish friend than about your tie. Did he check the tag on your shirt, too? The bars he mentioned don't indicate quality.

They are used by manufacturers to denote the weight of the lining. You can't grade neckwear while it's around your neck. Instead, suspend the tie by the narrow blade—it shouldn't twist. Stretch it slightly to see if it maintains its shape. The finest ties come in three sections instead of two, with both ends of the loop on the larger blade held securely under the center seam. The most important ways to judge a tie are the fit and feel. If it looks good on you, it's a good tie.

Leather pants

When is it acceptable to wear leather pants?—D.M., Detroit, Michigan

When you're trying out for the Village People. Leather belongs on shoes, belts, coats and cows.

Launder or dry clean?

Should I launder or dry-clean my dress shirts?—C.F., Toronto, Ontario

We prefer to launder with light starch and have the shirts hand-pressed and placed on hangers. It's better at removing ring around the collar and generally helps the shirts last longer. They may last even longer without starch, but that's how we like it done. Dry-cleaning results in less shrinkage but leaves the fabric too stiff for our taste.

Traveling with clothes

I've noticed that it's difficult to travel any great distance without looking as if you've slept in your clothes. Which fabrics are most likely to come out of a suitcase looking reasonable?—L.H., Juneau, Alaska

Polyester, rayon, wool and acrylic. But there's no need for a new wardrobe— just refine your packing technique. Ours is to roll our trousers, carefully fold our shirts and find a laundry when we arrive. We had a shirt pressed in Italy that looked so good we were reluctant to wear it.

What can I do to flatten a crease in a tie?—B.D., Boston, Massachusetts

Usually you can hang the wrinkles out. If that doesn't work, fold the tie in half, roll it around your index finger, slip it off and let it sit overnight.

Fashion faux pas

What do you think about guys who wear thongs?—J.H., Dallas, Texas

We try not to.

What is your position regarding men who wear short-sleeve shirts with ties but no jackets?—A.M., London, U.K.

They come around once a month to fix the copy machine.

The right jacket

Is it okay to wear a black overcoat with a navy or brown suit, or should I get camel hair?—J.W., Boston, Massachusetts

You'd be better off with a dark gray or vicuña coat that you can wear with blue, black, gray or some browns. Camel hair goes with anything, but it's dressy.

Translating the invite

My wife and I were invited to a wedding that will take place at 3 PM. The invitation reads "black tie optional." My wife says this means you should wear a tuxedo if you own one. I don't think it's right to wear a tux in the afternoon unless the host insists on it. Who's right?—J.K., Owings Mills, Maryland

We would wear a dark suit, but it depends on your personal taste—you won't be overdressed in a tux, and we suspect it might also get you laid. For the record, "black tie optional" and "black tie invited" are a notch below "black tie preferred" and two notches below "black tie required". In the last two cases we would wear a tux. With "optional" or "invited" you risk being the only man in a suit, but we've never been to an event at which that was the case. "Creative black tie" means you can have some fun.

The war on pleats

What's with the war on pleats? I've read three different admonitions in *Playboy* against wearing pleated pants. For example, you advise readers, "If you're size medium to skinny, you'll look better in flat fronts." Better in what way? I have two pairs of pleated slacks I wear for dressy occasions, and I frequently receive compliments from women on how dapper and urbane I look. I'm six feet tall with a 32-inch waist.—R.W., Pasadena, California

Did we say better? We meant hipper. Some of our best friends are pleats. But according to STS Market Research, which tracks apparel trends, more than half of all pants sold to men under 40 have flat fronts, up from 35 percent just two years earlier. Sales among older men have been more consistent; about 58 percent of the pants they buy have folds. Pleats definitely look better on guys who are heavier or have a barrel shape, but a medium or skinny build can go either way. The only real test is to see if women react the same way to a flat front. It may not be your trousers that impress them.

Panty hose for men

My boyfriend wears panty hose in public, even with shorts. He says panty hose on men is a trend. Is he goofy or in style?—J.T., Grand Rapids, Michigan

He may be ahead of his time—except for the shorts. Thousands of men wear panty hose for nonsexual reasons (that is, they aren't cross-dressers). One major supplier is G. Lieberman & Sons, whose chief executive, Steve Katz, began marketing to men in 1999 after trying on dozens of pairs of women's nylons and noting what he didn't like about their fit. The result is a durable hose with a fly, longer legs, a lower waistband and more room for the male package. Katz and his wife launched comfilon.com to sell hose as a fashionable alternative to socks and long underwear for men who have the "nylon gene," or as a practical one for warmth, circulation or to avoid contact with itchy wool pants. They also market to cops, truckers, construction workers, athletes and soldiers in Iraq (to protect against sand fleas). In fact, a pair kept us ventilated and compressed while answering your letter. That's startling only in that we usually go commando.

THE FEMALE BODY

Navigating her curves.

Finding the clitoris

Every woman I've been with has told me I do an amazing job going down on her. I even got a bloody lip once because a girl bucked so hard during orgasm. But I've found that right when a woman seems to reach the peak of her arousal, I always lose track of her clitoris. It just disappears. What's going on?—R.T., Tallahassee, Florida

In its Guide to Getting It On, *the staff of Goofy Foot Press notes that clitoris is Latin for "darned thing that was here just a second ago." As a woman becomes aroused, her clitoris swells. As she reaches the plateau phase just before climax, it may disappear beneath its hood of skin. Some researchers now believe this is an optical illusion: The clit stays put but the labia swell, hiding it. Whichever the case, the retreating clit is nature's way of reminding you to stay focused. If you lose track of her clitoris, you have two options. Dig deeper (get your nose in there), or gently explore her vulva and labia until she becomes just slightly less aroused. This will give the clitoris a false sense of security, and it will peek out to be captured by your tongue or finger. Have you noticed how teasing someone into oblivion is often the same thing as bumbling around? Just keep it moving.*

I used to have the same problem. Then one evening I decided to use my tongue to map my wife's vulva. I began gently spreading her labia with my fingers and thumbs, then licking her upward from the perineum, across the vaginal opening, between the parted labia, over the clitoris, and up the clitoral shaft. She went crazy, so I did it again, bottom to top, one long slow stroke. I found that by using her inner lips to guide the tip of my tongue, I could follow them like the banks of a river until they came together at the top, where her clitoris was quivering expectantly. After a few more strokes, I stayed put, giving her clit a few feathery strokes and then licking it more firmly with my tongue. Needless to say, I've had no trouble finding it since.—S.C., Boston, Massachusetts

Thanks for the tip. You're the Lewis and Clark of cunnilingus.

One breast is larger

My wife's left breast is larger than her right. This makes her feel self-conscious, so I searched online for photos of women with different-sized breasts to show her she's not abnormal. I found many, and most are like my wife— the left breast seems larger. Is there a reason for this?—K.H., Melbourne, Florida

Many women have noticeably different breasts, just as many guys have noticeably different testicles. We can't say why the left breast more often seems larger, but a study of 598 women in Akron, Ohio confirmed your perception and "the generally accepted clinical impression of left-breast dominance." In 54 percent of the subjects measured by the Akron team, the left breast was larger. In an earlier study of 248 women, however, the split was 50-50, so who knows? The researchers found only one woman among the 846 who had breasts of equal volume.

Vaginal odors

Whenever I finger my girlfriend and sniff my fingers, I smell a foul odor. It isn't horrible, but it sure isn't great. Is there a way to decrease the smell?— V.T., Tucson, Arizona

Yes. Don't sniff your fingers. Every woman smells different, but we'd describe the odor as pleasantly musky. Your girlfriend may have an infection such as bacterial vaginosis, but usually that produces itching, burning, a discharge and an odor that you would recognize as unquestionably bad. If you're concerned, tell her, "You know I love how you taste, but lately I've noticed it's different. I want to make sure you're okay." You may be the best friend her pussy's ever had.

Why is it that on the mornings after my husband and I have sex, I have a terrible odor coming from my vagina? I asked my sister if she had experienced anything like this and she said no.—A.K., Cherry Hill, New Jersey

There is a chance this is caused by your husband's semen. In 1995 a female patient of a family physician in Oakland, California complained that her genitals smelled fishy, but only after sex. She showed no other symptoms of bacterial vaginosis. Curious, the doctor asked the woman to return to his office every morning for a month so he could take cultures. He confirmed that she didn't have an infection and noted that the smell occurred only on mornings after she'd had unprotected intercourse.

I had this problem and found that it helps to sit on the toilet after sex and push the semen out. I also wear odor-absorbing panty liners. I've talked about this with my girlfriends, and we all agree that semen causes the odor.—L.K., Pittsboro, North Carolina

So while the guys talk about sports . . .

Finding her G-spot

My husband has searched for my G-spot without luck. How can we find it?—T.W., Cleveland, Ohio

You may already have. Not every woman finds stimulation of the Grafenberg spot all that memorable. In fact, an Italian scientist conducted anatomical studies that suggest some women either don't have a G-spot or have one so small that it can't easily be located. Others have wondered if it exists at all: A psychologist who reviewed the medical literature concluded that, without more definitive studies, the G-spot will remain a "gynecologic UFO." The idea of a pleasure spot, he says, puts undue stress on women who can't find theirs. The spot is easier to find if you're turned on, because it swells. In The Good Vibrations Guide: The G-Spot, *Cathy Winks suggests that you lie on your stomach, position yourself on your hands and knees or squat. "Reach your fingers an inch or two in from the vaginal opening and crook them toward the front wall of the vagina in a 'come hither' motion. The G-spot is responsive to pressure but not to light touch. If you brush lightly around the inside of the vagina, you probably won't feel anything. Instead, press firmly into the vaginal wall. Remember, the G-spot isn't on the vaginal wall; it's felt through the vaginal wall. As you explore from the pubic bone up toward the cervix, you should feel a slightly ridged area that begins to swell. You may find it helpful to take your other hand and press down on the outside of your belly just above the pubic hair line—sometimes you can feel the G-spot area swelling between your hands." Women have described the spot to Winks as "a spongy circle about the size of an almond," "a small cushion nestled against my pubic bone" and "sort of like a ripe strawberry." Happy hunting.*

Feeling her tail

While making out with a girl, I felt a nub at the top of her butt crack. I've heard that every human has a gene for a tail. Do some people actually have one?—E.W., Washington, D.C.

You're complaining about getting a little tail? Your date has an extended coccyx. No big deal.

How do your labia hang?

Our neighbor owns a porn store, so he knows a lot about sex. The other day he asked me which way my labia hang. He said that whichever way my lips hang is the way my husband's cock hangs. I ran home, dragged my husband into the bedroom and put a little throat on him. Sure enough, his erection bends slightly to the right, and my right lip is larger than my left. By the way, my neighbor is gay. Is this for real, or is he just trying to get a visual on my husband's cock?—M.M., Myrtle Beach, South Carolina

There's absolutely nothing to what your neighbor told you, although we're sure he'd love to hear the details. And your husband would love if you checked again.

I am dating a new guy and I'm afraid he may not like my pussy. My labia are prominent, and I'm worried that when he touches me or goes down on me, he will be turned off. I don't know why I'm hung up on this; none of my other boyfriends have said a word about it. I guess I need reassurance. What do guys think of women with large labia?—L.K., San Antonio, Texas

The right guy will think they're hot. We were sharing a limo with Juli Ashton and Tiffany Granath, the hosts of Playboy TV's Night Calls, when, believe it or not, this topic came up. (It was 6 AM, so you can imagine how the rest of the day went.) Tiffany expressed concern that her "meaty fins" might turn off a new beau. Juli chimed in that her left fin hung lower than her right and pointed out that women with long fins often can more easily reach orgasm. That's because typically a woman's clit is not stimulated enough during intercourse to bring her to climax without outside intervention (such as a finger or vibrator). But long fins wrap around the guy's erection, and his movement causes them to tug on her clit. The Advisor reassured our favorite redhead that any man who finds his face in her pussy is not thinking, This babe's too meaty. He's thinking, I can't believe that I'm going down on Tiffany Granath.

During interviews for our book, *Threesome: How to Fulfill Your Favorite Fantasy*, women with smaller "fins" said they stopped three-ways because of abrasion much more often than the well-endowed women. Larger, protruding lips retain vaginal lubrication, extend the vagina through the pubic hair and provide a longer, wetter tube. Men should be thankful for their partner's large labia, because they're better suited for extended intercourse.—Lori Gammon and Bill Strong, West Palm Beach, Florida

We've adjusted our fantasy accordingly.

My girlfriend's labia hang down almost an inch. When I discussed it with the guys at work, they all said it's because she's a slut. "Look at the porn stars," they said. I don't want to ask my girlfriend about this, but the guys have put this idea in my head, and I need reassurance.—J.A., Pullman, Washington

Sexual activity has nothing to do with the size of a woman's labia, nor does it affect her breasts, lips, eyes, nose, teeth, feet, buttocks, legs, fingers or toes. When you have a good thing going, it's always wise to share the particulars of your girlfriend's genitals on a need-to-know basis, which is to say—never. You're putting a lot of trust in these guys to keep their mouths shut.

My wife wants to have her inner labia trimmed. I tell her that I like hers the way they are. When she pulls on them, they stretch out to about two inches. Is there a doctor in his or her right mind who would do this type of operation? This is really bothering her.—S.W., Louisville, Kentucky

A plastic surgeon can trim the ends, or, in a technique developed by Dr. Gary Alter of Beverly Hills, remove a V-shaped wedge from the middle so the labia keep their natural edges. Alter says about 90 percent of the women who ask him to perform the surgery do so for cosmetic reasons; like your wife, they dislike the appearance of their genitals. Some are so hung up on it, they have a hard time enjoying sex. The other 10 percent, he says, complain of discomfort because the labia rub together or against clothes and become irritated, or get pinched. As with any surgery, there are risks, and the one-hour procedure will cost several thousand dollars or more (don't expect insurance coverage). Before your wife decides on surgery, buy her a copy of Femalia, *which includes 32 photos of vulvas with labia of all shapes and sizes. Its editor, Joani Blank, says she is troubled that any woman would have herself trimmed. "The scientific names we give the lips are unfortunate," she says. "Labia minora means 'little ones,' which implies to some people that they shouldn't show." Blank suggests that your wife speak with other women, who might have more luck convincing her that her labia are normal and natural. And you should keep reassuring her that her lips are as beautiful to you as the rest of her.*

Clit pumping

What is clit pumping?—B.J., Seattle, Washington

It resembles penis pumping, but you need a better eye. The practice draws blood to the clitoris, which increases sensitivity and lubrication. The FDA has approved a $360 device called Eros-CTD to assist women with sexual arousal disorder. It consists of a suction cup and a palm-size, battery-operated pump. But some women have been pumping for years. You'll find details in The Ultimate Guide to Strap-On Sex *by Karlyn Lotney, who reports that women have pumped their clits up to four and a half inches long and five inches around. That's the extreme; in most cases, pumping is viewed as occasional kinky fun. "Most men have about six inches of erectile tissue, and so do most women. It's just not as easy to see," she writes. "Pumping makes the clitoral shaft stand out in broad relief, which makes it easier for a partner to find and caress." Some women reach orgasm from the pump's sucking sensation; others find it intensifies the pleasure of oral sex after the cup is removed. Clit pumping can be hazardous, so women who attempt it should proceed carefully and stop immediately if they feel pain. Lotney suggests that beginners experiment with the yellow rubber suction cups found in snakebite kits. "Lubricate one of the suckers, squeeze it together around the flesh of your clitoris, and let go. The sucker will stay in place until you squeeze it again to break the suction." While a snakebite sucker is less intense than vacuum pumps, Lotney recommends not leaving it on your genitals for more than a few minutes at a time until you have more experience with the sensation.*

How deep is the vagina?

How deep is the average vagina? If you were to slide a yardstick into a woman, how far would it go?—C.C., Grand Ledge, Michigan

The ones we've measured have been about four inches. But we used our tongue.

Breaking the hymen

Can a woman lose her hymen before sex and not know it? I met my wife as a freshman in college, and she swore to me that she was a virgin. I believed her, but months later, when we finally had sex, there was no blood. In fact, she seemed very loose. What's your opinion?—S.B., Dallas, Texas

The notion that virgins always bleed is an ancient, stubborn and bogus belief. In many cases, the hymen doesn't produce much blood (if any) when it breaks, or

it stretches but remains intact, or it breaks naturally before sex, or the woman doesn't have one to begin with. There's no reliable way to tell if a woman is a virgin.

Spot the fake

My buddies and I often disagree on whether the Centerfold is all natural. Is there any surefire way to tell?—B.H., Chatsworth, California

Natural breasts aren't exactly the same size, they aren't perfectly round, they're in proportion to the woman's frame and weight and they don't defy gravity when she lies on her back. Many of the breast implants we see on women who believe "that's what Playboy *wants" can only be described as grotesque, which is why we never recommend the procedure. (Seventy percent of the women who submit photos to the magazine are rejected simply because they have bad boob jobs.) According to one of our photographers, only about 5 percent of the women he sees who have implants leave him guessing, which he sees as a sign of quality.*

Larger breasts through herbs

My fiancée has tiny breasts. I would love them to be larger, but I don't want her to go under the knife. I've seen magazine ads for herbal breast enlargement products such as Isis and Bloussant. Should I get her a supply?—R.T., New York, New York

Have you asked your fiancée about this? She may be happy with her size, which means she shouldn't change a thing. Regardless, enlargement pills and creams don't work. In fact, the Federal Trade Commission cracked down on the makers of Isis for false claims, including the company's assertion that its concoction had no side effects. (The FTC heard from hundreds of users who experienced headaches, nausea and allergic reactions.) A medical device called Brava has been shown to increase size in some women, but it has to be worn 10 to 12 hours a day for three months. A pump suctions air from plastic domes secured over the breasts with a mesh bra. This stretches the tissue, causing new cells to form. Not everyone is sold on the device, which costs $1,250 online or up to $2,500 if you buy from a doctor and Brava throws in a guarantee. Visit home.comcast.net/~drmomentum/bravargh for cautionary tales.

Ice-cold remedy

My friend told me to put ice packs on my breasts because they are stimulated by cold. Does that work? Also, if you have small breasts, how do you make yourself look sexy? Most guys want girls with large breasts.—S.S., Scarsdale, New York

Most guys aren't that picky. They may have quicker reflexes around large breasts, but they need more to keep them interested. We know plenty of women whose sex appeal makes their breasts exactly the right size. Ice packs will make your nipples hard and your breasts numb, but that's it.

FITNESS
The best shape of your life.

Free weights vs. machines

Which provide the better results—free weights or machines? I say there is no difference; my father says that a barbell and a bench are all he needs.—K.O., Chesapeake, Virginia

Studies have not shown a significant difference—your muscles don't care what provides the resistance. Free weights engage more muscles than a machine because you must balance and control the load. They also give you more flexibility to design exercises specific to your sport, especially for the lower body. They're less expensive, take up less space and work with every body type. However, they take more time to adjust, which can slow down your workout, and usually require a spotter. Machines are more comfortable for most people; free weights seem riskier to beginners. Some people prefer hybrids such as Bowflex, which provides resistance through flexible rods and handles.

Balancing the weight

A buddy was telling me about a theory that says if you strengthen your left arm and left leg, your right arm and right leg will grow equally strong. Sounds like bunk, but maybe I'm working with only one side of my brain.—B.N., Venice, California

You're talking about the concept of bilateral transfer, also known as cross-education. Studies have shown that when you train one side of your body, there can be improvements in the other side as well. But these changes are minor at best. Still, some research suggests that exercising one side of the body one day and the other side the next can lead to quicker strength gains (and allow you to hit the gym daily). It also can be helpful for athletes who continue light training after injuring an arm or a leg. As a regular routine, however, it ignores muscles that bridge the two sides and does nothing to develop balance or coordination. Generally, total-body conditioning with 48 hours' rest between sessions is the most efficient way to go.

Getting rid of chin flab

After being tossed back into the dating pool, I started working out. Running, biking, push-ups and sit-ups have worked wonders everywhere except my chubby face and double chin. What exercises can I do to tone those areas?—B.B., Los Angeles, California

Along with love handles, the chin and face are the toughest areas to slim. If you were only 10 or 20 pounds overweight, keep up your workouts and you should see slow improvement. If your weight loss was more than 30 pounds, liposuction may be the only option. Or you could grow a beard.

Butt, seriously

I'm in good shape, but my wife says my butt is starting to sag. How can I tighten it up?—K.B., Little Rock, Arkansas

At least she's still looking. To solidify your glutei, lie facedown on the bed or a workout table with your pelvis on the edge. Place the ball of one foot on the floor. Keeping that leg relaxed, lift your opposite foot toward the ceiling until you feel your butt muscles engage. Don't extend any further than when your hamstring is parallel to the floor. Do 10 reps with each leg, three sets total, which should take about five minutes a day. Once the exercise becomes easy, add ankle weights for resistance and go to three days a week.

Lift before or after workout?

Is it better to lift weights before or after your cardio workout? My buddy says to do cardio first because otherwise you burn lactic acid instead of fat when you lift. What do you think?—F.C., Spokane, Washington

If your goal is to burn fat, it makes no difference. The key to eliminating flab is a cardio workout designed for endurance, not speed. Lifting strengthens the muscles you'll need to endure the longer workouts.

Dangerous bike seats

A few years ago you warned that prolonged bicycling can lead to impotence. How much riding is too much?—W.D., San Francisco, California

It's hard to say. Some men ride for many hours per week and never have problems, while others are injured after one ride. One study of 1,800 cycling club members who averaged 118 miles per week on narrow racing seats found that 60 percent reported genital numbness and 13 percent experienced impotence. The more biking a man did, the more numbness he reported. Other studies suggest that racing seats can cause problems for women as well. The problem is that the nose of a saddle seat forces you to place your weight on the arteries and nerves that supply your genitals with blood and feeling, rather than on your "sit" bones. One study found that these seats cut the amount of oxygen reaching the penis by 70 to 80 percent within three minutes. Even newer ergonomic seats don't always relieve the pressure enough from this area. It's better, researchers say, to have a seat that doesn't have a nose. Whether you're riding outdoors or on a stationary bike, rise out of the seat every five or ten minutes. Lower your seat if your legs are fully extended at the bottom of the pedal stroke. The top tube of the bike should be positioned three or four inches below your crotch when you stand over the frame (better yet, pad it). Finally, lift your butt when you ride over railroad tracks or bumpy terrain.

Steam vs. sauna

What are the differences between a steam room and a sauna?—D.K., Brookline, Massachusetts

The difference you'll notice immediately is that one is hotter. A sauna is typically 170 to 180 degrees and has very little steam (dry heat). A steam room is typically 100 to 110 degrees and will have more steam (wet heat). Saunas are constructed of porous material such as cedar, while steam rooms are sealed off. There's no evidence that sitting in a hot room for 15 minutes rids your body of toxins, cleans pores, sheds pounds or offers any other longterm health benefits—even the diehards at the Finnish Sauna Society will tell you that. But it can be relaxing. Because saunas and steam rooms increase your heart rate dramatically, decrease your blood pressure and dehydrate you, doctors say they shouldn't be used before or after strenuous exercise.

Calculating heart rate

What is the proper method to calculate the heart rate you should maintain for a good cardio workout? I've read that you subtract your age from 220, then multiply that by 50 percent to 80 percent, depending on the intensity of your workout. That equation gives me 139, which I reach almost immediately when I exercise. The trainer at my gym said to push myself slightly past my comfort level and keep that up for 30 minutes. When I did that I had a heart rate of 172 beats a minute.—J.A., Tampa, Florida

Many exercise physiologists instead suggest a different formula, known as the Karvonen method: Subtract your age from 220, then subtract your resting heart rate; multiply the remainder by the percentage of intensity and add your resting rate back to the result. But perceived exertion—your trainer's suggestion—is a better guide. That's because some people's hearts apparently push blood with speed, and others' use volume. For example, some Olympic rowers in their twenties have a maximum heart rate of 220, while others who are the same age and just as fit have a maximum of 160. Monitoring your heart rate can be useful in checking for disease. Studies have found that people whose rate falls fewer than about 12 beats within a minute after stopping vigorous exercise are four times more likely to die within six years than those whose rate falls more rapidly.

Raise or lower weight?

The trainer at my gym set me up with a strength routine that includes two sets of 10 lifts for each of eight exercises. He told me to increase the weight on the second rep. But a gym regular who has been a bodybuilder for 50 years told me that's all wrong. He says I should lower the weight on the second rep. Who's right?—B.W., Mishawaka, Indiana

Raising the weight sounds too much like lift failure—that is, you lift until you can't lift anymore. That can lead to injury and hasn't been shown to increase strength any more than just lifting until it's difficult. According to Phil Wharton, who trains many top athletes and is co-author with his father, Jim, of The Whartons' Strength Book, *research has shown that each set after the first delivers only an 11 percent gain in benefit. So a second set is worth the effort after two to three minutes of rest, but the first is where you should focus your energy. A team from the American College of Sports Medicine reviewed 264 studies of resistance training and concluded that novices should start with 8 to 12 reps at 60 to 70 percent of the most weight they can lift. When you are able to complete two reps more than your maximum during two consecutive workouts, increase the weight for that exercise to the point at which the final reps are again difficult. This will typically be a jump of 2 to 10 percent.*

The only known aphrodisiac

According to the *Kinsey Institute New Report on Sex*, published in 1990: "The search for an herb, drug or potion that enhances sexual desire has been under way for centuries. No such substance has yet been proven effective, despite claims to the contrary made by companies that advertise such products." I can't believe that there is still no effective aphrodisiac. Does the Advisor know of any?—T.Y., Boise, Idaho

The only known love potion is sweat—your own, about three times a week. One study found strong evidence that men who exercise regularly have the least risk of impotence, and another concluded that as a man's waist size increases, so do his chances of erectile dysfunction. A British study found that men aged 55 to 65 who exercise have an average of 25 percent more testosterone, the hormone that fuels the sex drive. Working out appears to have the same effect on women. In one experiment, female subjects who had just finished 20 minutes on the bike at 70 percent of maximum heart rate had a stronger sexual response to an erotic film clip than those who had been sitting around. That's one more reason to hang out at the gym.

Swimming lesson

Since I'm in my mid-30s, I thought it was time to get serious about exercise. Swimming seems to be a great all-around muscle and cardio workout, plus I was on the swim team as a kid. On the second day, I pulled a muscle, and now I'm sitting here with a heating pad on my crotch. It seems easy to overdo it. Can you suggest a good daily workout?—D.J., Denton, Texas

The last time we swam, it was across the Grotto to get another drink. So we called our favorite pro, Allison Wagner, who won silver in the 400-meter individual medley at the 1996 Olympics and is now coaching and training for 2008. We especially like Wagner because she paints nudes in her spare time. You pulled your groin because of poor technique, probably while doing the breaststroke. So first get a refresher course from either a trainer or a video, then during each workout spend some time stretching and concentrating on form. Use the first 5 to 10 minutes of each session to warm up. During the 30 to 60 minutes you spend in the water, try to use all four strokes—breast, freestyle, backstroke and butterfly— so you hit a variety of muscles. For cardio, Wagner suggests intervals, i.e., swim a lap, pause 10 seconds to slow your heart rate, then swim another lap. FYI: Kicking on your side is good for your obliques (love handles), as is rotating your hips during freestyle.

GAMING

It's not luck, it's skill. And luck.

Placing your bets online

When betting online, how do you avoid getting ripped off?—R.M., Seattle, Washington

With more than 1,400 online casinos to choose from, you're going to encounter a few bad cherries—especially since you have little recourse if you get ripped off (whether it's even legal to gamble online is a gray area). Because word spreads rapidly online, the Internet provides a relatively easy way to identify dubious operators. Visit the discussion boards at winneronline.com and bet2gamble.com, where players share their best and worst experiences. Crushing the Internet Casinos, by Barry Meadow (available at lvago.com), can also shorten your learning curve. While it's devoted mostly to the strategy of playing for deposit bonuses, the $50 report includes tips on how to minimize losses to fraud. For example, Meadow says he gets suspicious if, over time, a virtual blackjack dealer winds up with 20 or better more than one time in four. Stick with casinos that use reputable software, such as that by Microgaming, BossMedia, Cryptologic or Playtech. The foremost challenge of gambling online is collecting your winnings. "It's better to have 20 casinos owing you $500 each than one casino owing you $10,000," says Meadow, who uses a database to track his plays.

You say that gambling online is a gray area. I always assumed it was okay to place a bet at Internet casinos because they aren't physically located in the U.S. What's the story?—P.T., Phoenix, Arizona

Most states ban gaming operations, online or off, but only about half specifically make it a crime to place a bet. Federal law prohibits accepting bets across state lines but not necessarily placing them. Nelson Rose, a professor at Whittier Law School who maintains the site gamblingandthelaw.com, says he knows of only one person ever convicted in the U.S. of placing an online bet—a car salesman in North Dakota who won thousands of dollars wagering on sports. "My guess is that the authorities noticed all these wire transfers of $10,000 or more going into his account and thought he was a drug dealer," Rose says. "When it *turned out he wasn't, they busted him for betting." The salesman paid a $500 fine and moved to another state. Other big-time bettors have contacted Rose saying authorities raided them but never filed charges. Many online casinos, including Playboy's Gibraltar-based operations, block visitors from creating an account if they live in a jurisdiction where gambling is illegal. But plenty of outfits take wagers from anyone. Rose says only about 25 people, mostly bookies also taking sports bets by phone, have been prosecuted in the U.S. for violations, so the odds are good for everyone involved, so far.*

Tipping a dealer

What is the proper way to tip a blackjack dealer?—C.J., Chicago, Illinois

You can hand the dealer cash, but the traditional method is to place a bet for him using casino chips. To do this, set at least a dollar chip above the betting circle. (When betting for the dealer, you don't have to observe the table minimum.) If you win, he wins. Bet a little more if you're winning, but don't overdo it. A buck every 30 minutes is reasonable on a five-dollar table. If you're losing, you can tip less frequently, or leave your last few chips on the table. You also can bet for the dealers at other games such as craps or roulette; let them know and they'll take care of it. Among dealers, a big tipper is known as a George. A lousy tipper is known as a Bruce, as in Willis. According to one dealer newsletter, other stiffs include Whitney Houston, Pete Rose, Howard Stern and Michael Jordan. That's a tough reputation to shake.

How to count cards

Can you explain how blackjack players count cards? How do they do it when a shoe has multiple decks shuffled together? Is it difficult to learn?—H.R., Duluth, Minnesota

It's not difficult, but casinos look unkindly on the practice, and counters must adopt elaborate strategies to hide their craft. In the most basic form of counting cards, you assign a numerical value to each card that's dealt from the shoe and add or subtract that value from the running count. Ian Andersen explains this method in Burning the Tables in Las Vegas: *"I start at zero, then add one when I see 2, 3, 4, 5 or 6, subtract one when I see 10, J, Q, K or A and do nothing when I see 7, 8 or 9. But most effective playing and betting decisions are based on what's known as the true count. You get that by dividing your running count by the number of decks left in the shoe. If I'm playing against a six-deck shoe and my running count is plus eight with four decks remaining, the true count is two. The higher the true count, the greater my advantage." As the dealer works farther into the shoe, the count carries more weight in determining whether the player should stand, take a hit, double down or buy insurance. More important, it guides his bets.*

Lay your money down

What are my best bets at casinos?—M.J., Michigan City, Indiana

We'll give you five, with assistance from Michael Konik, gaming columnist for Cigar Aficionado. (How's that for a job?) You'll find the best odds at video poker machines that offer deuces wild or double bonus. Played perfectly, these "full pay" machines can return more than a dollar for every dollar wagered over the long run. When playing craps, make a line bet on the come-out roll with (pass) or against (don't pass) the shooter. Back up your bet with the maximum "behind the line" wager, known as full odds. In baccarat, betting with the bank is slightly better than going with the player, but both give you pretty good odds. The casino advantage in basic-strategy blackjack (described below) can be reduced to nil or better if you can find a single-deck game in which the dealer stands on a soft 17, or you have an effective card-counting strategy. Avoid the tie bet in baccarat or "any seven" in craps. And we don't have to tell you that the absolute worst bets are those big six wheels, Keno and the bonus side bet in Caribbean stud poker.

Did you hear about the guy who sold everything he owned, including his clothes, rented a tux and stood with his family at a roulette wheel in Las Vegas to bet his \$135,300 savings on a single spin? He won and doubled his money. If you're going to take that kind of risk, is roulette the best game for it?—D.C., Phoenix, Arizona

No, baccarat is better. Michael Shackleford, an actuary who runs wizardof odds.com, notes that the banker bet gives the house an edge of only 1.06 percent and that the player bet isn't far behind, at 1.24. Blackjack, for those wondering, would be best if you could double or split your bet, but that's not possible when you put everything you have on the initial wager. If the tourist (whose stunt was filmed for a reality show) was determined to play roulette, he should have chosen a friendlier venue. He placed his wager at the Plaza Hotel, which uses a wheel with two zeros; this translates to a house edge of 5.26 percent. Had he gone to the Bellagio, the Mirage or the Aladdin, he could have bet on a single-zero wheel and benefited from a European rule that returns half an even-money wager if the ball lands on zero. In that case the house edge is 1.35 percent.

Basic blackjack

Does the Advisor know any simple blackjack strategies?—R.W., Oakland, California

Here's a common one: (1) Always split 8s and aces. (2) Double 10 or 11 if your total is greater than what the dealer shows. (3) Hit on a "hard" 11 or less (i.e., no flexible aces), unless doubling. (4) Stand on a hard 12 to 16 when the dealer shows 2 to 6; hit if the dealer shows 7 to ace. (5) Stand on 17 to 21 unless you have a soft 17. (6) Never take insurance. Played perfectly, these six rules will cut the casino's edge by more than half.

Who's smarter: bettors or oddsmakers?

The Nevada Gaming Control Board says that in a typical year casinos keep 2.9 percent of the money wagered on professional baseball. That's lower than any other sport. (The house keeps 5.9 percent of the money bet on basketball and 4.7 percent on football.) What is it about baseball that makes it less profitable for casinos? Are the bettors smarter or the oddsmakers dumber?—A.K., San Francisco, California

The oddsmakers are never dumber. Relatively few people bet on baseball. That creates intense competition among the casinos, especially since baseball is the only major league sport played for most of the summer. So while football has a 20-cent line, baseball has traditionally been a dime. A few casinos have edged that up to 15 cents; some online bookies have dropped it to five.

Recognizing a tell

My buddies and I have started a weekly poker game. I know that pro gamblers have studied the game this way and that, looking for advantages. Has anyone ever taken a closer look at classic tells? I'd like to add more of my friends' money to my take-home pay.—W.P., Duluth, Minnesota

Inexperienced players have numerous tells. A common tip-off, according to Mike Caro, author of the Book of Tells, *is an opponent who reflexively holds his breath. "Because bluffers are aware that anything they do may trigger your call, they have learned not to tempt fate by being conspicuous," he explains. "Often their breathing will become shallow or sometimes stop altogether." A player with a strong hand may feign indifference. "An opponent who looks away when it's your turn to act is almost always more dangerous and more likely to raise than a player who looks at you. He is trying to make your bet seem safe. This is especially true if the opponent's head is turned away but he is looking back at you through the corners of his eyes." Caro also watches for shaking hands ("this tell is usually misunderstood—bluffers force themselves to become rigid; a shaking hand often indicates an unbeatable hand"), an opponent who reflexively touches his chips or cards (he's antsy to bet), a bluffer who stares you down or cavalierly tosses in his chips, or a bluffer who won't exhale clouds while smoking (again, to avoid being conspicuous). Finally, Caro has observed what he calls pokerclack—a player who makes a subconscious clicking sound with his tongue after viewing a strong hand for the first time. Championship players have been known to fake tells, which can become a tell itself.*

When can you leave a game?

What is the best way to quit a poker game early, especially if you're way ahead in chips?—J.K., Phoenix, Arizona

You should be able to cash out anytime. "The notion that you can't quit while winning is silly," says Doyle Brunson, author of Poker Wisdom of a Champion. *"If you think you're outclassed, quit. If you're tired, quit. If you're feeling unsure about the honesty of another player, quit. But most of all, if you feel like taking your winnings home, quit. It should be understood that every player has the unquestionable right to leave at any time without being ridiculed." In practice this may not happen in a game with your buddies, but theoretically it's supposed to.*

Poker police

During a poker game, one of my buddies had a few too many and, upon laying down his cards, didn't realize he had won the pot. Another player scooped in the chips, but I stopped him. I said the cards speak for themselves. The other player insisted the individual is responsible for minding the action. Who's right?—Y.R., Ypsilanti, Michigan

We think that if you're so intoxicated as to be oblivious to winning, it's past the time to bow out. That said, the cards always speak. In fact players are obliged to assist the dealer and call attention to errors of this nature, including the misreading of a hand or an insufficient bet. In this situation, Jake Austen, editor of the anthology A Friendly Game of Poker, *notes that you should never show your hole cards unless you're sure you have a shot at the pot, because it reveals too much about how you play certain hands. He also notes that in games such as seven-card stud an oblivious winner may beat an eager pot scooper with only his up cards, and anyone at the table is more than right to point that out. "A more odious faux pas is the habit of announcing what cards are needed for the nut hand during play," Austen says. "While there is an obligation to inform the table of errors, terrible players shouldn't be discouraged from folding winning hands by a Chatty Cathy."*

House rules

My buddies and I get together every few weeks to play poker. We'd like to make the games more interesting by allowing each host to set some of his own rules. I'm going first. Any suggestions?—L.R., Washington, D.C.

Jake Austen suggests a standing ban on TVs, radios, cell phones, spouses and dates, as well as these variations: (1) At the end of the night, whoever brought the six-pack that has the most bottles or cans left has to cover everyone's last ante. This dissuades people from bringing cheap beer, and it encourages anyone who brought bad beer to drink it himself. (2) Allow for a straight in which the ace is both higher than a king and lower than a 2 (for example, Q-K-A-2-3), with the hand ranking below a real straight but above three of a kind. (3) If one of the up cards is a Black Maria (queen of spades), everyone throws in $5. (4) Fine players an extra ante for misdealing, flashing cards, splashing the pot or saying or doing something stupid. The table determines the fine, and any protest calls for another fine. (5) According to a 1986 study in American Mathematical Monthly, *before a deck can be dealt it must be riffle-shuffled seven times to achieve an acceptable degree of disorder.*

I'm too good

About a year ago my friends and I started a weekly poker game. For the past few months I've won every time we've played. I worry that my winning is going to break up the game. Should I lose on purpose to keep things going?—J.H., New Orleans, Louisiana

That's no fun, and your friends would feel insulted if they found out. A better strategy is to invest your winnings in the game. Rather than having the host rake the pot, offer to pay for the food and booze yourself. Contribute a bottle of premium whiskey (e.g., a $200 bottle of 25-year-old Talisker single malt) as well as cigars (e.g., Zino Platinum Scepter Grand Masters, at $156 a tin). The game may also benefit from a set of all-clay chips. If a good percentage of your winnings never leaves the room, your friends won't mind losing nearly as much.

The limits of Hold 'em

I'm planning a Texas Hold 'em party, and I'm not sure when and at what rate to raise the blinds. What do you suggest?—P.Z., West Seneca, New York

Hosts typically raise the blinds by some percentage (e.g., 25, 50, 100) every 30 or 60 minutes. Make sure everyone knows the schedule before play begins. How often and how much depends on whether you've invited janitors or lawyers; you want everyone to be comfortable with but challenged by the limits. We all love watching the cowboys check their hands on ESPN2, but have you considered hosting a game that involves actual card play, such as Omaha Hi-Lo or Seven-Card Stud? They call it Hold 'em for a reason—you spend a lot of time doing nothing.

GETTING HITCHED

Committed to the idea of committing.

Should I get married?

I am engaged to a woman I have known for 10 months. I love her, but we keep going through a vicious cycle of fighting, talking about a breakup, then deciding to commit. She's insecure, touchy-feely, fairly immature and has no interest in anything I'm into. She hasn't gone out with her friends since we started seeing each other, and she throws a fit when I go out with mine. I have never made love to her without fantasizing about someone else. My problem is that I'm conflicted about going through with the wedding. I know I just rattled off an astounding list of negatives, but I have feelings for this woman. She is the first girlfriend I've had in four years. I keep thinking I love her, I should be mature, that we ought to work things out and make a life together. I'll be 28 soon, and I don't want to break someone's heart so I can comb the city for the next however many years for someone who might be better for me but may not exist. Can you help?—L.J., Louisville, Kentucky

That is an astounding list of negatives. Lots of guys talk themselves past obstacles and do something they regret. Don't be one of them. The fear of being alone is not a reason to get married.

If not the fear of being alone, what is a reason to get married? Most married guys I know are miserable. And don't say love. Anybody who lives or works in Manhattan knows that it's possible for a man to fall in love every 20 feet while walking down Sixth Avenue in the summer.—A.C., New York, New York

Every 20 feet? You must be farsighted. We've never been champions of marriage except to raise children. Typically a man marries because the woman wants it and he isn't creative enough to imagine life without her. Is that too cynical? A few great minds, such as Socrates, have been more optimistic. "By all means, marry," he wrote. "If you get a good wife, you'll be happy. If you get a bad one, you'll become a philosopher." If you ever find yourself thinking, Maybe things will get better after we're married, step away from the edge. Marriage counselor Jeffry Larson reviewed social research from the past 65 years to develop a detailed questionnaire that helps couples decide if they'll be happy. You'll find it in his book Should We Stay Together? *Larson includes marriage myths (e.g., "you're my one and only" and "opposites attract") and ways to tell if getting hitched may not be the best idea, such as (1) Your fiancée asks relentlessly, "Are you sure that you love me?" (2) She says she's okay with your interests but also says you spend too much time on them. (3) When you consider breaking up, your first thought is that you'll miss the sex. (4) You are irritated by the idea of spending an entire day alone with her. (5) She's an addict. (6) She's a perfectionist. (7) You break up and reconcile repeatedly. (8) You're depressed (you'll be a depressed married person). (9) You think marriage will make you a better man.*

Can I get the ring back?

About six months ago, I asked my girlfriend to marry me. Now I've changed my mind. The ring cost me a small fortune, and I would like to get it back. Where do I stand?—G.F., Philadelphia, Pennsylvania

She should return it. The modern woman doesn't need a consolation prize. Legally, she has to return it: Numerous state courts, including the Pennsylvania Supreme Court, have ruled that an engagement ring is a "conditional" gift—the condition being that the marriage take place. But take a deep breath before you pursue this. If her family has to eat any deposits on canceled wedding arrangements, the ring is your contribution. If that's not the case, it still might be wise to consider the ring as you would a stock pick that didn't go your way. Say goodbye, then take a fresh look at the market.

Disinvited to the wedding

Two weeks after attending a bachelor party for a friend, I received this letter: "You attended a party that was meant to be a last night out for my future husband with his friends. Instead you turned it into something horrible. While we have decided to go ahead with the wedding, we request that you no longer be a part of it. I do not want to celebrate my marriage with men who encouraged my fiancé to take off his clothes and touch a whore. I would never make him stop being friends with you, but I will insist that you not attend." My girlfriend says I should lose this guy as a friend, but I'm not sure what to do. For the record, nothing distasteful happened at the party.—M.S., Montclair, New Jersey

This won't be a wedding. It will be a wake. You could insist that your buddy, rather than his dominatrix, disinvite you, but it appears he doesn't know what hit him. Sadly, being his friend just became a huge chore.

What a letter. Most men in their 20s don't have the common sense, foresight or balls to end a relationship like that. Their marriage ends in five to 10 years after much misery. That's because as the woman gets stronger-willed and more dominant, she grows frustrated by her pushover spouse. If your girlfriend has you whipped, it will be less painful to leave now than to wait until she divorces your sorry ass and takes the kids, the house and the money. Been there. Done that. Sorry now.—M.D., Kansas City, Missouri

This seems like a lesson that has to be learned the hard way. Guys who are whipped aren't able to take your advice.

I don't think you put much effort into your answer, Advisor. You can't blame just the girl. If the guy knew it could be a problem, he should have prevented it. For example, they could have had a mixed bachelor-and-bachelorette party, which is all the rage. They could also have set down rules, such as "I won't touch tits if you don't grab cock." When my husband and I had our parties, I told him I didn't want him near naked women because I knew his friends might set him up. I was right: They tried to pay a streetwalker to pose with him. Just because I don't want him around that sort of thing doesn't make me a controlling bitch. And it doesn't mean this girl was, either. She has the right to invite whomever she wants—it's her day. The problem is his being afraid to grow up and realize that real men listen to the women they love and try to see the woman's point of view.—A.T., Lancaster, Pennsylvania

Real women get over themselves. Your advice is all good—couples should talk—but to suggest that the woman had a right to disinvite her fiancé's friends is just incorrect.

Is she "the one"?
My girlfriend and I have been dating for several years. I'm 26 and many of my friends are getting married. I also would like to get married someday, but I'm not certain this girl is the one for me. I think the best thing for me to do is see other people. How do I tell my girlfriend this without losing her for good? What if I do this and she hates my guts, then I realize she is the girl I should marry? Do my doubts about spending the rest of my life with her mean anything? Please help.—J.K., Milwaukee, Wisconsin

In our view, any guy who doesn't have doubts about committing to one woman for the rest of his life needs to get to know her better. But you're overlooking an important player in this drama—your girlfriend. She may feel the same pressures

as she watches her friends get hitched, and the same uncertainty about marrying you. If you don't feel comfortable discussing your relationship with the other person involved, what sort of marriage can you expect? Every couple reaches a place where they know enough about each other to make long-term plans or go their separate ways. Rather than suffer regrets, remember that timing is everything. Your girlfriend may be the right woman at the wrong time or the wrong woman at the right time.

An elderly friend once told me a simple way to decide whether to get married: Ask yourself if the thought of living without her is worse than the thought of living with her.—R.C., Boyertown, Pennsylvania

You never stop asking that question.

My girlfriend and I started dating three years ago, when I was 19. I considered proposing but had reservations because I hadn't dated anyone else. I didn't want to cheat down the road, so I broke up with her to date more. After some soul-searching (brought on by her having met someone else), I decided she's the one. I told her I wanted her back, but she says she's still angry with me. We've talked only by e-mail; she won't let me call her. What should I do?—R.B., Ann Arbor, Michigan

Stop writing to her. Before you'll ever get your ex back, she has to miss you. You're pining because she hooked up before you did. You have a good plan, now follow through.

Engaged without engagement
A friend of mine and his fiancée have agreed not to have sex until their wedding night, even though they've been sleeping together for several years. Have you ever heard of this?—R.W., McLean, Virginia

Reclaiming your chastity is a great way to build anticipation. Here are some ground rules: The couple can kiss and caress so long as they avoid the genitals. They can't masturbate (harsh!). They should talk dirty and tease each other silly. Imagine the longing you'd feel after a few months (or, God forbid, a year or more) of that. If this idea catches on, expect a lot more shotgun weddings—with the groom supplying the shotgun. *

---

* After this appeared, an anonymous reader responded by tearing out the page, circling the response and writing in bold letters, "You bastard!"

How to propose

I'm ready to propose to my girlfriend. Do you have any suggestions?—R.B., Nashua, New Hampshire

Because the women in our lives always do the asking (without success, natch), we don't have any experience with this. So we called Michael Webb, who solicited 7,300 real-life proposals for his e-book The Romantic's Guide to Popping the Question *(online at theromantic.com). Webb's general tips: "(1) Don't do a public proposal unless your girlfriend is a public person. That is, if she does everything with her family and friends, she's less likely to feel on the spot if you ask her at a gathering. (2) Many guys ask around the holidays, but that's expected, and no matter what a woman says otherwise, she wants to be surprised. (3) Many guys think that the more money they spend, the more romantic the proposal. But women rarely mention the limo, the roses or the fancy dinner. They remember the personal details. The less money you spend, the more creative you tend to get to compensate. (4) The more complex the proposal, the more likely something will go wrong. Someone will forget their lines or, worse, squeal. A lot of guys plan a big weekend—if you do that, ask her on the first day, because you'll be nervous and it will make her think something's wrong. Assuming you get a yes, it also lets you enjoy the rest of the weekend together. (5) Learn from the mistakes of others. Examples: The guy who left the ring in the wet diaper of their baby, the guy who asked in front of the casket at his brother's funeral, the guy who had a messenger deliver the proposal and the romantic who presented the ring over a meal at McDonald's. (6) Finally, if you start the proposal by saying 'We need to talk' or 'You win,' reexamine what you're doing—quickly."*

When can you object at a wedding?

What are grounds for making an objection at a wedding? I love this girl and believe she's making a huge mistake. We have a history as friends, so I may have a chance. I know making an objection in front of 300 people isn't the most subtle way to get my point across, but I finally want to take a stand.—C.B., Providence, Rhode Island

It would be your last stand. Objecting at a wedding rarely works as a pickup line. If you think the marriage is a bad idea, let your beloved know well ahead of time. If she's persuaded, she'll need time to change course. Besides, in most ceremonies the presiding official doesn't ask for objections—it only leads to trouble, and unless it's a legal challenge (the bride is already married, for example), the proceedings continue anyway. More important, should you object, you'll diminish your chances with the bridesmaids.

The last hurrah

The last member of our group of 20 college friends is getting married, so we are planning a bachelor party. We have been all over the world for previous send-offs—Amsterdam, Las Vegas, South Beach, Daytona, Fort Lauderdale, New York, Los Angeles, D.C. and London. We are debating either going to Montreal, where none of us has been, or returning to Vegas. Thoughts?—M.A., Washington, D.C.

Montreal is an excellent choice. It has great restaurants, the Casino de Montréal and full-contact, all-nude strip clubs filled with gorgeous women. You will want to stay within a few blocks of Crescent and Ste. Catherine, and it's probably wise to hire a company such as MontrealVIP (montrealvip.com or 800-371-1224) to make arrangements and offer advice. Marc Tadros, one of the company's partners, says the dancers in Montreal aren't as aggressive as those in the States; you have to ask them for a private lap dance, which typically costs about U.S. $7.50 a song, with no tip required. (The girls keep everything they make.) The only thing you can't touch is her vulva. Tadros says most groups number about a dozen guys, but he has arranged trips for as few as four and as many as 50. You can't go wrong with Las Vegas as a plan B, says James Oliver Cury, author of The Playboy Guide to Bachelor Parties. *"Because the city is growing so fast, there's no way you can exhaust everything in one visit," he says. "If you go back, you can hit all new clubs and restaurants." The new Scores is gaining a reputation as the best strip club in town. In Europe, Cury suggests Dublin, which is where Londoners play and host their own stag parties. Cury's guide, which we recommend, includes a planning list, help with calculating everyone's cut, tips on how not to get ripped off at strip clubs, and a great bit of advice: "Always do what's best for the groom."*

My new wife's plan

I'm engaged to be married, and everyone in my family says they love my fiancée, but she has a huge problem with them because they are still in contact with my ex-wife. My ex and I have a good relationship, in part because we share custody of our six-year-old son. My fiancée, who is divorced as well, believes my family should cut all ties with my ex out of respect for our relationship. How do I convince them that by staying in touch with her they are hurting my future wife as well as me?—J.M., Milwaukee, Wisconsin

Are you kidding? Neither you nor your fiancée has any right to demand this, especially as it involves the mother of your family's grandchild and nephew. We hope your third wife has a better attitude.

GROOMING
Hair today, gone tomorrow.

Shaving your face

I've shaved with hot water, cold water, in the shower, after a shower, before a shower and with every brand of foam I can find, and I always get razor burn. Any suggestions?—N.R., Las Vegas, Nevada

We feel your pain. The most common cause of razor burn is shaving against the grain. So don't do that. The rest of our advice you've probably heard before. Prep your face with a hot (but not too hot), slightly soapy washcloth that you push against the grain to get the whiskers to stand up. Try a shaving brush to apply foam; it also helps the whiskers stand up and looks cool if any babes walk in. Use a razor that has a pivoting head. Don't press too hard, especially around your neck. Experiment with gels or natural oils. One oil we passed around the office has received rave reviews. It was developed by Bill Hamilton, a former roofer and frustrated shaver who as a teenager began concocting lotions with household products such as baking soda, vinegar, cooking oil and shampoos and conditioners. In 1987, after consulting with a pharmacist, Hamilton had his eureka moment. You can request a sample of Total Shaving Solutions by writing Total Solutions at 2400 S.W. Jefferson, Peoria, Illinois 61605 or through allabout shaving.com.

Shaving down there

My wife of five years likes the clean-shaven look on her genitals. What is the trick that so many of your models use, or is that just the magic of airbrushing?—J.E., Milwaukee, Wisconsin

Our models have professional help. Shaving your genitals is tricky business. The poor man's method is to cut the hair close with a blunt-nosed scissors, apply a warm wet towel to soften the stubble, spread shaving cream and carefully stroke each area no more than twice—first with the grain and then against. Even if you're careful, she'll probably suffer some irritation. She also may have to shave at least daily, or the combination of sharp hairs growing back and sensitive skin will be unbearable as she walks around. You might want to upgrade to the $10 Ladyfair shaver to trim *the hair to stubble and the $50 Seiko Cleancut to shave and for touch-ups. The bat-tery-powered razors are imported from Hong Kong and Japan by Ian Mark, a pussy-shaving evangelist who sells them at 2sensualproducts.com or 210-558-7262. Using depilatories such as Nair are always a bad idea.*

I recommend waxing instead of shaving. Waxing is necessary every three to six weeks, depending on hair growth. I'm an aesthetician, and many of my customers, men and women, come in monthly for a wax. Just make sure the hair isn't too long. Ouch!—F.B., Venice, California

That's an option, though the prospect of someone pouring hot wax near our genitals sounds . . . well, actually, it sounds great. It's the part where the pubes are ripped out en masse that give us the chills. Shaving will always have its appeal, especially when a partner is involved. First, it's much easier to do at home. Second, it can build trust in a relationship. Third, you need to shave often, and that tends to put your partner's face near your fun parts on a regular basis.

Your advice on how to avoid razor burn when shaving a woman's genitals is a little off. Most soaps, foams and gels contain alcohol, which will irritate the skin. We sell dancewear to strippers throughout the Carolinas and work primarily in the dressing rooms. I happened on a terrific remedy that most of my customers swear by. It is Vaseline Intensive Care Lotion Advanced Healing Formula, which contains vitamin E (for healing) and petroleum jelly (for a smoother "lather"). Pour a capful, spread it into your skin (it also can be used for legs and under-arms) and shave with a two-blade razor. The razor burn should disappear soon enough.—John Greene, Naughty Naughteaze, Greensboro, North Carolina

Nice gig.

Doing the Brazilian

What is a Brazilian bikini wax? Why are guys so hot over it?—J.W., San Francisco, California

They're hot for it because it reveals more woman. It has a reputation for enhancing oral sex and intercourse by uncovering acres of sensitive skin. (Gwyneth Paltrow once thanked the J Sisters, seven Brazilian siblings who run a New York salon, for changing her life.) The Brazilian involves using hot wax to remove every hair, including those in the butt crack and on the taint and labia, with the exception of a landing strip above the vulva. The process is unpleasant and must be repeated monthly. Also known as a Playboy because of its popularity among our models, it originated with thong bikinis. According to stylists at another New York hot spot, Completely Bare, the trend lately is to leave nothing behind, because some shorts and jeans ride low enough to reveal the tip of the strip. The salon also offers glue-on crystals or hand-painted graffiti, including some that glow in the dark. If you'd rather not spread for a stranger, visit JustKittyng.com, which offers home-stencil kits. Or visit the Archive and Alwyn Salon in London. It specializes in merkins, which are pubic wigs made from nylon or hair (human or yak) fashioned into logos, targets, hearts or other shapes and affixed with a G-string or glue. We wear one over our bald spot.

Hairy women are sexy

Playboy once published a photo of a beautiful woman described as "hirsute Samantha." How dare you! As an endocrinologist, I know this girl is normal, as is any woman who doesn't shave her armpits, including the majority in Europe and Latin America. Don't you understand that axillary hair represents in many ways a sample of what is in the crotch? That's something Spanish dancers know as they raise their arms.—C.S., Chevy Chase, Maryland

What can we say? The model is hirsute—and sexy, which is why we ran the photo. There's something to be said for body hair. First, it captures pheromones. Second, it means she won't be borrowing your razor.

My wife won't shave for me

My wife just gave birth to our second child. I asked her nicely if she intended to wax, shave or trim her pubic area anytime soon. She became upset that I even mentioned it. How do I bring up the topic again without annoying her? I would love her to "clean house" because a lot of pubic hair is a turnoff to me.—S.M., Nutley, New Jersey

We admire your focus, but your timing needs work. Your wife blew up because she's managing a newborn while you redesign her pubic hair. Put down your sketch pad, warm a bottle and wait for her to calm down. It usually takes about three years.

I shave my entire body

Some co-workers noticed that my arms are shaved. They asked if I shave other parts of my body. When I told them I shave everything, they decided that I must be gay. I'm not gay, just hairy. I even tweeze my eyebrows. My girlfriend says she loves my hairless body. So why do my co-workers have such a problem with it?—C.B., Clarksville, Tennessee

Because they're hairy and they aren't getting laid. You must be slippery in the shower.

Shaving for the toga party

My fraternity brothers and I have scheduled a toga party with a hot sorority. We can't decide whether to shave our chests. If we don't, the women may be turned off. If we do, we may get teased for being unmasculine. What should we do?—S.W., Buffalo, New York

It depends—do you want to look like a fraternity of gladiators or bathhouse servants? The real Romans wore togas over tunics (which resembled T-shirts with no sleeves). Try that. In the later years of the empire, the only women who wore togas were prostitutes. Should be a good time.

The battle against bald

I'm 29, and my hairline is receding at a frightening rate. The hair-restoration industry has ads everywhere claiming the days of hair plugs are gone. Is there any truth to this?—J.S., New York, New York

Transplants have become smaller (hair follicles are transplanted from the back or side of the head in groups of two or three rather than 15 to 20), which means they can be placed closer together to provide a more natural look. But the smaller and more numerous the grafts, the more delicate the operation and the greater the chance the follicles will be damaged. That's why the procedure costs thousands of dollars. Nonsurgical solutions include Rogaine (rubbed on your scalp) and Propecia (a daily pill), which slow hair loss by blocking the production of DHT, a form of testosterone that causes male-pattern baldness. These treatments are most effective on the crown. Meanwhile, science marches on. Researchers have discovered that manipulating a gene in bald mice causes their hair to start growing. The gene also exists in humans, so the hope is that it could eventually lead to a cure for androgenetic alopecia, or inherited baldness—by far the most common type. Researchers are also working on cloning hair cells in the lab that can be injected into the scalp. But in a University of Toronto experiment that tried this, only four of 23 subjects grew hair, and only one ended up with what the lead researcher called a "nice tuft." Nevertheless, the transplant chain Bosley Medical and the British biotech firm Intercytex promise to have "cellular-based hair-multiplication technology" available soon.

On the clock

I shave and brush my teeth in the shower each morning to save time. My girlfriend says this is uncivilized and barbaric. What does the Advisor think?—C.L., Huntington Beach, California

Don't tell her about the peeing.

Getting rid of dark circles

I have started to notice dark circles under my eyes. Is there a cream that can do everything from moisturizing to eliminating wrinkles?—M.D., Miami, Florida

A cream can't fix the circles, but it can hide them. As we age, the thin skin beneath our eyes becomes thinner and wrinkles, making the veins beneath appear more prominent. People with allergies, eczema, hay fever or asthma may have darker circles because the veins swell. (The traditional cucumber treatment is designed to reduce the swelling.) Our skin care writer, Donald Charles Richardson, suggests Surface Optimizing Skin Cream by Aramis as a cover-up.

Stop making scents

How much cologne is too much?—S.C., Columbus, Ohio

We could smell it on your letter. That's too much. The best advice we've heard is, "Spray enough that people know you're there, but not enough that they know you're coming." No one should smell you until you're within about an arm's length—what the fragrance industry calls your "scent circle"—and you shouldn't smell yourself unless you check your wrists. If you're using a standard bottle, don't splash. That happens only in commercials. Instead, apply a dab on one or both wrists, and/or the neck. Some guys also add a dab to their thighs, chest or back, for that all-over freshness. With spray bottles, limit yourself to two spritzes. A good cologne will last all day, especially if you have oily skin, which holds it better. If you're headed out for the evening, ask your girlfriend's opinion before applying a refresher dab.

HEALTH

Keep your body in mind.

Is sex good for you?

My wife heard somewhere that frequent intercourse can take years off a person's life. The theory is that rushing hormones speed up the aging process and knock down the immune system. Is that true? Please respond soon.—T.C., Green Bay, Wisconsin

We've heard the opposite. Research suggests that the more orgasms a man has, the longer he'll live. Scientists reached this conclusion after studying 918 middle-aged men from the Welsh village of Caerphilly. Between 1979 and 1983 they gave each man a physical exam and included questions about how often he had sex. Ten years later the scientists found that the men who said they had sex twice a week were half as likely to have died as those who had sex once a month. The researchers joked that "intervention programs could be considered, perhaps based on the exciting 'at least five a day' campaign aimed at increasing fruit and vegetable consumption." If you're tempted to use these findings to get laid ("Baby, I can't live without you"), keep in mind that they may only prove that healthy people have more sex than sick people do.

Power naps

When I feel tired at work, I close my door, take a 15-minute nap and awake feeling recharged. How is it possible to be able to rejuvenate my system so quickly? Why don't I feel that alert when I wake up in the morning?—R.C., Wallkill, New York

Because you need more sleep. Most adults require at least eight hours each night (excluding the two hours you have sex) and a regular schedule (same time to bed, same time to wake, including weekends). People who can't manage that nod off when their body temperature dips about eight hours after they get up, typically between 3 PM and 5 PM. That's why half the world takes a siesta. It's best to get enough sleep at night, but if you don't, take a 20-minute power nap. If you have a cubicle, use the trick we learned from Dilbert: Put your forehead on the desk and a pencil on the floor. If someone wakes you, pick up the pencil.

Is pain bad for you?

Is pain bad for the body? I don't like it, but at the same time I'm reluctant to pop a pill every time I feel discomfort.—J.P., Las Vegas, Nevada

In the sense that it keeps you from touching a hot stove, it's not bad. (Those rare people born without the ability to feel pain—a mutation known as HSAN V—tend to die young.) Pain sends a message we often don't want to hear: You're working too hard, you have to come out of the game, etc. The risk is that acute pain may become chronic. One hypothesis for why this occurs is that when acute pain isn't treated, your nerves get more time to practice transmitting pain signals to the brain, and that makes them better at it.

Is it healthier to sleep nude?

About 30 years ago I saw the French film *Shoot the Piano Player*. In one scene, the lead character is awakened by a knock on the door and he answers in the buff. The visitor asks if he always sleeps in the nude and he says, "It's healthier that way." The film inspired me to sleep nude, and I've done so ever since. My wife of 20 years also sleeps nude and we have great health, so obviously it's not unhealthy. I can't imagine wearing anything as constricting as underwear to bed. I have read that approximately 20 percent of men and 6 percent of women sleep naked. But is there any evidence that sleeping in the nude is healthier?—J.W., San Diego, California

Not that we could find, though it certainly does wonders for your sex life, and it also might help you get a better night's sleep. Your body temperature drops as you nod off, and researchers have found that if a person remains too warm, the depth and continuity of his or her sleep suffers. In that instance, losing your pajamas could be a good idea. We also located one highly questionable study that claims up to 60 percent of gynecological problems in Japan are caused by tight underwear worn to bed, but we'll endorse the research anyway, for the sake of Japanese men. You're also in good company: Famous nocturnal nudists include Al Gore, Pablo Picasso, Marilyn Monroe and, at one time, Alyssa Milano. "I used to sleep nude," she once explained, "until the earthquake in Los Angeles in 1994, when I saw a neighbor in his underpants and was like, okay, that's gross. I don't want to be that guy. I'm going to put on clothes now." For her male neighbors, that was the day's second disaster.

Snoring problem

I leave on vacation in three weeks and will be staying with friends and family, mostly sharing rooms. I've been told by my girlfriend that I have a serious snoring problem. Should I look for my own lodging? Should I mention this up front to the people I stay with?—E.S., Newport Beach, California

If you're sharing rooms, you may meet your match—about 50 percent of men and 25 percent of women snore. Most are over 40. We suggest you see a doctor, because serious snoring may contribute to heart disease, diabetes, stroke or hypertension. The most dangerous form is obstructive sleep apnea, characterized by heavy sawing interrupted by moments of silence when you temporarily stop breathing, followed by a snort as you wake yourself up. The most common treatments are to lose weight, treat allergies, get more sleep, attach nasal strips, avoid alcohol, tobacco and sedatives before bedtime or sew a tennis ball into the back of your pajamas to force you to sleep on your side. If none of that works, a doctor can fit you with a mouthpiece that holds your jaw forward to open your airway, or a cumbersome breathing mask that pushes air into your throat. You also may want to investigate laser-assisted uvulopalatoplasty or somnoplasty to remove tissue from your soft palate.

Cracking knuckles

Has any research been done on whether cracking your knuckles causes arthritis? I've been doing it a dozen times a day for 30 years but haven't had any problems.—T.C., Tallahassee, Florida

There's no evidence it leads to arthritis, but it may harm ligaments. A study of 74 habitual knuckle-crackers found they had less grip strength and more hand swelling. However, the ability to crack could be a symptom of existing damage rather than its cause. The sound is actually the popping of a carbon dioxide bubble that forms in the joint when it's pulled out of position. We know this because of an experiment in 1971 by the Bioengineering Group for the Study of Human Joints at the University of Leeds. The team glued a ring to the right middle finger of each of 17 volunteers, attached twine (so it could be tugged to create a crack) and had the subjects place their hands under an X-ray machine. It found that the carbon dioxide, which is released from the fluid that lubricates the joint, takes about 20 minutes to be reabsorbed, which is why you can't crack your knuckles in succession. That's nature's way of keeping the rest of us sane.

A case of heartache

After my girlfriend dumped me, I had a heavy feeling in my chest. I feel better now, but I wondered: Is heartache a psychological or physiological response?—D.K., Homestead, Florida

It's a bit of both. A doctor might say you were suffering from psychosomatic symptoms, or that you "somaticized" your grief—your body reacted to the emotional stress. This may not be much solace, but the most productive periods of our lives have been between girlfriends.

Why does her leg twitch?

Sometimes my girlfriend's leg twitches as she falls asleep. It always startles me. What causes it?—M.P., Stowe, Vermont

The twitches are known as hypnic jerks. It's not clear what causes them; your girlfriend's body may be reacting to the mistaken belief that she's falling rather than simply falling asleep. A more serious problem is periodic limb movement disorder, which is when a person's legs or arms jerk at regular intervals, sometimes for hours, after he or she has fallen asleep. Some people never realize it occurs until their partners complain. The condition is relieved with the same drugs used to treat Parkinson's disease.

Whiskey as disinfectant

Let's say you were deep in the wilderness and you cut yourself. Would whiskey work as a disinfectant?—E.D., Terre Haute, Indiana

In a pinch, sure. Sip the rest to ease your pain. Whiskey also has been recommended for toothaches and insomnia and as an elixir (mix it in hot water with sugar). In an experiment at the Georgetown University Medical Center, whiskey and scotch killed bacteria better than gin, rum or vodka, but the booze had to be at least 80 proof. In a similar study at Oregon State, scientists found that wine—in this case, a chardonnay and a pinot noir—killed salmonella and E. coli within an hour. Researchers began the study after hearing about a food-poisoning outbreak aboard a cruise ship on which guests who'd had wine with dinner didn't seem to get sick. The alcohol in the wine apparently weakens the walls of the germ cells, allowing the acid to penetrate and kill them.

Spotting a concussion

How can you tell if you have a concussion?—R.T., San Antonio, Texas

Too many weekend athletes make the mistake of thinking they have to be knocked out to get a concussion. Common symptoms are a persistent low-grade headache, vision disturbance, dizziness, confusion, amnesia, ringing ears, nausea and difficulty concentrating. You may also have a stiff neck, convulsions, unusual sleepiness and/or difficulty speaking or using your arms. If you believe you've suffered a concussion, stop playing immediately. As one doctor says, "You can ice your ankle, but you can't ice your brain." Most concussions are treated with rest and Tylenol, and full recovery can take a month or longer. There are no strict rules as to when you can compete again, but your doctor will give you guidance. You want to avoid having multiple concussions—after one, you're three times as likely to suffer another. One study of 2,500 retired NFL players found that those who suffered multiple concussions have a greater risk of developing clinical depression. It's not clear if there's a connection to Alzheimer's or stroke.

When to get a physical

How often should a guy get a physical? I'm 38, and my wife wants me to go every year. Also, what are the best tests to ask for?—R.L., Chicago, Illinois

You should have a physical every other year in your 40s and every year starting at 50. The American Heart Association recommends that men and women have their fasting lipid profile (which measures cholesterol levels, an indicator for heart disease) checked at least every five years after the age of 20 and their fasting blood glucose (which helps predict the risk of diabetes) checked every three years after the age of 45. Dr. Raul Seballos of the Cleveland Clinic, who specializes in preventive medicine, says an important gauge of health is your waist circumference, measured over your belly button. It has been found to be a better indicator than body-mass index (weight in relation to height) of an increased risk for heart disease and diabetes. A waist of more than 40 inches in men or 35 inches in women is cause for concern. Seballos suggests that each exam also include a prostate-specific antigen test, which screens for prostate cancer. The test is sometimes inaccurate and no one agrees on the best treatment if your PSA is high, but Seballos says it's useful to establish a baseline to make sure levels don't spike (see below). He also recommends a test for highly sensitive C-reactive protein, which your liver produces. An elevated result indicates you have inflammation somewhere in your body; the location can be pinpointed with further tests. Finally Seballos suggests having the level of vitamin D in your blood checked. It helps absorb calcium, and a deficiency can indicate trouble.

The finger of life

I'm due for a physical but am reluctant to get the prostate exam. Is it absolutely necessary that the doctor stick a finger up my ass?—K.L., Farmington Hills, Michigan

Most tumors begin in the area of the gland he can feel with his finger, so he's looking for lumps. As an alternative you can request a PSA test. Whether either method is necessary is a topic of debate among physicians because there's no way to tell if a tumor will kill you quickly or hang out for years, and aggressive treatment can have serious side effects. In 2002 a government task force noted that "screening is associated with important harms, including frequent false positives and unnecessary anxiety, biopsies and potential complications of treatment of some cancers [such as impotence or incontinence] that may never have affected a patient's health." According to the Centers for Disease Control and Prevention, of every 100 men over the age of 50 who have a PSA screening, 85 have a normal reading (including a small number who have a tumor that is missed) and 15 have a high reading that requires further tests. Of those 15, three will have cancer. Clinical trials are under way to determine whether men screened annually are less likely to die of prostate cancer than those who never get tested. On a related note, a study of 1,453 men by researchers in Seattle found that those who reported drinking four or more glasses of red wine each week had a 50 percent lower chance of developing prostate cancer.

Sweat problem

I perspire too much, but only when I'm not in a relationship. Whenever I have a girlfriend, it stops. Is this extra sweat designed to send out pheromones, or am I just insecure? Do you know how to correct it? It can be embarrassing.—W.L., Dallas, Texas

That's an interesting hypothesis. Do single guys sweat more? A substance in men's perspiration, androstenol, has been found to be pleasant to women, but it appears only in fresh sweat, and the woman must already be in your personal space to smell it. Once your sweat hits the air, it releases a steroid, androstenone, that has been shown to turn women off or, at best, has no effect. More likely, you're suffering from hyperhidrosis, which is thought to affect three percent of Americans. It can be caused by anxiety or a variety of conditions, such as diabetes and nerve damage. Usually it occurs all over the body. Primary hyperhidrosis, believed to be genetic, typically affects only the armpits, palms, face and/or feet.

It occurs whether you are nervous or relaxed. Sweathelp.org describes some treatments. For example, getting Botox shots in each armpit every six months has been found to be effective in treating excessive sweat there. In your case, a stronger antiperspirant such as Certain Dri or Secret Platinum may help, or you can get a prescription for Drysol. One trick: Apply antiperspirant at night to your dry pits, then add another coat in the morning. For some reason this seems to improve the protection.

Ordering Viagra online
Some websites will mail you a supply of Viagra without your having to see a doctor. Is it legal to get the drug that way?—P.L., Roanoke, Virginia

Many states have cracked down on doctors who write new prescriptions without seeing patients, but just as many allow it. That's why so many websites are able to offer Viagra and other drugs. Typically, a site will ask you to fill out a questionnaire about your medical history, which is forwarded to a physician for review. If he doesn't see (or chooses to ignore) red flags such as heart disease, he writes the prescription and charges you for the "visit." The scrip can only be filled by the site's pharmacist, who isn't offering any bargains. Sites based entirely overseas may not bother with the prescription, but because they're outside the jurisdiction of the FDA, you have no assurance of what you're actually getting, or its quality. Before you buy any prescription drug online, check with the National Association of Boards of Pharmacy at nabp.org to determine if the site is legitimate. The primary reason to see a physician is that your erection difficulties may indicate a more serious problem. Because an Internet consultation is a one-way conversation, an online doc could miss important symptoms.

Can Ecstasy harm your sex life?
Are there any good things to say about Ecstasy? Does it benefit sick people the way marijuana does?—J.B., Knoxville, Tennessee

Before the drug was outlawed in the 1980s, some psychotherapists experimented with X on severely depressed patients. As you may know, it's a warm, energetic high, but it has dark lows, which is why you hear talk after rave weekends of "Suicide Tuesday" hangovers. Used regularly, Ecstasy may hurt your love life. A survey of 768 young adults in Italy and England found that those who had taken Ecstasy more than 20 times were three times as likely as nonusers to report a loss of libido. This may be because the drug, over time, damages the neurons that regulate the production of mood-elevating serotonin. Researchers can't say precisely how much is too much and how often is too often, or even what the long-term effects might be. Also remember that because it's illegal, you're dealing with a street drug. While Ecstasy is relatively easy to make, it's harder to purify. Pills sold as Ecstasy have included amphetamine, ephedrine, caffeine and ketamine. Proceed with caution.

Marijuana and fertility

I smoke one or two joints a day. Should I stop so that my wife and I have a better chance of conceiving?—M.L., Pasadena, California

Yes. It's well established that long-term, regular use of weed leads to decreased sperm production. A study in 2003 of 22 men who smoked at least twice a day for five years also found that their sperm swam too fast too soon and had trouble attaching to the egg. Researchers believe it could take four to six clean months for things to return to normal. Here's a possible antidote: A study of 750 Brazilians suggests that guys who drink coffee have more energetic sperm.

Does male menopause exist?

Is there such a thing as male menopause? If so, what can I do about it?—T.L., Pittsburgh, Pennsylvania

While women's hormone levels drop dramatically, usually in their early 50s, men experience a more gradual decline. One study found that men's testosterone levels drop about one percent annually from age 39 to 70. As men age, their bodies sag. They take longer to heal from illnesses or injuries. They have less physical endurance. They may feel depressed, anxious, irritable or indecisive. They have less interest in sex, less forceful ejaculations and difficulty achieving and maintaining erections. What role testosterone or other hormones play in this remains unclear. That's one reason to be cautious about testosterone therapy, which can increase your risk of prostate cancer and may not cure erectile dysfunction if the problem is high blood pressure, arteriosclerosis, diabetes, depression or another illness. Scientists are studying the effects of various hormones on the symptoms of middle age. In the meantime, exercise, good nutrition and regular medical exams are always a good idea.

IN THE BEDROOM
Let's keep the lights on.

Sky high

I'd like to make an important point regarding the mile high club. The only people who can join are the pilot and his or her partner. Passengers, a.k.a. self-loading freight, do not qualify. A purist like myself also says the autopilot should not be used. Am I a member of the club? No, I am simply a pilot who hates to see what began as an exclusive club watered down for groundlings. I'll earn my wings one day, and I will do so in a way I can be proud of. — P.J., San Leandro, California

Now, now—we're all in this together. Your standard is much too strict, and making love in the cockpit of an airborne plane is foolhardy. In our view, a pilot who's having intercourse is freight on a pilotless plane. You fly, and let passengers take care of the sex.

Since Denver is the Mile High City, could my boyfriend and I join the mile high club if we screwed like crazy in a hotel room there? The thought of having sex on an airplane is arousing, but I can't risk getting caught. What do you say? Would we qualify?—J.L., St. Paul, Minnesota

Sorry, no. However, you would be eligible for the less exclusive "Fucked in Denver" club.

How about if you have sex on Mount Everest?—B.W., Portland, Oregon

We'd give you credit, but you might piss off the Sherpas—and the mountain. The Buddhist guides do not take kindly to anyone "making sauce" on Chomolungma, as they believe it insults and angers the mountain (same with killing animals, getting drunk and burning trash). One photographer caught during a private moment with his girlfriend told National Geographic Adventure *that a Sherpa warned, "The weather is bad, and I think you are adding to it. No taki-taki on the mountain." But at least one climber says the raunchy Sherpas are half-kidding and themselves sometimes hook up with Western women during expeditions. In 2004 a professor of international relations at New Zealand's Victoria University of Wellington, as an exercise in organizing a global social movement, created a website inviting people to assemble at the Everest base camp. He hopes to show support for Sherpa efforts to counter the "most spiritually erosive effects of mountain tourism," including sex.*

Have you heard of the mile low club? To qualify, you ride the Eurostar through the "Chunnel of Love" between Britain and France and do it in the roomy washrooms during the 20 minutes or so that the train is in the tunnel.—C.V., London, U.K.

Sounds like quite a ride, but you're far short of a mile. The Eurostar reaches a depth of 377 feet below sea level about 11 minutes after it enters the tunnel. You'll need at least 14 more trips to reach a cumulative mile, which might be fun but can't be considered an official qualifier. To join the mile low club, figure out a way to claim two of the three seats on a deep-sea research submersible. We're already in training.

Some of the Witwatersrand Reef gold mines around Johannesburg offer tours that take you down a mile or farther below ground. You just need to figure out a way to lose the rest of the group. That's what might be called going down with someone.—J.B., San Antonio, Texas

Traveling a mile below the surface doesn't qualify. You have to be a mile below sea level. By that account, the Witwatersrand mines extend a third of a mile down. However, it can be done. The Western Deep Levels mine southwest of Johannesburg reaches a depth of 2.5 miles, allowing miners to descend at least a mile below sea level. Peter Bunkell of the Chamber of Mines of South Africa points out that "conditions for lovemaking at that depth, though not prohibitive, would be far from ideal." For starters, he says, "it is very, very hot."

Dirty thoughts

A co-worker closes his door for 20 minutes every day so he can meditate. He says I should give it a try, but it seems like a hassle. Is there any advantage to meditation?—N.G., Detroit, Michigan

Buddhists have thought so for at least 2,500 years, and they may be onto something. Researchers at the University of Wisconsin wanted to see if meditation caused physical changes to the brain, so they used an MRI machine to monitor eight Tibetan monks who had each practiced meditation for 10,000 to 50,000 hours over 15 to 40 years. While meditating on unconditional compassion, the monks produced the highest level of gamma waves—the brain impulses associated with happiness, mental awareness and coordinated thinking—ever recorded in healthy people. Even when they weren't meditating, the monks had more gamma activity than a control group of novices. This and other studies indicate that meditation sharpens the mind in the same way that exercise tones the body—a radical concept, as scientists have long believed that connections among the brain's nerve cells become fixed in childhood. Can meditation lead to better sex? In her book Sex for One, *Betty Dodson describes taking her daily 40-minute meditation to a new level by chanting her mantra while touching herself with a vibrator. She calls her sessions, which conclude with orgasm, transcendental masturbation. Researchers at Rutgers University who monitored Dodson's brain while she meditated in a lab found that she entered a daydream-like state during her extended masturbation and a deeper, trancelike state just before she came.*

Bad language

While reading the Advisor's responses to a few questions about sex, I was surprised at your use of the word *fuck*, which degrades the writers' sexuality and makes you appear cheap. It seems that you don't know the difference between having sex and fucking.—G.R., Tempe, Arizona

Sure we do. You fuck when you're sweaty; you have sex after a shower. You fuck in a cheap motel room; you have sex in a master bedroom. You fuck on a hardwood floor; you have sex on carpeting. You fuck on a swing set; you have sex on a porch. You fuck in the woods; you have sex on the beach. Or vice versa on any of those, depending on your mood. The difference between fucking and having sex is between your ears, and everyone's love life should have a little of both.

All-natural sex

Is there such a thing as a natural-born lover?—T.S., Lufkin, Texas

Everyone fumbles at first. But some people get a head start because they have parents or a school that provides realistic sex education, and they masturbate, which teaches them how and where they like to be touched before anyone else does the touching. They also read and watch erotica for ideas, never run out of lube, aren't afraid of fantasies and understand that good lovin'—like any skill—takes practice.

What's your move?

On an episode of *Seinfeld*, Jerry refers to "the move," a sexual technique that he uses to bring unspeakable pleasure to his partner. What do you think the move is?—M.W., Maryville, Tennessee

If it works, it's the move. If it doesn't, it's the move over.

How do lesbians have sex?

My girlfriend and I are fascinated by the idea of two women together. We've speculated on how lesbians achieve mutual sexual satisfaction, and we thought the Advisor could fill us in. What are the most common lesbian sexual activities?—F.G., Beloit, Wisconsin

What makes you think we're experts on lesbians? We're experts on porn lesbians— the kind who have sex with each other only until the guy arrives. Felice Newman, author of The Whole Lesbian Sex Book, *confirms the obvious here, that lesbians are like anyone else: They love sex in all its varieties, with the exception of the variety that involves a man. Lesbians kiss, lick, caress, rub against each other, play with each other's breasts, penetrate with fingers, fists or sex toys. Susie Bright has written that the nicest thing she ever said to a man was, "You use your hands like a dyke." The gay woman and straight man who compiled* Lesbian Sex Secrets for Men *note that foreplay as preparation for intercourse is a foreign concept to most lesbians—it's all play. There's a lesson in that: The next time you want to make an impression in bed, stretch your fingers, soften your touch, take your time and pretend you're a lesbian. That shouldn't be too hard—you're already attracted to women.*

Making dirty movies

My boyfriend and I have been living together for seven months. A few weeks ago I found a tape of him and his ex having sex. I watched a few minutes of it out of curiosity. Three weeks later I decided I wanted to tape us having sex. During the session he kept saying things either to me or the camera that he had said in the tape with his ex. In some instances they were verbatim. Should I be offended, or should I assume he says these things when there's a camera on regardless of whom he's with?—L.A., Orlando, Florida

We prefer fantasies for which we've seen the script and have a speaking part. If you tape again and he spouts the same lines, you'll need to step in with creative suggestions.

Sensualist vs. sexualist

I just started dating a guy, and he's already driving me crazy. He's into setting the mood whenever we have sex: candles, incense, music, the works. Sometimes I want to be ravaged, or ravage him, but if I start grabbing at his clothes or kissing him hard to get things going, he says, "Hold that thought," and scurries around to get things just right. Most guys I've dated have no interest in any of this stuff—they're ready to go whenever. Should I be concerned?—R.T., Duluth, Minnesota

Your boyfriend sounds like what one of our favorite cultural observers, Lisa Carver, would call a sensualist. You, on the other hand, are a sexualist. "Sexualists are into sex," explains Carver, who edits a fanzine called Rollerderby. *"Sensualists are into eroticism—things that aren't sex but that involve the thought of sex. Sensualists are romantics; they like to set the mood. Sexualists aren't waiting around for someone to light some damn candles." Foot fetishists are sensualists, as is anyone who experiments with tantric sex, writes erotic e-mail or fusses over dimming the lights. Henry Miller and Marilyn Monroe were sensualists; Jack Nicholson and Xena the Warrior Princess are sexualists. Like you, Carver is a sexualist. "I had sex with a sensualist once. He hung his hair around my face like a tent, cutting off all light, and said, 'How does that look and feel?' I realized he was waiting for me to compliment him on his eroticism, and until I did, he was withholding his thrusts. So I lied and said, 'That's so cool.'" The issue isn't your different approaches to sex, but the lack of variety. Unless your new boyfriend is willing to set aside his sensualism once in a while and let you take charge, this relationship may be a challenge.*

Condom rally

I slept with a guy who said he hadn't had sex in a year. After one stroke he came and said he needed another condom. He put it on, slid inside me, pumped once and came again. Another condom, another stroke and he was done. This "lovemaking" took two minutes, and he never made any effort to please me. The next morning we made out. Without my touching him and while fully clothed, he creamed himself. Again he made no effort to satisfy me. I thought I liked the guy, but now I'm pissed. When he asked me later if I missed him, he showed no sign of embarrassment. He has told our mutual friends that he thinks sex is overrated. Does that mean he doesn't enjoy it either? We are not talking about a teenager. This guy is in his mid-30s and was married for four years. Should I tell him that he has a problem or let some other poor woman suffer?—L.R., Jacksonville, Florida

Your multiorgasmic pre-ejaculator needs a sex-ed class and perhaps medication. Do you want to provide the former? It sounds like no.

Sex and the older man

As a man in his mid-70s, I'm troubled when I read that we "older" people presumably have reduced sex lives. Growing older has its advantages. In our mid-50s, my wife and I went from having sex three weeks out of the month to four weeks—no more blackout periods. When all the kids had moved out, my wife and I had complete control of the house for any and all activities 24 hours a day. Two years ago I agreed to my wife's suggestion that every night was a bit of a strain. So we do it every other night, with the exception of special events such as Father's Day. You may wonder what keeps our interest so high. Good health, good diet, vitamins and hot fantasies. Adult movies also help. So never assume that us older types aren't enjoying sex to the fullest.—R.H., Litchfield, Connecticut

Who's assuming? The Advisor often hears from readers of an advanced age (i.e., older than us), and they seem to know what they're doing. In one survey of singles over 70, two-thirds reported being sexually active. In another study of healthy 80- to 102-year-olds, half said sex was at least as interesting and important to them as when they were younger. You'll enjoy an anthology edited by Joani Blank called Still Doing It: Women and Men Over 60 Write About Their Sexuality. *While sex later in life may not be as frequent or intense, Blank's contributors show that it's often more tender, satisfying and kinky. Many people come to realize, usually by necessity, that sex can occur even when a penis doesn't get hard, a vulva doesn't get wet, and no one reaches climax. Speaking of aging, we were startled by the title of another book that crossed our desk:* Great Sex After 40. *Is it that time already?*

Exploring her second nature

My best friend gave me a massage. She rubbed and sucked my breasts and put her fingers inside me. This almost happened once before, but she stopped herself. This time I said it was okay. I like men, but I also enjoyed exploring my bi curiosity. Is it all right for two friends to have sex every so often?—K.K., Tampa, Florida

Okay by us. Personally, we're tri-curious. We'll try anything that involves two women.

Bumping the baby

My wife is five months pregnant. Everything I've read says having sex won't harm the fetus. I am sure that's true, but psychologically I can't get turned on knowing my penis would be in such close proximity to my child. I also worry that her orgasms might trigger a miscarriage. Am I being paranoid?—C.S., Dayton, Ohio

Not at all. Your intellect is battling your emotions—welcome to parenthood. Sure, your erection will be near the fetus, but think of it as staying in adjacent rooms at the same resort. The only opening to the womb is the cervix, which at this point is the size of a pinhead and plugged with mucous, so there's no danger of poking your kid in the head. If you're uncomfortable with intercourse (some guys are okay with the penetration but dislike the idea of a kid between partners during missionary), think outside the box. Get your fingers and tongue involved, or use a dildo—straight on, it looks like a rattle. Although the baby may kick or move each time your wife comes, it's highly unlikely the contractions will cause problems. Doctors routinely caution women who have had miscarriages or premature labor in the past to be careful. Ask yours for reassurance.

My husband doesn't have fantasies

I asked my husband to tell me his sexual fantasies, and he claimed he didn't have any. When I persisted, he said pleasing me is his fantasy. Is he saying that to stop me from asking or because he's afraid to share? Can a man actually not have any fantasies?—S.M., Denver, Colorado

Doubtful. We suspect your husband has a few kinky ideas but believes you would judge them harshly or fail to understand, and he has no interest in hurting you or making himself vulnerable. For example, a natural fantasy for a married guy is fucking another—usually younger—woman or having a threesome. But some wives take even the idea of variety as an insult ("I'm not enough for you?"). Rather than push him on this subject, ask if he'll indulge you. While your fantasy is playing out, his desires may reveal themselves. The simplest way to do this is to experiment with role-playing—for example, the classic doctor-patient or teacher-student scenarios that cater to our base desire to be dominant and/or submissive. Weave your tale for him—simply calling him Professor in a sweet voice as you unbuckle his pants may unleash the beast. In her book Fantasy Made Flesh, *Deborah Addington suggests other offbeat pairings, such as bandit and victim, deity and worshipper, dorky teen and Playmate, drill sergeant and private, pet and owner, and president and intern. Have fun.*

An ex-girlfriend once asked me the same question, and I honestly gave her the same answer. She offered to set up a threesome, but I said no. Why didn't I have fantasies? Because she took care of all my needs, sexually and otherwise. For example, if I was watching football on TV, she would prepare food, bring me beers and give me head at halftime. When I got home from work she'd say, "I know you're tired, but can we please have sex?" She even went to the gun club with me to learn to shoot. Anything I could do for her in return wasn't enough. This idea that I must have routine fantasies became such a point of contention that it damaged our trust, and the relationship ended. She fulfilled all my desires but wouldn't believe it. Now I have fantasies about strangers but only memories of her.—J.P., Liverpool, New York

Did you consider that your ex's fantasy was to share a fantasy with you? Given her willingness to explore boundaries (yours and hers, known or yet to be discovered), you showed an amazing lack of creativity. She deserved better.

A cheap fuck would be good for us

My girlfriend and I have been going out for nine months. We have sex four or five times a week, which to me is similar to Social Security—you can live on it, but barely. Whenever she goes down on me, it's usually only after I ask her to, which ruins the anticipation. I feel a little guilty asking her to do something that she doesn't seem to enjoy. One night she began stroking me. I wanted her to make the first move, so I laid back and made it clear I was enjoying myself. She kept stroking me with her dry hand. After 10 minutes, I told her I was getting raw. But instead of getting lube or going down on me, she just stopped. The subsequent conversation brought out a lot. She says that oral sex makes her feel slutty, and that she's just a dud when it comes to sex. I had bought some sex toys and she's been able to use them to reach "really good" orgasms (she's told me I'm the first guy to make her climax). But she's never lost it, gone crazy, etc. All we ever do is "make love." I've told her that some cheap fucking could be good for us. I try to be creative but she never likes one thing more than another. I tell her she hasn't discovered her underlying sexual animal yet. Any suggestions for finding it, or are there some people who have no libido? I've been able to make every other girl I've been with do whatever I want her to do, so long as I promise to do for her what she likes.—W.H., Seattle, Washington

Your girlfriend isn't a dud. She's a beginner. Cut her some slack. We appreciate what you're saying—you want her to fuck your brains out. But you also can't get caught up in the porn ethos that says a woman isn't satisfied until she's clutching the bed and screaming for more. You've made the right moves—buying sex toys, talking to her about your desires, asking what she likes. Don't get discouraged. It may take time for her to gain enough confidence to "go crazy." You might try a different approach—instead of daily sex, rev her up slowly. Tease her. View everything you do together as foreplay. Whisper to her what you have in mind. Be kind to her. Promise her mysterious pleasures, and give her a date and time to be ready. Once you're there, don't play mind games by making her guess what you want. If you're after cheap fucking, explain yourself. Does it mean you want her to grab you at the door and, without saying a word, use your cock as a dildo? Make that request. Eventually, she'll be better at anticipating and start to surprise you. If all else fails, stick your tongue up her ass. Keep searching for that inner slut.

Sleep sex

After an evening of energetic sex with my girlfriend, I awoke at 2:30 AM to find her lips on my cock. I said, "I can't believe this, baby," at which point she pulled away, looking startled. Turns out she was asleep and had no idea what was going on. My girlfriend is a sleepsucker! We both are wondering if this is common.—R.C., Vermillion, South Dakota

It's not common enough, that's for sure. In 1996 we ran letters from two women who claimed their husbands had made love to them while asleep. We had our doubts, but a respected sleep expert, Dr. Michael Thorpy of the Sleep-Wake Disorder Center at Montefiore Medical Center in New York assured us that people are capable of doing many unusual things while slumbering. We called him for an update. "There's now more awareness among doctors that this occurs," he says. "It's part of a process known as confusional arousal. It occurs while people are in a deep sleep—deeper than even the dream stage—usually during the first half of the night. Something rouses them, but they don't wake up. Instead they enter a half-sleep, half-awake state." That leads to sleepwalking or other odd behavior. One study at Stanford University involved two sleeping women who would moan loudly as if being aroused, a woman and a man who would mas-turbate furiously, and six men and a woman who would make unwanted and sometimes violent advances on their partner. A 26-year-old would fondle her hus-band and talk dirty to him. When he responded, she would wake up and accuse him of trying to seduce her while she slept. Her husband wouldn't believe she had been unconscious. They went to a counselor but didn't make any progress until a sleep lab revealed what was going on.

My new boyfriend told me he falls asleep after he climaxes. I thought he meant likes to hit the sack, but he passes out for 30 seconds. I laugh or tickle him and get no response. He also told me he can't have sex in the shower because he might injure himself. Is this for real?—P.L., Miami, Florida

It's unusual but not unheard of. Dr. Thorpy suspects your boyfriend may suffer from a combination of narcolepsy (sudden unexpected sleep or sleepiness) and cataplexy (the extreme muscle weakness or temporary paralysis associated with narcolepsy). The two conditions usually appear separately but sometimes merge. The emotional stimulus of orgasm can trigger cataplexy, which can lead to sudden, brief REM (dream-state) sleep. According to Dr. Thorpy, cat-aplexy occurs at orgasm in about 40 percent of narcoleptics. And about 30 per-cent suffer from sleep attacks during sex. Certain antidepressant medications can help.

Lingerie secrets

I'd like to buy my wife some lingerie but have no idea what to get her. Any suggestions?—P.R., Providence, Rhode Island

The best lingerie is comfortable enough that she'll want to put it on and revealing enough that you'll want to take it off. If you see an item of lingerie and think "slutty," she won't like it. If you think "elegant," she will. Check your wife's underwear drawer for her bra and panty sizes. The number one reason—or excuse—for returns is poor fit.

My friend says a woman should wear her panties under the garter. I say they are worn over the garter. Who's right?—L.C., Bridgeport, West Virginia

It depends on your date. A good girl wears her panties under the garter, so they're harder to remove. A bad girl doesn't have the patience to unhook her hose.

What is tantric sex?

I have been seeing the term "tantric sex" lately and have to plead ignorance. (Or is it innocence?) Quick description, please?—D.P., Omaha, Nebraska

Tantra is a spiritual movement that views prolonged, ritualistic sexual pleasure as a path to the divine. Why can't more religions be like that? It dates from about the sixth century, when it arose within both Hinduism and Buddhism. To extend lovemaking, male tantrists teach themselves to withhold ejaculation during climax, which allows them to maintain their erections. The method takes practice and is accomplished by pressing a point along the perineum or through superior muscle control. Interlocked couples also typically gaze into each other's eyes, searching for enlightenment. (They may not find it, but eye contact can be an incredible turn-on.) In the West, the word tantra *has come to describe any type of meditative sexuality, especially among marketers, but traditional tantra covers a wider range of beliefs and rituals. You'll find an introduction online at the Church of Tantra at tantra.org. There, Swami Nostradamus Virato introduces tantra this way: "There is a most beautiful word for sex in the Sanskrit language, and that is Kama, which means sex and love indivisible. Almost everyone is familiar with the* Kama Sutra, *a tantric treatise on lovemaking. Kama is also the name of the Hindu goddess of love. And love is what tantra encourages—total unconditional love, including the mind, the spirit and the body. In tantra, the orgasm is with the universe." Talk about a big bang.*

Is sex magic the same as tantra?—J.H., Cleveland, Ohio

Sex magic has been used to describe a variety of practices that merge the sexual and spiritual, including tantra. One basic ritual is to create a symbol for a goal, then concentrate on that symbol during sex. At the moment you climax, say something like, "I dedicate this orgasm to finding a new job." As one manual explains it, "The power of your sexual energy becomes a vehicle for your will." Like most spiritual beliefs, sex magic is poetic yet vague and occasionally ridiculous. Then again, there's no doubt that orgasms are a powerful force of nature. Sex diva Annie Sprinkle described one of her experiences with sex magic this way: "When my house burned down, a friend sent out an e-mail suggesting people dedicate an orgasm to me. A lot of people did. The erotic prayer provided an amazing cushion. I felt so little pain." Others have taken the concept to the streets. A book called The Psychic Investor *recommends sex magic to beat the market. Carve a stock ticker symbol into the side of a white candle. Focus on the symbol with your partner, then face each other, remove your clothes and build the sexual energy. Once fully aroused, begin intercourse with the man sitting and the woman on top. Delay your orgasm as long as possible. Concentrate on the stock, not her tits. Reflect on the company's impressive board of directors, its inexpensive workforce in Honduras, its promising P/E ratio. Chant. As you reach climax, envision the stock going up, up, up. The book advises that you split any profits. It takes two, after all.*

KINK

It takes all kinds.

Panties against my balls

Last week, after I had brought her to orgasm, my wife got out of bed, reached into her dresser and pulled out a pair of silk panties. She told me to put them on. I asked why, but she said to trust her. I pulled the panties over my hard-on, and she straddled me to rub my cock and kiss it through the silk. She slid over me and began grinding her hips, telling me how good my cock encased in silk felt against her pussy. I had one of the most intense orgasms I can recall. I would love to repeat the experience, but does enjoying it so much classify me as a weirdo?—T.B., Anaheim, California

Some people might consider you weird if you wore her panties to work, but what guy hasn't done that?

I am totally turned on when my boyfriend wears panties for me. My favorite move is to go into the bathroom at the office (we work together) and remove my thong panties. I then slip them into his pocket when he's on the phone or standing at the copier. Minutes later he'll walk by my desk with a big smile, and I'll know he's wearing them. Sharing this intimate secret drives me wild. By the end of the day I can hardly wait to fuck him. I also love doing this at restaurants, theaters and family dinners. In my opinion any girl who isn't open to this kind of foreplay isn't worth dating.—L.B., San Diego, California

Next time leave anal beads in his pocket and see what happens.

Turning her on

If I were to touch a nine-volt battery to my girlfriend's clitoris, would she get a charge out of it? How about if I tied a wire around my big toe (+) and a wire around her big toe (–), and attached them to the terminals of a lantern battery? Would sparks fly when my tongue touched her? What if I hooked up the apparatus to a power source such as my stereo? Please advise.—W.B., Los Angeles, California

Good grief. Your battery test would only produce an unpleasant burning sensation, and the toe contraption wouldn't do anything. Your stereo is another matter. A few mad scientists have figured out a way to have sex with their hi-fi equipment, which combines two of our favorite interests but also gives us the willies. One online manual, Erotic Electronic Stereo Sexual Stimulation Techniques, *describes an intricate experiment in which you connect speaker wire from an amplifier to solder probes molded to fit around the penis (and into the urethra), cradle the testicles or penetrate the anus. "Be careful of high bass settings," the manual warns. "In the beginning, do not play classical music, as it can be explosive. Use soft rock or talk radio. Another method some users have enjoyed is to connect their TV to their stereo and play porno videos." The author of a similar guide recounts an incident in which he touched a lamp while hooked up; the shock dislocated his shoulder. You sound like the experimental type, so we'll caution you against juicing up your sex life too much. Even modest amounts of electricity can be dangerous, especially if applied above the waist. Besides killing you, a surge could destroy your stereo.*

This little piggy

I thought I'd share a discovery my husband and I made in the bedroom: toe sex. I was straddling his leg while giving him a blow job and began to rub my clit against his shin to stimulate myself. I slid lower until I could feel his foot. He wiggled his toes to play with my pussy, then slid his big toe inside me. He could feel how wet I had become and enjoyed the sensation of me rocking toward climax on his foot. This could change the way women look at men—we'll want to see them in sandals before taking them to bed.—T.D., Knoxville, Tennessee

Before you know it, someone will introduce a toe extender.

Smoke before fire

My girlfriend smokes. The problem, if you can call it that, is that I am incredibly turned on when she lights up. Against my better judgment, I told her this. Now she has become almost obsessed. She smokes during foreplay. She wears dark red lipstick and alternates sucking on her cigarette and my cock. If we happen to be out with friends, she'll always get my attention before she lights up because she knows it makes me hard. Two of her co-workers told her during a cigarette break that their boyfriends also are turned on by watching them smoke. One of these women told my girlfriend to buy Virginia Slims 120s because the foil inside the pack has small ridges. She said to empty the box and then squeeze the foil to fit around my penis. My girlfriend did this and gave me an incredible hand job. Now she wants to invite one of her friends to smoke a cigarette in front of me while she (my girlfriend) gives me head. I told her I don't get turned on by watching anyone smoke but her, but she promises that it would just be an experiment. Apparently the friend is okay with it as long as she only has to flirt and show her tits. Meanwhile, my girlfriend has purchased a velvet-lined cigarette case to stroke me with. It's torture because she says that unlike the cigarette packs, the box is too expensive for me to come inside of. We also have a normal sex life that doesn't involve her habit. But this has happened so fast that I guess I'm overwhelmed. Is this normal behavior, or does one of us have a problem? I'm slightly worried about it but also don't want her to stop.—M.D., Memphis, Tennessee

We've always been warned not to smoke in bed, but it sounds in your case like there's no danger of anyone falling asleep. Your preference is far from unusual; the Internet is full of sites such as smokesigs.com that cater to butt men. Since you also have what you consider normal sex—which apparently occurs when your girlfriend decides to put out her cigarette—we wouldn't worry about it. It's a game: You told your girlfriend how to take control of your desire, and she obliged. The question is, where will the relationship go if she quits? And can you share a cigarette after sex, or does that get you all revved up again?

Sex in space

Has anyone ever had sex in outer space? What were the results? Surely someone must have tried it by now.—G.S., Austin, Texas

Sex in space—the final frontier. NASA says no one has become a member of the 250-mile-high club on an American mission. The Russians are another matter. There has been speculation—but no proof—that sex occurred after an adventurous female cosmonaut joined the two-man crew of a Soviet space station in 1982. We're skeptical, but that may be our patriotism showing. Space agencies in both countries have shied away from the topic, yet it's becoming relevant now that missions can last months. (A manned trip to Mars would take six months each way.) Weightless sex would be a challenge—without restraints, a couple would drift apart as they pushed against each other. On the upside, as Arthur C. Clarke once observed in Playboy, *"the absence of gravity would certainly make the more acrobatic performances outlined in the* Kama Sutra *less likely to invoke the urgent services of a chiropractor. Consider, for example, the notorious daisy chain—hitherto, merely two-dimensional. In zero gravity, all the regular solids and many highly irregular ones could be constructed." Pity the poor sap who has to be strapped down to get it started. Gene Meyers of Space Island Group, which hopes to build a space hotel sometime sooner than later, says he expects the crew sent to build the $15 billion structure will be the first humans to copulate in space. The hotel itself will include "zero-gravity romance rooms, each with a window" and "the walls will be padded and elastic cords and harnesses will hang from the ceiling."*

What about masturbation? In its literature about the space shuttle, NASA points out that "the bathroom on the orbiter is a private room where the curtain is drawn, with a normal-looking toilet, a light over the right shoulder to read by and the hatch window to look down at earth." The toilet includes a flex tube that uses airflow to pull urine (or come) into a receptacle. Unfortunately, NASA doesn't provide specifics on the force of this airflow, or suction created by this tube, or how closely it fits the penis.—R.B., Miami Beach, Florida

It is difficult to believe that at least a few astronauts haven't yanked their emergency cords in-flight. Over breakfast, the cosmonauts aboard Mir would reportedly ask each other, "Dognal devushku?" ("Did you catch up with the girl?") And a former NASA flight surgeon reported "anecdotal evidence" that arousal and ejaculation can occur in zero gravity. As if every guy on earth doesn't already know erections can happen anywhere.

Whence fetishes?

What is the root of fetishes?—L.R., Columbia, South Carolina

We're all fetishists at heart. Social scientists believe that fetishes are the result of brain chemistry, conditioning and/or early sexual experiences. In the most entertaining theory we've read, Freud suggested that fetishes in men arise from the last impression a boy has of his mother when he discovers she doesn't have a penis. Thus the popularity of foot and shoe fetishes—you're on the floor as a toddler, you inadvertently look up your mother's skirt and, shocked, find yourself staring back down into her leather boots. Bam! You're hanging around shoe stores. Others argue that fetishes stem from whatever object or body part played a role in your first orgasm. Are fetishes healthy? If your preoccupation with a woman's shoes, breasts, butt, earlobes, lips, belly button, leather pants, stockings, legs, tattoos, smoking posture or piercings becomes so consuming it keeps you from seeing her as a walking, talking, sexual being, that's a problem. If your fetish is nothing more than a launchpad, then you're no different from most. If you fetishize an entire person, sentimental types call it love.

Drink it in

My girlfriend is always willing to try new things. Recently we began to experiment with pee play, and it turns out it's a major turn-on for both of us. As part of our fun I sometimes drink from her. The problem is I am subject to random drug testing at my job and my girlfriend is an occasional pot smoker. Am I flirting with disaster?—W.M., New York, New York

We only have any expertise in one of these activities, so we asked Wilkie Wilson, a professor of pharmacology at Duke University, to ponder the possibility. "It's not inconceivable, depending on how much she smokes, how much he drinks and the sensitivity of the test for THC and its metabolites," he says. "In this situation I would worry most about marijuana. Other illegal drugs are metabolized by the body into inactive components." Dan Savage, in his column Savage Love, *has printed testimony from at least one guy who claims to have tested positive in this manner.*

Hair-raising experience

I find haircuts an erotic experience, especially when electric clippers are used to get close to the scalp. I rarely get an erection in the barber's chair, but I almost always masturbate when I get home. I suppose this is a "true" fetish in that it's the experience itself that arouses me rather than the attractiveness or even the gender of the barber. I remember hating haircuts as a child, and it wasn't until I was in the military and getting frequent buzz cuts that it turned me on. Perhaps it makes me feel more manly or virile. What does the Advisor think?—B.P., San Diego, California

We never have a sexual thought—not one—when Fat Charley cuts our hair. His assistant, however—her shampoo massage could go on forever. We've heard from guys who fantasize about bald women ("naked from the neck up," as they say), but never from anyone who gets turned on from sitting in the chair. It's not surprising that you find the experience arousing; the scalp is overlooked as an erogenous zone.

(Try massaging your lover's head, or rubbing her hair, and gauge her response.) If a haircut is the only way you can get turned on, you have a true fetish. That's not healthy, or much fun. May you never suffer from male-pattern baldness.

Nipple sex

When I was younger, I attended a boarding school for girls. I'm now 21 and married to a great guy. My husband and I read *Playboy* together in bed, and he suggested I write you. My roommate at school was a lesbian. We became good friends and, after a time, lovers. She led the way. It was mostly kissing at first, then fondling, shared masturbation and oral sex. There was one thing she taught me that I haven't seen or heard of since. She would have me suck her nipples to hardness, then, as I lay on my tummy, she would part my bum cheeks with her thumbs and (one at a time) press a stiffened nipple into my rectum. When she gave the word, I would begin a rhythmic clenching of my bum. It felt gorgeous, like I was sucking her into me, and she would masturbate me while bringing herself off on my leg. We took turns, but she always preferred "getting" the nipple to "giving" it. I enjoyed both roles. I've told my husband about it (no secrets, right?), and he loves the idea. And although he can't reciprocate with a swollen nipple, he more than compensates with his penis. Is this a common lesbian practice?—D.D., Kelowna, British Columbia

It's not common, but it's inventive. Where will the world's nipples go next? You were fortunate to have had such an adventurous lover. Now maybe it's time to put your husband on his tummy.

All tied up

My girlfriend claims she needs to be dominant to enjoy sex, so she ties me up a lot. I don't mind her being in control, but it also means I can't touch her. This past week she left me bound in the bedroom. When I called out, she came back and gagged me. I was angry and a little afraid. I spent 90 minutes trying to get free. When she saw that I had tried to escape, she lit into me, then devoured me. The sex was amazing, but I am worried. What if she decides to leave me for longer periods? When I tell her how I feel, she calls me a sissy and asks if the sex isn't good.—D.T., Kansas City, Missouri

The sex may be great, but the setup needs work. Before you do this again, establish a safe word that ends play immediately when uttered by either partner. This ensures that no one crosses boundaries, and it can also prevent injuries. For

example, if your girlfriend ties her knots so tight that they cut off your circulation, you have no way of convincing her that you are not just being a "sissy." If she won't agree to a safe word, or if you agree on one and she then ignores it, you should not allow her to bind you in any way.

How exactly does one utter a safe word while gagged?—M.P., Defiance, Ohio

Our safe word is "mmmmph," so it always works out. If you're planning to be gagged, you need a safe move. Your top might give you a bell to ring or a ball that you can drop if the scene becomes too intense. The couple had a larger issue to address, which is that the bottom didn't trust his top. A safe word or move is pointless without that. In his book SM 101, *Jay Wiseman offers more tips for bondage that we found helpful the last time we couldn't get away for lunch: "(1) SM is something you do with someone, not to someone. (2) You almost never get into serious trouble by going too slowly. (3) If you want to know what they're into, watch their eyes. They can't fake their eyes. (4) Experience it yourself before you do it to someone else. (5) Never tie a submissive into a position that would require his cooperation in releasing him." And finally, "(6) If you don't have a current CPR card, you cannot call yourself a responsible dominant." Youch.*

Hand fetish

Have you ever heard of anyone having a hand fetish? I asked my girlfriend what first attracted her to me, and she said she loved my hands. Is she pulling my leg?—H.G., Baltimore, Maryland

Every woman will develop a hand fetish if her lover uses his digits wisely. Lisa Carver, editor of the fanzine Rollerderby, *once interviewed a hard-core hand lover about what turns her on. "The thumb is very important," she explained. "It represents strength. My father has great hands—they're honest. The puffy part of his thumb is big. That indicates kindness. Anyone with hands like his—especially older men—I'm drawn to. I trust them. I want to be safe under their hands. Another quality I look for is the handling of small things, like stereo knobs. I know he'll treat my nipples and clit the same way. If he's subtle and articulate in how he adjusts the volume knob, then I'm his for the asking." Don't crank that dial, fellas, caress it. If your girlfriend says she adores your hands, cup every part of her body with them.*

Erotic spanking

Is there a subtle way to ask how a new lover feels about spanking? Also, are there any signs that someone enjoys this type of sex play?—P.R., Trenton, New Jersey

Besides the fact that they never sit down? It's hit or miss. In general, the better the sex, the more likely your partner will experiment. One spanking fan hints to new lovers that he enjoys "a little more slap than tickle"; another lays it on the line as soon as the relationship gets intimate. To test the waters, initiate a discussion about erotic likes and dislikes, or share an adult video that includes a spanking scene and study your partner's reaction. Naturally, the simplest way to find a spanker or spankee is to hang with them through organizations such as Shadow Lane (shadowlane.com), which sells spanking erotica, publishes a magazine of lonely-butts ads and hosts frequent parties.

During foreplay my female friend was lying across my lap while I gently spanked her ass. After a few minutes she spread her legs, raised her ass to expose her lips and asked me to spank her vulva. After six spanks she was soaking wet and after a few more she squeezed my hand between her thighs and had a shuddering orgasm. Is this unusual or had I just missed something?—G.H., West Palm Beach, Florida

Nothing is unusual if you have the right woman, the right position, the right teacher, the right timing and the right pressure. Don't think about what you may have missed. Think about what you've found.

Fight club

I am a housewife, age 34. I've been happily married for 10 years. Our sex life is satisfactory but hardly what you'd call adventurous. (He begs me to try lingerie and oral sex but I have done so only on rare occasions.) Something happened recently that made me feel ashamed. My husband and I had gone to a mall. As we loaded our car before leaving, a young woman pulled into a space nearby. She opened her door and hit the car next to her. The man in the car jumped out and began screaming profanities and threatening her. When two construction workers came to her aid, the idiot began to verbally assault them. A fistfight broke out. One of the workers pulled a pair of pliers out of his tool belt and pinched the man's groin. He screamed in pain. By the time we arrived home a few minutes later, I was so horny I couldn't stand it. My husband unloaded the car, and I ran to the house to relieve myself. I had two of the most satisfying orgasms I've ever experienced. Since that day, I have enjoyed masturbation as never before; every time I think of that scene at the mall I become extremely aroused. But I also feel incredibly guilty. Have you ever heard of such a thing? I've never enjoyed pain or seeing anyone suffer.—C.W., Cleveland, Ohio

Here's our hypothesis as to why you became so turned on: Besides the menace in the situation, which would get anyone's blood flowing, you observed one person clearly demonstrating carnal power over another. You've always been a passive participant in sex; your husband has told you what he wants, but you aren't sure how to express your desires, or even how to discover what they might be. That's why you retreated to masturbate when you should have thrown your husband on the hood of the car and told him, "I am so turned on. Fuck me—now." In a way this incident may be a godsend, because it's helped you get in touch with your inner dominatrix. Tell your husband that he can have his lingerie and oral sex, but only after he's on his knees.

Catfight

For as long as I can remember, I have been outspoken and in control, but now I need some serious advice. Recently I went to my ex-husband's house to see him. He wasn't there, but his 24-year-old fiancée opened the door. I made myself at home, against her wishes. To her credit, she was polite when she asked me to leave, but I never missed a chance to take a cheap jab. I told her to hush, that she was just a piece of ass to him, and that what he needed was a real woman. That pissed her off, and she proceeded to jump me and thoroughly kick my ass. I told her I gave up, but she was too mad to let it go. To cut to specifics, soon I was licking her pussy through her underwear until she came. She then brought me to climax with her fingers, telling me that now I would know who was the piece of ass. When we were finished, she forced me to wear her panties. That was seven months ago. I have been wearing her panties ever since. Three weeks ago she came to my apartment and showed me two pairs of panties—one mine and one hers—and told me to choose. If I chose mine, it meant I had learned my lesson. For reasons I can't explain, I chose hers. Am I getting what I deserve? Please help.—M.S., Des Moines, Iowa

You met your match, and it turned you on. That's hardly surprising. The most enthusiastic submissives are dominant in every other area of their lives. This is a tricky situation. It begins with the fact that you're having an affair with your

ex-husband's lover. Given the other complications here (such as not changing your underwear for seven months), that almost seems quaint. Your ex will find out eventually, and you have a better idea than we do how he'll react. Your priority should be to agree on a safe word—a signal that you want an encounter to end. No responsible dominant refuses to establish one. If yours won't, we suggest you wear your own panties. That's not such a bad idea anyway. You've discovered something new about your sexuality; now find a more suitable partner to share it with.

Sex education

My lover and I enjoy moderate S&M. Lately his kid brother, who attends college nearby, has been asking questions about the more exotic and erotic aspects of sex. My lord and master has decided to give his brother a sex education course, using me as a demonstration model. Lesson one will show how to gently and passionately strip a woman. Lesson two will cover foreplay and a variety of positions. Lesson three will include the delights of oral sex and some pointers on S&M, if that interests him. I'm proud of my body and don't mind displaying it, but I'm concerned about my lover. Although he says he loves the feeling of owning me completely, I don't think he could help but regard me as a whore if he saw me with another man. We've agreed to let you decide if we should go ahead with the plan.—L.R., Washington, D.C.

Let's be honest. This isn't about sex education. It's about fulfilling your sexual fantasies. The only thing the kid will learn in your bedroom is how to fuck his brother's girlfriend. That's not particularly useful in the dating scene. Arranging a threesome—or, technically, a twosome and a voyeur—is complicated enough without involving relatives. Besides, you're overlooking the third heart in this scenario. Your lover's brother may want more than a demonstration model to teach him about sex.

Yeah baby

My boyfriend of two years and I have started talking about marriage. Recently he told me a secret that he has kept for 15 years from his friends and family: He enjoys dressing as a baby once or twice a week, complete with diapers. Sometimes he wears them overnight. He says it relieves stress. He has tried to stop, but after seeing other adult babies on daytime talk shows he decided that there isn't a problem as long as he's not hurting anyone. He wanted me to know about it before things progressed. I love him and am not sure what to do. Should I encourage him to change? This isn't the way I imagined becoming a mother.—C.F., Austin, Texas

It's good to see you've kept your sense of humor about what's certainly a stressful situation. Your boyfriend showed courage revealing his secret; he risked losing you but chose to be honest. That says something about your relationship. Realize that you aren't going to wean him from this fetish—it's not a hobby. However, many couples manage to integrate a variety of offbeat tastes into mutually satisfying sex lives. Infantilism is common as uncommon tastes go; there are support groups online and companies that sell giant diapers, rubber pants, pins, rattles, pacifiers and bibs for adults. Most ABers are men, though some women also enjoy dressing as infants or young girls. The act of becoming an infant can be a stress buster: It allows the submissive partner to take a break from the responsibilities of the adult world. At the same time, he can demand without guilt that every whim be fulfilled, which gives him control. We see no harm in this sort of sexual play as long as you're willing to participate and it's not the only way your boyfriend gets off. Find an open-minded therapist for premarital counseling. Your boyfriend can explain his desires; you can voice your concerns and set limits. Couples in love have negotiated greater conflicts than this. Look on the bright side: If you have a kid, you'll both already have experience with diapers.

Our kids saw me tied up

One of my turn-ons is to be bound and gagged. With my husband due home from work in half an hour and my teenage daughters at a sleepover, I had a girl-friend tie me up (fully clothed) and leave me in a kitchen chair. My husband was late, but after 45 minutes my daughters appeared. Their sleepover had been canceled. After they untied me I told them their father and I were playing a game. They seemed to accept that but could they now think I'm weird? Should I attempt a better explanation?—L.L., Philadelphia, Pennsylvania

All teenagers think their parents are weird; you just confirmed it for your daughters. We like your explanation, and it's none of their business beyond what you offered anyway. But take a lesson from your misadventure: It's never a good idea to be tied up and left alone. Bondage requires safeguards, including supervision and safe words or signals. Your girlfriend should have hung around until your husband returned, even if she had one foot out the door. You should also send your daughters to camp.

Honey, I'm home . . .

Three weeks ago, I got home from work to find my wife dressed in leather and holding a whip. She said I was to be punished for arriving home late. I didn't know what she was talking about, but I went along with it. I went upstairs to shower as I always do. Two of my wife's friends were waiting, and they ambushed me, stripped off my clothes and tied me to the bed. My wife beat my ass with the whip until I could barely stand it anymore. Then she made me perform cunnilingus on her friends. She stood over us, telling me that today she was the boss and that I would do as I was told. I got so hard I thought I was going to burst. Then came the real surprise. My wife loves anal intercourse, but she turned the tables, strapped on a dildo and gave me what I had been giving her. She knew enough to use a lot of lube, and it felt great. I've had to wear panties to work every day since, and I'm never sure what to expect when I get home. Is there something wrong with my wife, or do a lot of women enjoy this?—G.K., Des Moines, Iowa

Did you get her permission to write us, dogmeat? Erotic female domination is a place most couples never go, but it's out there. Keri Pentauk, who edited a magazine for the scene called Whap!, *says "a lot of women reach the point where they feel they have no choice but to put their foot down. You should thank your lucky stars you have such a fantastic wife."*

Give them a foot . . .

My girlfriend has gorgeous feet. For some reason, hot-pink polish on her toenails drives me nuts. I also love to see wrinkles in her soles, especially when she's sitting in a chair and curls her toes on the ground. My girlfriend once met a fellow who begged to rub her feet. Another guy commented on her painted toenails, and even had the guts to say, "I'll bet he does your feet," referring to me. Does the Advisor hear from many foot fetishists?—K.T., Fort Worth, Texas

Sure, including a number who can't understand why we don't publish close-ups of the Playmates' feet. That's not to say we can't appreciate the graceful lines, suckable toes and delicate balance of a woman's cloppers. We've even heard image consultants complain that open-toed shoes reveal too much "cleavage" for the office. Some theorize that men fixate on women's feet because they're harder to reach than the genitals. Feet are also less demanding sexually—you don't have to arouse her toes—which may appeal to men with performance anxieties.

In a recent issue *Playboy* featured several models displaying their beautiful feet. In the event this becomes a trend, I thought I would share my ideas about what constitutes a hot foot. It should be rounded instead of angular, as if diagrammed using a compass. The toes should be orbs of diminishing diameter, aligned in an arch, with none protruding above or retracting below this line. They also should be free to wriggle, not scrunched together or pressed into angular shapes. The balls of the feet should be well defined, with a high instep and a broad heel. I don't personally meet the definition of a fetishist, because it's not necessary that a woman's feet or any other body part match my ideal. But it's nice when it happens.—R.B., Miami Beach, Florida

Once you start looking for barefoot women, they turn up everywhere. Playboy Special Editions has published several volumes of Barefoot Beauties, *and many adult movies now seem to include at least one sole-searching scene. One hypothesis is that the relative safety of foot sex becomes more appealing during epidemics of sexually transmitted diseases. A study published a few years ago in* Psychological Reports *argued that each of the three major STD epidemics during the past millennium was accompanied by a surge of interest in the female foot in art, literature and fashion. To see if the pattern continued with AIDS, the researchers counted the number of photos featuring bared female feet in* Playboy, Penthouse *and six other adult magazines between 1965 and 1994. They found a fourfold increase.*

Bondage 101

I grew up in a small town but recently moved to Chicago. I feel fairly unsophisticated. For example, I met a woman at a bar who told me she was into bondage. Does that mean she wants to be tied up or that she wants to tie me up? The women in Chicago seem much more confident and aggressive than those I knew growing up.—D.T., Chicago, Illinois

Tell us about it. Turn your back for a second around here and you'll find yourself handcuffed to the bed. When you see this woman again—if she doesn't find you first—ask if she's a top or a bottom. This will reveal your casual knowledge of the topic; Jay Wiseman's Erotic Bondage Handbook *can provide a more thorough education. A top generally likes to control the sexual situation, though the control is a fantasy, since both partners can end the game at any time. As a top, she would tie you up and discipline you. If she's a bottom, she'll want you to take charge. Or she may enjoy playing either role.*

At Realmstone.com, we avoid the terms *top* and *bottom* because everything we do is considered a consensual power exchange, and sadism and masochism are not always necessarily so. It's better, especially for the novice, to use terms such as *dominant* (or *dom*) and *submissive* (or *sub*). If D.T. enjoyed the sensations of being dominated in a social setting, he can safely explore the sensations online before he considers a real-life encounter.—M.S., Anaheim, California

Isn't every relationship a consensual power exchange?

Rape fantasy

I fantasize about being raped. Is that normal? If it is, how should I request playing out this fantasy? To tell my fiancé would ruin the element of surprise that turns me on. I'm also not quite sure how he would handle it.—K.M., Houston, Texas

Being overpowered is a common sexual fantasy, though calling it rape is a misnomer. Rape is an act of violence over which the victim has no control. You always retain some control over the fantasy, because you can end the situation with a single word. It isn't going to happen spontaneously, because your fiancé isn't going to force you to do anything. You'll have to explain yourself. Tell him you want to be "taken." Ask him to make demands, and repeat them, and ignore your protests unless you utter a preestablished code word. (Use something like yellow or red rather than stop or no.) Then he can surprise you.

Sorting it out

What is the difference between a transvestite, a transsexual and a hermaphrodite?—M.O., St. Louis, Missouri

New to the dating scene? A transvestite is a person (usually a man, and usually heterosexual) who is turned on by wearing the clothing of the opposite sex. A transsexual is a person with gender dysphoria (i.e., he or she feels trapped inside the body of the opposite sex), a situation that often leads to hormone treatments and surgery. A hermaphrodite is born with male and female genitalia and may identify with either sex. These days a transsexual is more likely to be referred to as transgendered, and a hermaphrodite to be called intersexed.

Pedal to the metal

Ever since I was a child, I have fixated on women in cars that won't start. I suppose you could call this a fetish, because it gets me incredibly turned on. Have you ever heard of such a thing?—A.K., Harrisonburg, Virginia

We don't recommend that you work as a mechanic.

Eating out

You may not believe this, but I fantasize about being eaten. I don't mean oral sex but full-scale devouring by a woman who gets so excited by my taste that she loses all control and consumes me, cleanly and painlessly. There are a few variations on the theme: being cooked for a feast held by a group of hungry women, or being eaten slowly, with each piece cooked in front of me. Some of my girlfriends have been amused by my desires, but others were horrified. Have you ever heard of this?—W.I., Cleveland, Ohio

No, but we're never surprised anymore. Katharine Gates opens her book Deviant Desires *with a story she heard from a New York dominatrix. One of the woman's clients had drawn knobs and dials on a large cardboard box to make it resemble an oven. Wearing only socks, he laid on his back inside the box, put his arms tight against his sides and lifted his knees, so he resembled a turkey. The dominatrix then described for him how the oven was slowly growing hotter, and how she couldn't wait to remove her roaster, carve him up and eat him. Gates thought this unusual until she investigated and found a universe of people who shared similar cannibalistic desires. (It is known as* vore, *which makes you a vorephile.) "It's a kind of rape fantasy that substitutes oral engulfment for intercourse," Gates writes. As to why this idea turns you on, there are theories that it has to do with separation anxiety or an early fixation with nature shows and fairy tales. To each his own. We're content to have a woman devour our penis, as long as she doesn't chew.*

He wants boobs

I have been a cross-dresser for many years. My wife has always allowed me to wear panties and bras and carry a purse around the house. I also wear a nightgown to bed. Now, after 25 years of marriage, my wife has suggested I get breast implants. She said that because I'm getting ready to retire and I often wear a bra under my clothes, "why not get some boobs for it?" She said she wants me to get big ones—"boobs you have to deal with." She wants them to bounce when I walk. I was flabbergasted at first, but now I think I'd like to do it. Can you help me find a good plastic surgeon?—D.P., Oklahoma City, Oklahoma

No, no, no, no. Breasts are like babies. They're fun to play with, but only when they belong to someone else. Even if we thought this was a good idea, a board-certified plastic surgeon wouldn't consider such a fundamental change unless you were living full-time as a woman and had a note from your shrink. Now, what's up with your wife?

Fired up

My boyfriend and I have a friend who told us he puts a gun in his girlfriend's mouth while they have sex. I asked him if the gun was loaded, and he said, "Of course. What would be the point of doing it with an empty gun?" He said his girlfriend insists the safety be off. I was horrified, but I'm wondering if most men would find this game erotic or exciting. My boyfriend admitted he would enjoy doing it if he had the chance. He won't—at least not with me. I would be so frightened that I wouldn't be able to enjoy the sex. Have you ever heard of this?—M.W., Brooklyn, New York

Yeah, we've heard of it—Richie Aprile and Tony's sister Janice did something like this on The Sopranos. *It was creepy as drama, and it's creepy in real life. If your boyfriend wants a thrill, he should try it first while masturbating.*

I think this activity is more prevalent than you'd expect. I had the joyous and miserable experience of dating a stripper. One day I took her to a shooting range to fire my Tec-9. She went through five boxes of ammo, then suggested we play out a fantasy she had of being overpowered by a man with a gun. She wanted to do this in public, but I thought better of it. We reached a compromise: I knocked on the door of my house carrying a coat over my arm to hide the gun. She answered the door pretending to be a real estate agent showing the house. The muzzle went into her mouth as soon as we got inside and the door was closed. She insisted that the gun be loaded, and that the safety be off. She even made me load it while she watched. I tried to discourage this fantasy, but her response was always "If you can't kill me, you can't thrill me." There is no way I would ever put a loaded gun into someone's mouth. Once I got outside the door, I would pull the active clip, put in an empty one, remove the round from the chamber and pull the trigger at least three times.

The scenarios that followed included her being held up against a wall while slowly shedding her clothes and being backed through the house to the bedroom with her hands up, then being told to strip and move to the bed. As long as the fantasy was intense, she was hot for it. You can bet your ass I never had a sip of alcohol before we played these games. If anything went wrong, can you imagine a jury buying my story? Our relationship ended after a year. I'm certain I will never again run my hands over such a beautiful body, but, unfortunately, the body was attached to a brain that was part bitch and part psycho. It was creepy fun while it lasted.—J.M., Tucson, Arizona

Your ex is lucky she had you. You'll enjoy this story: A resident of Hamburg called the police after hearing gunshots, followed by moaning. Turns out a guy was shooting at his girlfriend to fulfill her cops-and-robbers fantasy. He practiced safe sex by using blanks.

Sit on my face, please

I've been blessed, or cursed, with an odd fetish. I love to have girls sit on my face and cut off my oxygen supply. I haven't figured out a good way to bring it up in conversation. Most of the time I just out and say it; other times I drop hints. Most women get squeamish when the topic comes up. How do I arrange this pleasure? I suppose I'm just one of those submissive, dominatrix-paying types and I'll never be able to enjoy this with someone I love.—J.S., Albuquerque, New Mexico

If you're a submissive, we can understand why queening turns you on. Controlling a person's breathing is as close as it gets to controlling his life, and when a person panics from lack of oxygen, the body responds with a surge of adrenaline. But there's another problem besides potential brain damage. If you can't get excited except when a woman suffocates you, she isn't going to find the sex that interesting.

Double fisting

In an interview, porn star Brittany Andrews was asked whether her job had introduced her to anything she hadn't tried before. She answered, "Double fisting." I assume she meant having two fists inserted into her vagina (or anus?) at the same time. Is that safe? Is it widely practiced?—J.C., Minneapolis, Minnesota

Widely is the only way it's practiced. A vagina can expand enough to accommodate a newborn, so a fist, or even two, is possible if a woman is sufficiently wet and relaxed. A supply of lube and latex gloves is essential. The practice is common enough that at least one sex manual—A Hand in the Bush—is devoted to the topic. Its author, Deborah Addington, suggests taking it slow (no kidding) and adding lube each time you insert a finger. When you've worked up to four fingers and a thumb (palm up), "add more lube. When you have a big, slippery mess and you're sure that you've used more than enough, add more. If she still feels tight, gently open and close your fingers as if you were making a hand puppet talk. Remind her to relax her vaginal, sphincter and PC muscles. When you're both ready, ease the bridge of your hand through and marvel as it's consumed by her cunt. Once inside, clench and unclench your fist, like a beating heart. If you've ever wondered what an orgasm feels like from a woman's perspective, fisting is a great way to find out." Power to the pussy. We recommend getting the book for more details before attempting this maneuver. Anal fisting is more popular with gay men and has a higher risk of injury.

The letter about double fisting reminded me of a clip I saw on the Internet that shows a man putting his entire head into a woman's vagina. Even if the clip was fake, could this actually be done?—S.S., Spokane, Washington

Most guys have had their heads inside a vagina once, but there's no going back.

Going full circle

Last week I came home earlier than expected and found my husband of four months naked on the living room floor with the stereo blaring. He was too involved to notice I was in the room. My husband is no contortionist, nor is he well endowed, but he was adeptly licking and sucking the head of his penis. I couldn't believe what I was seeing and finally yelled at him to let him know he had an audience. He told me that he had been doing it since high school, that it isn't abnormal and that most guys would do it if they were able. He swears that he has no homosexual tendencies. It seems kinky to me—and not necessarily in a good way. How common is this, and do I need to be as concerned as I am?—G.S., Columbus, Ohio

We assume you're less concerned with the masturbation than with the method. Autofellatio is uncommon but doesn't indicate anything except that your husband will always have a job in the porno circus. Alfred Kinsey found that two or three

males out of a thousand could suck their own penises, with many others acknowledging that they had come up short. Completing the circle is a habit among chimpanzees, rhesus monkeys and other primates, prompting Kinsey to observe, "In his psychic drive, the human animal is more mammalian than even his anatomy allows him to be." We heard this month from a reader who said he had leaned over and licked his penis while his new girlfriend was giving him head. How's that for a freak-out? You have a special guy there. Don't let him roll away.

Touch me, feel me, heal me

My fiancée is studying to become a nurse. The other night when I got home from work she was in her naughty nurse outfit (a short white skirt, see-through blouse, garter, stockings, sexy panties). She took me to our bedroom and said, "It's time to prep you for surgery." She laid me on the bed and removed my clothes. After telling me to relax, she gave me an enema. As she did, she straddled me in the 69 position and gulped my cock and worked my balls with her free hand. I had the most intense orgasm of my life. I'd like to ask her to repeat what she did to me, but I'm afraid she'll think I'm a pervert. What do you suggest?—S.D., Madison, Wisconsin

Your girlfriend already thinks you're a pervert—that's why she brought the enema. Find out when the naughty nurse is next available and make an appointment.

I was having sex with an escort, and she asked me to perform CPR on her. I asked if she was okay, and she said she was fine but that having a guy pump gently on her chest and give her mouth-to-mouth turned her on. Later she told me that six months earlier she had had a heart attack and been zapped back to life. Have you ever heard of anything like this?—A.A., Brooks, Alberta

Simulated CPR is part of a medical fetish that includes people—overwhelmingly guys—who like to listen to heartbeats or give fake injections (check out the site medicaltoys.com for a taste of the variety). Did you at least get a discount?

Aroused by loud shoes

I find it arousing to see or hear a woman walk in loud shoes. I also love to hear them tap-dance. Is this normal?—J.F., Houston, Texas

It's uncommon. In his online history of foot sex, podiatrist Cameron Kippen of Curtin University in Australia references a case "in which a man reached orgasm

by following women whose shoes creaked (known as acousticophilia, *or arousal from sound). It was thought the origins of the association related to an early experience having standing sex on a staircase—his partner's shoes had creaked with each thrusting." This may be impossible, but you need to find a woman who likes new shoes.*

Snake eyes

My girlfriend wants a tattoo—two eyeballs, one for each butt cheek. I don't want to look at that bullshit every time we're doing it doggy style. What should I do?— B.Z. New York, New York

Pretend you're getting a blow job. If she's serious about this (which we doubt), keep her sober. If she goes through with it, stock up on crotchless panties.

He likes to watch her being watched

I get turned on when my wife is the object of other men's desires. She is generous about engaging in this behavior. We visited a restaurant recently with the idea in mind. My wife got her order and sat down opposite a guy who began staring at her legs. Before she had a chance to make it a show, he dropped his napkin and looked up her skirt. My wife is reluctant to admit that this turns her on, but we always have great sex afterward. Does this fetish have a name? Do many couples engage in it?—M.W., Myrtle Beach, South Carolina

You're both exhibitionists. Your wife enjoys showing off, and you get a vicarious thrill watching your wife show off. Most people flaunt it once in a while, but the fact that you plan these encounters puts you in a select group. The reaction of other men affirms to your wife that she's desirable to strangers; it affirms to you that you're with a desirable woman. Many couples play this game—for evidence, consider the numerous websites that post images of women furtively exposing themselves in public. The boyfriends and husbands who snap the shots are not aroused as much by the flash (as a voyeur would be) as they are by the imagined response of other men to the flash.

Is sucking toes dangerous?

Many women like to have their toes sucked. Does nail polish have anything in it that would be harmful to the sucker?—B.T., Chicago, Illinois

If you can suck the polish off a toenail, it's too bad you're not a woman.

You shouldn't have blown off that toe sucker. Most brands of nail polish contain phthalates, a family of industrial chemicals commonly used in cosmetics to make them more flexible and durable. In animal studies phthalates have been found to wreak havoc on the reproductive, endocrine and immune systems. For men, an overload of phthalates may lead to atrophied testicles, low sperm count, overdeveloped breasts, immune deficiency and testicular cancer. One phthalate in particular tends to leech onto the skin every time the polish comes into contact with water or, presumably, saliva. Practice safe sucks by asking your partner to eschew polish or use phthalate-free ones such as those by Urban Decay or products in L'Oréal's Jet Set line.—D.R., Salt Lake City, Utah

This is one reason we stick with cunnilingus. The cosmetics industry insists its products are safe. And you'd have to suck a ridiculous number of toes to duplicate the level of phthalate exposure in animal testing.

The ties that bind

Whenever I watch porn I play with my nipples. I sometimes attach binder clips to get them hard. Is there any risk to this?—J.T., Pittsburgh, Pennsylvania

Besides not having anything to hold your documents together? There's little danger unless you're wearing the clips for hours at a time. The interesting thing about nipple clips is that they pinch when you put them on and ache while they're there, but the real pain doesn't come until you take them off and the blood rushes into the crushed flesh.

I'm a guy who also likes to stimulate my nipples, but I use the suction cups sold at nipplefunwear.com. I wait until my nipples fill 80 percent of the cups and then squeeze—the pleasure is exquisite. When the cups are removed I always have large, hard nipples.—B.B., Thousand Oaks, California

Thanks for the pointers.

My husband dresses like a woman

I started playing a dress-up game with my husband. He looks good, or as he says, "passable," as a woman. He's growing his hair long and has shaved his body hair. He's starting to look more and more like the women in your magazine. Recently he volunteered to drive me to Chicago for a business trip. I was flabbergasted when he showed up at my job dressed as a woman. (He told my secretary he was my cousin.) On the way to Chicago he asked for a blow job—it was the first full erection I had seen him get in a while, so I complied. He wore women's clothing around the city all weekend without any problem, and we had great sex. I think this game has gone to his head, and I'm trying to get him to stop before he gets too serious. Please help.—A.B., Cedar Rapids, Iowa

He's already serious. Your husband has come out as a cross-dresser after what has probably been many years of hiding his behavior. The practice is more common than you'd think and widely misunderstood. Dr. William Stayton, a professor at the University of Pennsylvania's Program in Human Sexuality Education, counsels cross-dressers and says most hesitate to tell their lovers because they fear it will end the relationship. In many cases, they're right. Women who stay cope by accepting their partner's female persona as a third wheel or friend. (One wife says she dishes to her new confidante about her husband.) Cross-dressers are usually not gay. They enjoy wearing women's clothing for a number of reasons: It gives them an erotic charge, it provides a sense of well-being, it helps them relax. ("You can't imagine how many politicians can't give a speech in Congress without wearing panties," Stayton has said.) Couples should establish boundaries. For instance, your husband went too far when he showed up unannounced at your office dressed as a woman. Or you may not feel comfortable making love when he's in his female persona. Visit the Society for the Second Self at tri-ess.org to join an online support group for the wives and girlfriends of cross-dressers.

Nipping and sucking

My husband has been hinting that he would like me to get my nipples pierced. The problem is that just before we go to sleep each night he sucks on one of them, which is so relaxing it promptly puts us both to sleep. He sucks off and on all night. I've heard that pierced nipples take six to eight months to heal, so I'm afraid that going through with it will put an end to this time of closeness. What is your advice?—K.B., Windom, Minnesota

Unless there are complications, such as an infection, these types of piercings heal within six to eight weeks, during which time your husband could suck on your clit. If you'd like to have your nipples pierced (don't do it for him), here's a Solomonic solution: Start with the one farthest away from him. That is, if he sleeps on the right side of the bed, do your left nipple first. Once that nipple heals, pierce the right and switch sides of the bed. That way hubby always has a nipple handy. The jewelry should be small so it doesn't get in the way.

Picky, picky

One afternoon I noticed my wife picking her nose as she read a book. I can't explain why, but I got an instant erection. I let her in on my turn-on, and now she picks her nose on purpose. Have you ever heard of this?—T.P., Westlake, Ohio

Nose picking is a social taboo, so it's not surprising that it would turn you on when a woman shows her nasty side. For wank material see snotgirls.com, where nude models "poke their brains" and "dig for gold." Hard yet? You know your fetish has reached critical mass when someone creates a website about it—a pay site, no less—although in some cases critical mass may involve as few as two guys (one to post material and one to find it). We're still searching for the "girls aroused by good advice" home page.

Flex appeal

I am overwhelmed by the urge to get toned, beautiful women to flex for me. I've asked for a flex twice, and both women said no. Now I just compliment women on their physiques and get my kicks that way. My obsession with getting a flex is interfering with my ability to socialize. What should I do?—J.R., Des Moines, Iowa

We love breasts, but that doesn't mean we ask every attractive woman we meet to lift her shirt. In the same way, you can't just ask for a flex. Besides, do you really want to date a woman who flashes her biceps for every guy who asks? It's more fun when she, like a 15-pound weight, offers a little resistance. Save the flex for sex. After you've become intimate your partner will be more likely to show off, especially when she sees the effect it has on you.

Seeing eye to knee

I consider myself a lucky little man. I'm small enough (five-foot-five) and light enough (138 pounds) to have kinky fun with my six-foot girlfriend. If I fall asleep on the couch, she'll carry me to bed. If I can't reach something at the supermarket, she'll lift me from under my arms. She does this at home so often that I've put away our step stool. Is there a name for this?—A.F., Salisbury, Maryland

Dependence? There's no particular name for this—you just have a thing for tall, strong, dominant women known in the fetish community as amazons. (For the record, your preference needs to be distinguished from men who fantasize about giantesses, pretend they're infants, lust after female wrestlers or chase female bodybuilders.) Amazons are appealing to the smaller man because, as one discussion board puts it, they can be either your "ultimate fantasy or worst nightmare." The eroticism lies in that dichotomy. You two should open a painting business.

THE MARRIED LIFE

Living with your choice.

How often do couples have sex?

What is the average number of times per week or month that a couple who has been married three years and who are 54 and 46 years old have sex? Everyone my wife asked said it was once a month. The two people I talked to guessed it was more like once a week.—P.C., Colorado Springs, Colorado

Your friends are right, or at least they're average. A survey of nearly 10,000 Americans found that most adults have sex 58 times a year, or once a week plus three holidays, two birthdays and National Sex Day (it's today). Married people have more sex than single people, and younger have more than older. Frequency remains steady through the mid-30s, then drops 20 percent before the age of 44, an additional 25 percent before the age of 54, another 25 percent before the age of 64. A survey of 65,000 male and 15,000 female Playboy *readers found that most reported discontent when frequency fell below weekly. According to the survey mentioned earlier, only five percent of American adults have sex more than three times a week. It also found that 42 percent of adults engage in about 85 percent of the sex and concluded that the more sex a person has, the more likely he or she will report having a happy life and a happy marriage. They needed to interview 10,000 people to figure that out?*

He doesn't get the laundry done

My wife stays at home with our three young children while I work 50 hours a week to pay the bills. I don't want to sound like a caveman, but I think stay-at-home wives have less trouble these days. Microwaves and dishwashers make it much easier to do housework, while VCRs keep the children occupied (two of our kids go to school part-time). My wife is tanned and in shape, and I am glad her lifestyle allows her to keep herself hot. I have trouble finding more than one or two days a week for a workout. She gets angry when I complain about not having clean laundry or the house not being picked up. My chores consist of lawn work and special projects. I feel I spend more time handling responsibilities than she does, and I usually take the two older kids when I get home. I don't want my wife to work, I just want her to run the house a little better. Am I the only one who feels this way? Do I have a legitimate gripe?—S.R., Philadelphia, Pennsylvania

If your wife looks that great after three kids, and she's not complaining, we wouldn't get too worked up about the laundry. Save that energy for the bedroom.

The thing with the ring

I wore my wedding ring for a few weeks after the ceremony but then stopped. When my wife asked me why I put it on only for family events (to avoid a confrontation with my mother-in-law, although I've stopped doing even that), I told her the truth: I have never worn jewelry, not even a watch, so I find the ring distracting and uncomfortable. I also found that it snagged on everything, and whenever I washed my hands the design would catch all the soap. We have a truce now (if you call not bringing it up a truce), so my only question is, Why does a wife consider it such a big deal if her husband doesn't wear a ring?—J.N., Seattle, Washington

Your wife is disappointed, as most women would be, because the wedding band is a recognized and powerful symbol that you showed up for the ceremony. Practically, she knows the ring doesn't mean a thing if you're having a fling. But she also wonders if you don't mind that people don't know you're married or, more specifically, that she exists. We're sure that isn't the case—when a cute woman flirts with you, you eventually mention your wife, right? You've already made many small sacrifices for your marriage; this is another one. In the spirit of compromise, visit a jeweler. If you get a band that looks good and fits well, you may find it enjoyable to wear. And you'll save single women some time at parties.

Your solution doesn't sound like much of a compromise. When my wife and I got engaged, I let her know that I don't wear jewelry. She insisted only that I wear one for the ceremony. Maybe I just have a cool wife, or maybe that reader's wife needs to unwind a little.—S.T., Austin, Texas

The reader should buy a chain and put his band on it, à la Frodo in *Lord of the Rings*. For symbolic reasons, it should not have a clasp. He should also tell his wife, "It's closer to my heart this way." It worked for me. I was surprised at how little the chain distracted me after a few days.—T.S., Dayton, Ohio

Why not call the situation what it is? The reader's wife, like most wives (and husbands), wants to mark her territory. It may not be the prettiest side of human nature, but it is what it is.—E.Q., Grand Rapids, Michigan

My husband has never worn his ring. He is an electrician, and we both feel it's safer that he doesn't. If the reader's wife is so uncomfortable with his not wearing a band, maybe he could get a ring tattoo.—A.G., Wakefield, Massachusetts

Daddy factory

About a year ago my wife started using unlubricated condoms with no spermicide when we had sex on Saturday mornings. After sex, she would leave in a hurry, saying that she had to go somewhere. After several months I asked her what she was doing. She paraded three women through the house in various stages of pregnancy and said she was helping them start families. Her idea was that she could be like a loving aunt or sister to the children. I would have been happy to help these women personally, but my wife said that would have been adultery. Since my wife donated my sperm, will I have to pay child support if one of these women goes to court? Is this something that's common—women helping other women start families through their husbands?—W.C., Little Rock, Arkansas

We suspect your letter is an attempt at humor, but there's a lesson in it. If a child is created by deceit using your sperm—even if you weren't an active participant in the insemination—a judge will still make you pay. We've never heard of an exception, regardless of the circumstances. Perhaps you should sell your story to the tabloids to finance your expanding family.

Anger management

My wife and I often argue by e-mail. I think it's better because you have time to think before you speak. Plus when we see each other again, the issue has been resolved. What do you think?—B.R., Riverside, California

We like it, as long as you aren't typing with your caps lock on. But it does limit the effectiveness of our favorite defense, which is "I never said that." What's important, however, may not be the medium but your approach. Psychologist John Gottman of the University of Washington has studied more than 600 married couples and how they fight. He divides couples who stay together into three types:

avoiders, who agree not to discuss their disagreements; attackers, who bicker about seemingly everything; and soothers, who choose their battles, listen respectfully and respond with gentle persuasion. According to Gottman, most marriages have trouble only when spouses have conflicting styles. For example, soothers overwhelm avoiders, and soothers and attackers reach a standstill. The worst combination is avoider and attacker. Gottman also found that among couples who stay together, the positive remarks they make to each other, during fights or otherwise, outnumber their negative comments by at least a five-to-one margin. E-mail certainly makes that easier to tally.

Is my wife a hooker?

From time to time, my girlfriend and I enjoy role-playing in bed. My favorite fantasy is to pretend she's a hooker, give her money and demand she do anything I want. The problem is that she keeps the money ($20 to $30, depending on the tip). Does that make her a prostitute?—T.G., LaCrosse, Wisconsin

She's not a prostitute unless she has other clients. You tip her?

Mercy fucks

Last month you ran a letter from a fellow who complained about his wife and their sex life. He asked, she gave, and that upset him. My wife and I are in our 60s, and she used to be like that. If I didn't ask, it didn't happen. I pointed this out, and she replied that she is no longer interested in sex. She said, "If you can find someone else to do it with, I don't think it would bother me much." I told her she was nuts, that it would destroy our relationship. Here was our solution: After I read the newspaper on Sunday mornings, I take a bath. When I'm finished, she takes a bath. Afterward, she walks silently past me on the way to the bedroom, I follow her and we have sex. I never ask, she never offers. We call it Pavlov's Poke. Sometimes if you don't ask, you shall receive.—R.T., Seattle, Washington

That sounds like some hot sex. Does your wife keep an egg timer on the nightstand? You have important issues to discuss outside the bedroom. Start by reading Passionate Marriage, *by sex therapist David Schnarch. In it, he describes the risks of the mercy fuck (definition: "You let your partner climb on top of you to get him off your back"): "People who accept mercy fucks can rationalize that it's better than no sex at all, but is it? If you accept mercy fucks 'until the good stuff comes along,' it never does and it never will. Your partner knows you'll settle for lousy sex, so there's no reason to deal with the problems blocking better sex." Let Pavlov's dogs run free! First, your wife's lack of desire may be caused by a medical problem that can be addressed by a physician. Many women lose interest in sex after menopause. Your wife may not be able to reach orgasm easily, or she may not generate suffi- cient lubrication. As in men, circulatory problems could be a factor, or hormonal changes may play a role—your wife should ask her gynecologist to check her testos- terone and thyroid levels (preferably early in the morning). She also could be clin- ically depressed, one symptom of which is low sex drive. Once any medical prob- lems have been addressed, consider visiting a sex therapist together. As the man who loves this woman above all others, make it your goal to encourage her desire. You may be comfortable with a weekly mercy fuck, but you're both missing out on the sex life you deserve.*

Do open relationships work?

Do you have any opinion on open relationships? By that I mean having a com- mitted emotional and sexual relationship with one person while also having lovers on the side with no strings attached.—M.B., Harrisburg, Pennsylvania

It sounds great, but for most people they don't work, at least not in the long term. Whether this is because we are naturally monogamous or simply socialized to have only one partner at a time is the subject of much debate. In our view, any intimate encounter has at least a few strings attached. That's what makes us human. The problem with open relationships is that many people who decide to have them neglect to inform their partners.

Two years ago my wife told me she is bisexual. She arranged several three- somes, which I loved. Ten months ago she met our current girlfriend, and the three of us are planning a commitment ceremony. The problem is, my wife has changed. For 14 years I thought she was straight; now I would say she is 75 percent gay and 25 percent straight. She and our girlfriend are inseparable; they are always holding hands and kissing. I love my wife but have a feeling she would choose our girlfriend over me. Do I have a reason to feel this way, or am I being petty?—A.J., Cincinnati, Ohio

This is a common issue among newly polyamorous couples. Your wife and girl- friend are enjoying the giddiness of a new romance. That will subside. The more important question is, where will the three of you be in five years? It is possible to maintain a triad (or even a quad) for decades, but only if each partner understands that no two are greater than the whole. For that reason you should not expect that you and your wife will be the primary relationship, with your girlfriend orbiting. They also should not expect you to orbit them. It may be too soon, after 10 months of dating, for any of you to commit. Many people in alternative relationships struggle with jealousy; to combat it they rely on the wisdom of those who have gone before. The poly community has support groups in most states and a national magazine called Loving More *(lovemore.com).*

There are many types of polyamorous relationships. I am in an MFM V-triad, which means that I am with both my husband and our male best friend, but they are not with each other. The three of us have chosen to become a family and raise our children together. I understand some people might find this impossible because of jealousy, or issues of safety, but if someone in a relationship is cheating, how safe is that?—L.W., San Francisco, California

Our question is, who controls the remote?

My wife drives me nuts

My wife is driving me crazy. We've been married six years and it's like my mother said, "The things you think are cute at the beginning will make you nuts later." When we got married, I loved that she had a strong personality. Since then she's become pushy, and we've been fighting. Does the Advisor have any suggestions to keep my marriage from falling apart?—L.K., Toledo, Ohio

Don't expect your wife to change. Besides the fact that it won't happen, you agreed six years ago to accept her as a package deal, and she, you—marriage doesn't come with a line-item veto. That's the counsel of Andrew Christensen, co-author of Reconcilable Differences *and director of a five-year study called the Couples Therapy Project. Every couple has incompatible traits that could destroy the relationship; those who survive learn to accept, rather than challenge, these differences. Your perceptions also play a role. You may have been attracted to your wife because she was outspoken, but now she's outspoken with you and you're blind to everything but the negative side of the trait. Like any effective therapy, acceptance puts the focus on the only person you have the power to change. Christensen suggests these strategies to defuse tension when you argue: (1) Figure out the "third side" of the story that incorporates your partner's views. (2) View the problem as "it" rather than something being done to you. (3) Summarize what your spouse says during the argument to show you get it (but without sounding like a smartass). (4) Focus on one problem at a time. (5) Don't insist you're right.*

Pulling a fast one

Three years after my wife and I were married, I went to Central America to help with my family's business. I stayed about a year and met another woman. We were married, and she returned with me to the United States. I told wife number one that the new woman was my cousin and would be staying with us. It has now been 12 months and wife number one wants to know when my so-called cousin will be moving out. What should I do? I guess I really screwed up this time.—A.R., San Diego, California

We'll say. One wife wasn't enough? Your spouse—the original one—knows something is up. If she finds out about the marriage, she could go to the police. Bigamy is a felony in nearly every state, including California. If you can't decide who it's going to be, the decision will be made for you. *

I've only slept with two women—am I missing out?

I am 30 and happily married. This is the second marriage for both of us. My problem is, the only two women I've ever slept with are my ex and my wife. Hell, they're the only two women I've been naked with. This bothers me, and I'm not sure why. Both my ex and my wife had multiple partners before we met. I don't feel that's a bad thing, just that I've missed out. How can I get over these feelings without putting my marriage in jeopardy?—C.T., Cypress, California

Look on the bright side—you're two steps ahead of the virgins. You won't "get over" these feelings any time soon. Even guys who have had hundreds of lovers wonder what it would be like to be with a woman besides their wife. Some men choose to cheat—and then wonder what sex would be like with a different mistress. That's why marriage can be exasperating and rewarding at the same time; you may only have sex with one woman, but you got your first choice. You could abandon your marriage and begin a Don Juanian quest for fulfillment, but we both know you'd

---

* In February 1999 the digital voyeur Spacewurm eavesdropped on a random cell phone call in San Francisco and transcribed the conversation for his book *I Listen*. A guy was reading this letter and our response to his girlfriend. After he finished, there was a five-second pause, and then the woman said simply, "Damn."

regret it. If you want wild flings, you're sleeping with a woman who knows better than any other how to turn you on. In the long run you'll have more fun with her.

A shell of a man

I don't like my husband going to strip clubs because of the way he treats me afterward. He says every man either has to watch dancers or cheat on his wife. Otherwise he becomes "a shell of himself." What do you think?—R.R., Colorado Springs, Colorado

Your husband sounds like a single guy living in a married man's body. There's nothing wrong with a guy visiting a strip club but only if it doesn't cause a rift in the relationship. When it does, he continues at his peril. Your husband is in a sad place indeed if he feels empty without strippers in his life.

The pain of childbirth

My wife and I are expecting our first child. She told me she had read that when a member of the Huichol tribe of Mexico goes into labor she ties a string around her husband's testicles. As the pain of the contractions increases, she tugs on the string so her husband can share in her agony. Please tell me this isn't true, because my wife doesn't need these ideas in her head.—P.T., Atlanta, Georgia

That's a good one. We checked with Stacy Schaefer, an anthropology professor at California State University at Chico who specializes in gender roles among the Huichol tribe. She says it's not true. If God wanted men to share in the pain of childbirth, she would have made it easier for us to have multiple orgasms.

Six tips for better sex

For those readers whose sex lives have dried up since the kids arrived, here's what works to keep my husband and me active five or six nights a week: (1) Hire a sitter once a week while you go for a walk, hold hands and talk. (2) Be a help-mate—there's nothing sexier than a man who folds socks or massages feet during *Monday Night Football*. (3) Clean house—if ear and nose hair was gross on your grandfather, they are not attractive on you, either. (4) Make sure your wife has time to read a Susan Johnson book once a month to keep the juices flowing. (5) Schedule a little romance—do at least one small thing each week (rose petals have lots of uses). (6) Be a lifelong learner—read the *Kama Sutra* or watch the Better Sex video series.—J.B., Santa Rosa, California

Admit it—you'd have sex with your husband four times a week even if he didn't do all this stuff. Most guys understand that they have to make an effort, but these lists feel like work. We always want to ask, when was the last time you fucked your husband for no reason at all?

My husband blabs about our sex life

My husband tells all the men he meets about our sex life. I suck, lick and swallow. I also like anal sex. I even asked him to arrange a threesome. It turns me on to see my husband get turned on. The problem is when he tells his friends how he gets anything he wants, I feel like our personal life isn't personal anymore. When they ask me if he's full of shit, I just laugh. Should I tell them, "Sure, I do it all" or deny everything?—K.B., Minneapolis, Minnesota

Have you told your husband about your concerns? He needs to know. You're sexually adventurous because you feel comfortable with him, but his boasting makes you uncomfortable. If he continues to be indiscreet, tell his friends something like this, within earshot: "I don't discuss my sex life. My husband can discuss his, but he may not have one soon." Not that you would carry out that threat, because it would deprive you. But it might get the point across.

I said okay, but now I'm pissed

A year ago I told my wife she had the freedom to be with other men. A couple of days ago, she took me up on the offer. The man is a friend, and I'm having a hard time with it. I asked her not to sleep with him again until I could accept it. My wife is disappointed, but understanding. Now I feel like an ass. How can I get over these feelings of inadequacy? I want to give my wife what she desires.—J.S., Lawrence, Kansas

Did she ask for her freedom, or did you volunteer it? Giving your wife what she desires should turn you on—if not, you're giving away too much. A large part of the problem is that she's sleeping with a friend, and you imagine they have or will develop an emotional bond. A guy may fantasize about his wife's fucking another man, but it's only her body he's sharing. Perhaps you can arrange to give your wife this freedom in a place where neither of you has anything invested but the pursuit of pleasure. Find a swing club where you can arrive and leave as a couple. You may feel more comfortable with this arrangement, especially if you're getting a blow job at the time.

I want my husband to have an affair

The thought of my husband having an affair makes me wet, especially the anticipation I'd feel before his return after a night out. The problem is that whenever he's in a position to meet another woman, he refuses to pretend to be single, or at least unhappily married. He won't even remove his wedding ring. Few women believe that this mature, sexy guy is being truthful when he says he has my permission to cheat. What should I do? Send a permission slip? Make a matronly phone call?—L.R., Phoenix, Arizona

We like your husband's approach because it's honest and keeps the third party in the fantasy from having any illusions about what she's getting into. It's not an affair—it's a threesome with the wife waiting at home. Next time your husband reaches the point where a prospect can't believe he has your approval, have him give you a signal. Introduce yourself. Explain that "we each do our own thing," or be more direct: "My husband is the best lover I've ever had—and I don't mind sharing." Then take your leave. You can't do everything for the guy.

Why stay married?

Are people generally happier in their second marriages than in their first?—B.J., Omaha, Nebraska

Not necessarily. One study of 1,400 families found that 40 percent of the spouses who divorced found new partners but reported the same problems. Another study focused on 645 adults who said they were unhappily married. Five years later, two thirds of those who stuck it out reported being content. Among those who divorced, only half said they were happy (a notable exception was people who had been in violent or abusive relationships). So while many marriages end in divorce, it could be said that many divorces fail also.

I can't stop thinking about Jenny McCarthy

I fantasize about fucking Jenny McCarthy. I told my wife about this, and she agreed to have sex with me while saying things like "You like the feeling of Jenny's lips on your cock?" and "Come on, fuck Jenny McCarthy!" The problem now is that I can't get turned on unless I'm looking at a photo of Jenny or my wife is pretending to be her. What should I do?—J.W., Baltimore, Maryland

You'd better do something quick or your wife will be a fantasy too. It's not unusual to imagine being with other people while having sex with your partner, but it's a bad sign when it's the same person all the time, everytime. (It's known

as allogynia, *or the inability to come without fantasizing about a more desirable lover.) We would suggest aversion therapy, but we don't know of any photos in which Jenny looks bad. The next time you have sex—if there is a next time—banish her photo and use "baby" and "honey" when encouraging your wife so you don't slip up. Concentrate on the sensations and think about Jenny all you want, but keep it to yourself. We suspect you'll get over this.*

My husband isn't much fun

My husband is a hardworking guy who provides for his family and so on, but when it comes to fun and romance he's at a loss. He's 30 years old but acts as though he's 50. He works all the time and stresses about the house, bills, money and everyone else's problems. How can I help him lighten up, enjoy his family and live life while he's young (and still has a wife)? I've begun to do almost everything without him.—C.S., Portland, Oregon

You need to tell your husband that his work habits are not working for you. We can anticipate his response: As do most workaholics, he sees his family's pleas for affection and attention not as a sign that he is loved and needed but as an intrusion or an interruption. Many men struggle with this. They feel immense pressure to provide, which can make them crabby and distant. They prefer the controlled environment of work to the chaos of a home with children. Changing these habits is difficult. Usually it requires a close friend to lead by example. That's what happened to literary agent Jonathon Lazear, who wrote a book about his experience, The Man Who Mistook His Job for a Life. *He told us, "Too many men abandon their families, and for what? Is there a financial crisis? Most likely no. They're probably doing as their father did. Men need to remember that they're less productive when they overwork; they make mistakes. A wife may have to say, 'We're out of here unless you examine what you want. You can find a balance—and we'll help you.'" With any luck your husband won't join the legions of men who realize only later what they missed, especially in the lives of their children.*

Wife says it's not true

In the beginning of our relationship, my wife readily told me stories of her sexual past. I felt obligated to share my own experiences. It made me feel good to be honest with the woman I love. But my wife now says she made up most of her stories. I have asked for the truth, but she says it's none of my business. I believe she made it my business by listening to my confessions. What do you think?—M.M., Franklin, Minnesota

What else has she lied about?

I like waiting on my man

I do everything for my man. I clean the house, prepare his clothes for work and have a meal on the table when he gets home for lunch and supper. Since the day we married he has never made his own meal or opened his own can of beer. He brags to everyone about our relationship. I love pleasing him. He works long hours almost every day to provide me with everything I need. The problem is that everyone tells me this is a bad relationship. They say he is too controlling and that I should leave. But I have always felt that a real woman takes care of her man. Am I wrong? He's happy, I'm happy, so what's the problem? How do I get people to stop judging our relationship?—J.H., Columbus, Ohio

Your husband needs to open his own beer. Also, people should mind their own fucking business.

Going back for more

My husband and I enjoy going to strip clubs. During our last visit he had too much to drink but wanted to drive us home. I grabbed the car keys, but he refused to get in. Exasperated, I told him to call a cab and left. We worked it out the next morning, but he also revealed that he had gone back inside the club and ordered a lap dance. He says he didn't think I would be mad about this, but I feel that if your pissed-off wife leaves you at a strip club, it's not the best time to pay for pussy in your face. Am I out of line?—S.D., Dallas, Texas

What better time? You were already mad at him. Actually we're smarter than that. Your husband's decision demonstrates how seriously his judgment was impaired, which proves your point that he shouldn't have been driving. A smart man would acknowledge this, grovel appropriately and count his many blessings, including a wife who gets upset when he goes to strip clubs without her.

I'm sleeping with my mother-in-law

For the past five months I have been having an affair with my wife's mother. She's 56 and has a great body. The affair began when she stayed with us while looking for a house. My wife works the night shift as a nurse, and I was home watching TV when my mother-in-law came out of the bedroom wearing a robe and smoking a joint! She sat down, offered me a hit and told me she hadn't had sex in three years (since my wife's father died). I told her she was high and should go back to bed, but she slid closer and started kissing me. We ended up in the bedroom and made love four times before I fell asleep. Then I had sex with my wife the next morning. (It wasn't easy, but I managed.) Two weeks ago my mother-in-law moved into her new house, and now we screw there. My wife thinks that I get along so well with her mother, but she wonders why I go to see her every night. I tell her it's to move furniture, but that won't work forever. I still love my wife, but the sex is too good with her mother. What should I do?—S.M., Orlando, Florida

Come clean with your wife, after which you will have her mother all to yourself.

Here's an update. I left my wife after I told her what I was doing. She hasn't spoken to her mother since. In the past few weeks my mother-in-law has worn garters, teddies, stockings and high heels for me. We also use plenty of whipped cream and honey. Magic Shell—that stuff you put on ice cream—works great too. She told me to quit my job and said she would take care of me. All she has asked is that I not fool around. The relationship has its drawbacks, though. While we were out dancing one night, a couple said, "Oh, how nice. A son out with his mother." But what do they know? I have never been happier. I don't know how long this relationship will last, but while it does I love my mother-in-law with all my heart.—S.M., Orlando, Florida

MASTURBATION

Love the one you're with.

The walls have ears

An attractive woman lives down the hall from me in my apartment building. We've exchanged small talk, but that's it. I often fantasize about her while masturbating. A few weeks ago the couple who live next door to me invited the woman to a barbecue. They asked her to bring me along. Puzzled, she asked why. The couple said they could hear us on some nights and assumed we were dating. When she told them we weren't, it dawned on all of them that what they had been hearing was my moaning this woman's name. A few days ago my neighbor—nice guy that he is—told me everything. I was speechless. He said the woman had seemed amused. I had wanted to ask her out, but now that seems comical. What should I do?—J.W., San Diego, California

The next time you beat off, put the other sock in your mouth. The only way to find out if the object of your affection was horrified, mildly amused or totally turned on is to ask her out for coffee. You'll have your answer in a nanosecond. For the record, the women in our office—an open-minded group, to be sure—universally agreed that this revelation would creep them out. If you can score in this situation, no woman will ever again seem like a challenge. You may have the balls to fess up, but a better strategy might be misdirection. That is, say hello, apologize for not introducing yourself earlier, ask her name as if you didn't know it, then lie: "That's funny. My ex has the same name." She may not believe you, but it could plant a reasonable doubt, and that's all you need for acquittal.

Uncharted waters

Last month my girlfriend dared me to act out a sexual fantasy, so I masturbated in her roommate's bedroom. Now she wants me to do it again. It's a little twisted and exciting, but I don't want to risk being caught. Should I just forget it?—R.G., Olympia, Washington

You completed the dare. Now it's time to challenge your girlfriend. Whatever you decide she should do, videotape it. Her double dare will be to leave the tape on top of the VCR over a weekend.

Keeping it real

Can you suggest new ways to masturbate? Getting laid is preferable, of course, but not everyone is so fortunate.—M.H., Sydney, Australia

As you've discovered, nobody ever got lucky thinking of new ways to beat off. If you promise to get off your butt, we'll share a resource you won't forget—Jackinworld.com, a compendium of advanced techniques, each rated with one to four palms. A visitor favorite is the Vagina: "Lie on your side and hold on to your penis with a backhand grip. Roll over farther and brace your hand against the bed, and thrust your penis in and out of your hand. It's a different feeling to masturbate by moving your pelvis rather than your hand. It's also fun to put your other hand down and feel your scrotum moving back and forth as you pump in and out." Another hit is the Rosy Palm: "With lubrication, rub the tip of your penis head against the palm of your other hand. The orgasm will be very powerful." The site is fun but also serves important purposes: Conditioning yourself to get off only in a certain way can be a problem when you're with a partner. Variety is also useful in learning to control your arousal. Finally, if you don't know how you like to be touched, it's difficult to tell someone else how to do it.

Try toothpaste lather for the same cool, tingly sensation you feel when brushing your teeth.—A.C., Grinnell, Iowa

By what process did you discover this?

I prefer bananabation. I wrap masking tape around a banana three quarters of the way up. Then I roll it between my palms to soften it. I cut the end off below the tape, squeeze the insides out and eat them. When it's all empty I have the next best thing to pussy. I lube my erection and then microwave the banana sheath for 23 seconds. I find it adds some excitement between dates. Have you ever heard of this? Is it dangerous?—P.P., Chicago, Illinois

It's dangerous in the monkey house.

Once you have an erection, spread the head to open the urethra. Push down on the hole with the index finger of your other hand. Repeat 170 times, then keep your finger over the hole as you slowly stroke your penis. As you reach climax the shaft will fill up with sperm, and the air inside will cause a pressure buildup. The stream of semen that erupts is incredible.—J.A., Los Angeles, California

Because we care about your well-being, we'll warn you of the remote chance that your technique could lead to an embolism. Then we'll get out of the way.

Desperate husbands

Last evening when I came home from work, I caught my husband in the bathroom trying to pull up his pants. I asked him if he had been taking a shower. He said no. While I was in the bathroom preparing for bed I heard him fiddling with the VCR. I can't prove it, but I think my husband was jerking off to an adult movie. Why do men do this? I don't have a problem with my husband's satisfying himself, but why does he have to sneak around? It's especially troubling because he's in the mood for sex only about once a week.—S.B., Fort Wayne, Indiana

Blow your husband every day for a week and see how often he masturbates. Your husband beats off for the same reason he did before you were married—it feels good and it doesn't require permission. He masturbates in private because he's always done it in private; by definition, it's a solitary act. If you're there while he masturbates, it's sex, and he's not always in the mood to negotiate that. For her Book of the Penis, Maggie Paley asked numerous men about why they masturbate. One guy noted that women's magazines often print letters from readers who have discovered that their husbands beat off and are now asking themselves, Am I not satisfying him? His response: "There isn't one person on earth who can satisfy any man. Men masturbate always. It's not a reflection on his relationship with his wife. He's shaving and suddenly he thinks, I'll jerk off. And he does." Your husband's masturbation would be less of a problem if you got laid more often. That's where to start the discussion.

You worked hard to justify the guy's behavior, but not only was your response insufficient, it was inconsistent with what you wrote back in 1994. Then, you advised a female reader to leave her masturbating man. A masturbating husband is not a big deal as long as he satisfies his wife. Those of us who enjoy sex find it to be a personal insult—he's choosing his hand over us. When a man reaches orgasm by masturbating, he has chosen another "partner." In my book, that makes masturbation cheating. A man may do it because it doesn't require negotiation, but I assure you that if a woman masturbates it is because she is not being satisfied. If your wife is begging for sex and you're jerking off in the bathroom, something is wrong. Don't take her for granted. She may not be around someday, and then your only choice will be your hand.—M.S., Atlanta, Georgia

Here is our response: (1) 1994 was a long, long time ago, in man years. (2) You're right: Masturbation is a problem when your partner isn't getting enough sex. (3) Masturbation isn't cheating. That's ridiculous. (4) You are misinformed if you believe that women masturbate only when they're not being satisfied. (5) A guy's only choice before she was around was his hand. He'd survive.

Ladies, we are all bothered by our guys' masturbating. It is a selfish act that makes us feel a variety of things, from rejected to worthless to unattractive to cheated on. However, guys are going to continue to masturbate. They can't help themselves. They say to themselves, "It's there, it feels good, so why not?" Women have more control. So what can you do? Confront your husband. Ask him how often he does it, what he thinks about, if it is a reflection on your relationship and what you can do to make him turn to you for pleasure. Your husband is not going to want to discuss this. Masturbation is something he has hidden since age 12 or 13 and he's going to feel you have invaded his private world. If he is like most guys, he will make a smartass comment and change the subject. This is where you will have to stress how deeply it affects you. If he loves you completely, he will listen and eventually the conversation will unfold. I'm not saying that he'll stop, but at least he knows how you feel. Then, if the masturbation continues and your sex life suffers, he won't be surprised when you move on.—R.R., Atlanta, Georgia

Who, exactly, are you going to move on to? A guy who doesn't masturbate, or just one who's better at hiding it from you? Women don't possess more control than men, or less desire. They're simply more often socialized not to explore "down there." Those who work past that taboo have a wonderful time. Many of our female readers will be amused at your notion that they should "confront" their partner about his lifelong habit, as if he needed an intervention ("Honey, your family is here because we feel you're wrestling the noodle a little too much"). In our world—and we're glad to live in it—a guy telling his wife what he thinks about when he masturbates is called foreplay.

My husband is free to beat off whenever he has the urge. I masturbate just about every morning in the shower, and the fantasies I invent often become part of our lovemaking. It never occurred to me that my attitude about jerking off was unusual.—E.O., Chicago, Illinois

I love watching my husband masturbate. Occasionally, if I'm not in the mood, he'll go ahead without me. Sex in a marriage isn't about keeping score and trying to ensure that your partner's orgasms are always directly related to or caused by you. Confronting your partner is not going to improve your sex life. You'll have a lot more luck tapping into that sexual energy in a positive, nonconfrontational way.—N.M., Silver Spring, Maryland

I'm a guy who doesn't masturbate. Never have, probably never will. I don't think there's anything wrong with masturbation, but I've always found it satisfying to have a woman do it for me. Lucky for me, I've never had a problem finding one. Does that make me a liar or a freak? I don't think so.—T.J., Atlanta, Georgia
Your day will come.

Guys masturbate because it's low maintenance and immediately gratifying. If you want your husband to stop, you need to offer something even more low maintenance and immediately gratifying. If you blow him every morning, that might slow him down. But if your goal is for him to stop completely, you'll have to provide at least three BJs a day. My husband of 19 years gets oral sex every day. Yes, he still masturbates. He also scopes out all the hot babes. And I'm happy he does.—M.P., Santa Rosa, California

Masturbation fantasies
My friends and I were the last guests at a party. Everyone was a little drunk. Someone posed a question to the group: "What's the oddest thing you've masturbated to?" One girl said NFL football, a guy said receptionists (not a particular receptionist, but the idea) and another guy said women who smoke calabash-type pipes. All of these answers passed without comment. Then I said, "Cartoon women"—notably Holli Would from *Cool World*, Julia Chang from *Tekken 3* and Rogue from *X-Men* comics. My friends all laughed hysterically. Am I as fucked up as they claim?—S.J., New Orleans, Louisiana
You're taking grief from those weirdoes?

Breaking old habits

From what I gather, I masturbate differently than most guys. Wearing underwear, I lie on my stomach, make my right hand into a fist and rub my penis with my knuckles. I've tried stroking my penis the normal way but I can't reach orgasm. It also affects me when I'm with a woman. Blow jobs don't do much for me, and I take forever to come during sex. Have you ever heard of this?—B.B., Santa Barbara, California

Many therapists believe that if you masturbate in an unorthodox way over a long period of time, you may condition yourself to respond only to that stimulation. Your situation is a textbook example of what has been called "traumatic masturbatory syndrome." Writing in the Journal of Sex and Marital Therapy, *therapist Lawrence Sank described four of his patients who had trouble getting erect or reaching orgasm during sex. He attributed this to their masturbatory technique, which was to lie on their stomachs and rub their penises against the mattress, a pillow or the sheets. One 62-year-old had used this method almost daily for decades to avoid touching his penis, which a priest had told him was the equivalent of "recrucifying Jesus." Another man used your technique, but with both fists. Sank calls for better sex education for young men to prevent these problems. A website devoted to fighting TMS (healthystrokes.com) recommends that boys be taught to masturbate only on their backs.*

One-two punch

Is it okay to masturbate while wearing boxing gloves?—R.G., Chicago, Illinois

Sure. Knock yourself out.

Jack-off clubs

While searching online I came across a site devoted to what teenagers once called circle jerks. A coed solo sex party sounds like a great alternative to a full-blown orgy, especially since it eliminates the risk of STDs. How would I find one?—N.T., Los Angeles, California

Since 1987 Tom and Lynda Gayle have been hosting parties at least monthly in Tampa and Orlando as part of their Club Relate (clubrelate.net). Couples and singles interested in attending must complete a two-hour orientation, during which they talk about their masturbation experiences, and they must agree to the club rules: no drugs, no smoking and always be polite by saying, "No, thank you, but thank you for asking." As many as 40 people attend each party, and the Gayles keep the ratio at no more than two men to every woman. There's also an annual Masturbate-a-Thon organized in San Francisco by Carol Queen as a fund-raiser for her nonprofit Center for Sex & Culture (masturbate-a-thon.com).

Porno party

My friends and I sometimes share porn clips by e-mail and joke about masturbation. Everyone has a good laugh. But once in a while we get together to drink, and the host will put a porno in the DVD player. That's when the awkwardness begins, because as the film goes on everyone gets horny and is dying to jerk off. The last time it happened I tried to end the silent tension by suggesting a circle jerk. Everyone called me a pervert. What do you recommend in this situation?—J.R., Boston, Massachusetts

Calling it a night.

Driving Miss Daisy

I drive a lot for my job, which is stressful. A friend suggested I touch myself to relieve the tension. I tried it, but it got a little dangerous, because as I rubbed my clit through my panties I stiffened my steering arm and wanted to close my eyes. During one trip I was eating an apple when I got an idea. I put it on the seat between my legs and started moving my hips in a circular motion. I got so turned on I couldn't concentrate. I pulled into a rest stop and rode the apple to an incredible orgasm. When I told my friend about it, he asked if I then finished the apple. Yes, I did. It was warmer and softer but still good. What do you think?—C.T., Chicago, Illinois

We've always liked apple with cherry.

Does masturbation prevent cancer?

Does regular masturbation reduce the chance that you'll get prostate cancer?—T.S., Harrison, Michigan

Apparently yes. You'll go blind and grow hair on your palms, but you'll live forever. Scientists at the National Cancer Institute examined, over eight years, the self-reported ejaculation frequency of nearly 30,000 men. Those who came most often—a lifetime average of 21 times a month—were one-third less likely to develop organ-confined or slow-growing prostate cancer than the control group of men, who came four to seven times a month. The study found a benefit in men who had more than 12 orgasms a month. Regular ejaculation may be beneficial because it flushes out carcinogens in the gland. Come for life.

MISCELLANEOUS

A little bit of everything.

Can men breastfeed?

My wife read a short story about a man who grew breasts to help nurse his girlfriend's baby. She asked if I would be willing to do that. I said, "Sure, why not?" Now she's six months along and expects this of me. I'm taking hormones to make my breasts grow, and I'm eating asparagus to stimulate my milk glands, along with licorice root, blessed thistle and black cohosh because she says they are primarily female herbs. I also use a breast pump for 10 minutes twice a day. My wife says men can produce milk but just never develop the ability. My breasts do feel softer and more sensitive. Will this work?—C.M., Detroit, Michigan

We thought no, but apparently men can, with considerable effort, produce breast milk. This can be accomplished by stimulating your nipples over days or weeks; it doesn't require hormones or herbs. It's unclear if the quality of the milk will be the same as a woman's or if a man can produce enough to sustain a child, but there are reports of men who have fed infants this way. We wouldn't take hormones except under a doctor's care, but what can we say otherwise? You're ahead of your time. Guys, if you know what's good for you, keep this quiet.

The rules of nudity

During our honeymoon, my fiancé and I plan to spend a week at a resort in Cap d'Agde, France. We're told nudity is encouraged throughout the village. Can you confirm this? Also, can you explain the etiquette for going topless or nude? We don't want to break any laws or offend anyone.—C.O., Chicago, Illinois

Cap d'Agde is a clothing-optional coastal town 50 miles southwest of Montpellier that began as a campground in 1956 and has since grown to about 20,000 residents. According to local lore, police ensure that clothing is not worn except in cases of severe sunburn. Here are some guidelines for any nude resort: Always sit on a towel. Don't leer. Don't be lewd. Don't shoot a lot of photos or videos. And don't show off your erection. (Instead, one veteran nudist advises, hide it in the sand, under a towel or in the water "until your steamy imagination adjusts to the reality that sex, as you know it, is not the reason that people are unclothed.") If you enjoy the experience, the American Association for Nude Recreation (800-879-6833, or aanr.com) can suggest nudist clubs in the U.S. that are close to where you live or vacation.

Does sex attract bears?

My wife and I went camping for a few days in Yellowstone. I wanted to make love, but she refused. She said that having sex in the woods might attract bears. Is that true?—T.Y., Boulder, Colorado

Unless you're covered in honey or make love while frying bacon, you aren't putting yourself in danger. Professor Steve Herrero of the University of Calgary, who has documented nearly 900 bear attacks over the past 30 years, has found only a few where a couple reported having sex before the bear showed up. "That's probably nothing more than chance," he says. He won't dismiss a connection completely—"a bear's sense of smell is as good or better than any bloodhound's"—but the chances you'll be attacked are almost nil to begin with if you observe the standard precautions of backcountry camping, such as keeping your food properly sealed and stored. (Most attacks occur when the animal is surprised by hikers.) Herrero has also recorded only three or four cases where a bear attacked a woman who happened to be menstruating, another common but exaggerated fear. Bears can be as unpredictable as humans, however, so triple-bag fresh and used tampons and sanitary napkins, scented soaps and colognes. Then again, if you're carrying cologne into the woods, you don't belong there.

Searching for work

What is the best way to prepare for a job search?—S.D., Milwaukee, Wisconsin

Have you checked your references? Many people are surprised to learn that past supervisors and co-workers aren't saying the nicest things about them. Job hunters typically become suspicious only after a few interviews go well but don't lead to offers. Companies such as Allison & Taylor (allisontaylor.com or 248-651-9299) will call your references, offer a vague explanation about doing an employment verification and make sure you aren't being dissed. The standard fee is $79 a reference. Heidi Allison says that although employers tell managers to provide only basic data—especially about an employee who was fired—many yak away. Even those who are relatively discreet may still make damning comments, such as "Let me get the legal file to see what I'm allowed to say" or, when asked to rate a skill, "Can I give a negative number?" Other screeners *echo Allison's advice to job hunters, which is never to omit a job from your résumé nor any of your past bosses from your list of references. Instead address trouble spots in the interview by saying such things as "He's not my best reference because we had some disagreements." That's one reason not to list references on your résumé; you'll have a better chance of making a good first impression before any calls are made. The latest trend among employers is to phone an applicant's ex-assistants. Says Allison, "They check under you instead of over."*

When a job application asks if I've ever been convicted of a crime, I check no. But the truth is that when I was 18 I got arrested for shoplifting $7 worth of stuff. Two years later I was charged with disorderly conduct. (My buddies and I got drunk and yelled at the cop.) These things happened 16 and 18 years ago, and I chalk them up to being a dumb, rowdy college kid in West Virginia. I paid the fines and cleaned up my act. I now have a great career. I hate being untruthful, but I think answering yes on an application would count against me. Will a background check bring my transgressions to light? Is there a way to clean up my record?—W.K., Cleveland, Ohio

Our instinct would also be to check no, but the human resources people we asked all said that's a bad move. A few suggested that you qualify your response on applications by writing "college pranks." The risk in answering no is that if a background check does uncover the crimes, a potential employer may wonder what other secrets you keep. It's unlikely that 20-year-old indiscretions will be a factor, especially if you've had a clean record and an impressive work history since. But don't spend any more time worrying about this without doing an investigation of your own. Contact the state police to request a copy of your criminal record. With any luck the incidents fell through the cracks. If not, you can petition a judge in the county where you were charged to have the infractions expunged. It's been done many times before.

Are people born lucky?

Are some people born lucky or does it just seem that way?—R.G., Dayton, Ohio

You have to wonder, especially when we read about someone winning the lotto twice, or dating successive Playmates. We've always suspected that luck is a combination of attitude and perception, and psychologist Richard Wiseman backs us up. In The Luck Factor, *he describes a 10-year study he conducted with 400 volunteers who considered themselves lucky or unlucky. His subjects kept diaries, took personality tests and submitted to interviews. Wiseman concluded that those who thought themselves lucky were more skilled at noticing chance opportunities, making decisions based on intuition, creating self-fulfilling positive prophecies and adopting a resilient attitude. "Personality tests revealed that the unlucky are generally more tense and anxious," Wiseman explains. "That mind-set disrupts their ability to notice the unexpected." Many lucky subjects went to great lengths to introduce variety into their lives, which increased their chance encounters. They also tended to react to misfortune by thinking, I'm lucky it wasn't worse. By having the unfortunate adopt the habits of the fortunate, Wiseman found that they began reporting more lucky breaks.*

Lump sum, or annual?

A few of us at work have talked about pooling our money to buy lottery tickets, but we can't agree on how we would take the winnings. Let's say that we win $20 million. Should we take a lump sum or annual payments over 20 years?—W.G., Cortland, Ohio

Lump sum, always. You'll make more investing the smaller cash-out than waiting for the full amount over 20 years. Assume you beat the odds—the equivalent of flipping a coin and having it come up heads 24 times in a row. First, you should have a partnership agreement and a federal tax ID number in place to avoid headaches splitting the pot. Almost half of your jackpot will be consumed by state and federal taxes. Choosing the lump sum will knock it down further, to about $6 million. Don't do anything brash such as quitting your job or buying a new house until you've hired a tax advisor and an investment counselor. Then take 10 percent of your share and blow it.

Cussing in Deadwood

I'm sure there was plenty of cussing in the 1870s but perhaps not as much as one hears on HBO's *Deadwood*. Did people living on the frontier really use words such as *fuck, cunt, cocksucker* and *motherfucker*?—B.G., Sparks, Nevada

Linguists who study the 19th century are forced to rely on printed evidence, so it's hard to say definitively which swear words beyond goddamn *and* damn *were used in Deadwood in July 1876. The show's creator says the crude dialogue is based on the fact that visitors who returned from the camp reported being shocked by the language. Simple blasphemies wouldn't jar the modern viewer, so creative license is probably in play to evoke the same sense of danger and lawlessness. Jesse*

Sheidlower, the American editor of the Oxford English Dictionary *and author of a dictionary devoted to the F word, says prostitutes and their customers probably used* fuck *in its literal sense and also may have referred to the vagina as a* cunt. *While residents of Deadwood conceivably could have said* cocksucker *(which dates at least to the Civil War), linguists say it's extremely unlikely to have rolled off the tongue as it does on the show.* Motherfucker *didn't appear in print until the 1910s.*

Yiddish for vulva

A Jewish friend was reciting all the Yiddish words that he knows for penis: *schmuck, putz, shvantz, schlong,* etc. But he said there was no word in Yiddish for vulva. That's hard to believe. Do you know one?—R.S., New York, New York

There's no widely used word, but that doesn't mean you can't get your point across. In an essay in The Ecstatic Moment, *Albert Stern describes his quest for the word after his Gentile girlfriend asked about it. Stern spoke to elderly Jews who suggested slang such as* loch, pirgeh, shmoonke, shmushka *and* shtalt. *A professor of Yiddish offered* oysemoken *("that place"),* dos vayberifher *("the female part") and* die mayse *("the story"). Stern found these choices decidedly unerotic and vague, but what can you do? Barbara Kligman, editor of* Plotz, *reports that many of the women she grew up with referred to the vulva as a* knish. *Sounds delicious.*

Exotic pets

I've had cats and dogs but want something cooler. Would a pig be a good choice?—C.F., Harleysville, Pennsylvania

Sure, if you like bacon. That's a joke, of course, because we know the owners of potbellied pigs take their duties seriously. If you want a pig, make sure it's okay by local ordinance and that you're ready to commit for up to 15 years. Most potbellied pigs weigh 90 to 150 pounds and require room to roam and a wading pool. That's one reason so many end up in shelters. If you want exotic, how about a tiger? That's also a joke, although there are twice as many pet tigers (10,000 or more) in the U.S. as there are tigers living in the wild. The cubs are cute until they grow into 500-pound killing machines that require 10 to 20 pounds of horse meat or beef a day. People also attempt to domesticate cougars, lions, monkeys, bears, wolves and alligators, which is legal as long as the animals aren't imported and you don't live in one of 21 states with bans. If you're looking for female companionship, a lapdog on a leash has a magnetic effect on women. We're not sure what reaction you'd get with a pig.

Charisma defined

What is charisma, and how do you cultivate it?—M.S., Raleigh, North Carolina

Charisma is the ability to make other people feel good about themselves. It requires equal measures of confidence and empathy. It also helps to have a good tailor.

Getting a roommate to move out

Why is it so hard to get someone to move out? A college friend moved in with me to help pay the mortgage, but he's a slob and I need him gone. I can't afford a lawyer, and I'm not sure what can be done short of throwing his stuff in the street and changing the locks. Any suggestions?—K.L., San Jose, California

You may have no choice but to go to court. Local laws vary, but in your county and others you must first give your roommate a written 30-day notice. The next step is to ask the judge for an "unlawful detainer action." The sheriff will deliver this document, then remove your roommate and his stuff. Don't do anything drastic, such as changing the locks, pitching his belongings or moving out and shutting off the utilities. That will put you on the defensive and only delay the proceedings. This is true even if the person is related to you. Many people assume that a long-term guest has no right to stay if there's no lease, but that's not how the law sees it.

Making a citizen's arrest

How does a person make a citizen's arrest?—H.N., Washington, D.C.

Rarely is it necessary to detain someone, which can be risky and lead to a lawsuit if you don't have your facts straight. Instead, the typical arrest involves calling the police, giving a statement and signing a complaint. The police must agree that a crime has taken place, which is why arresting a politician for voting to invade Iraq or a police officer for speeding usually won't get you far. (In 2004 at San Francisco City Hall a citizen attempted to arrest a volunteer conducting gay civil unions but couldn't find a cop who would help.) You can make a citizen's arrest in every state and D.C. if you suspect that a felony has taken place. A few states, notably California, allow citizen's arrests for misdemeanors if you witness the infraction. That's in part why the LAPD processes more than 6,000 citizen's arrests annually, while D.C. seldom has one. Police say they appreciate citizens getting involved but find that some get a little too involved. For example, a motorist in Wisconsin pulled a gun and handcuffed another driver for playing his music too loud and squealing his tires. In Oklahoma, a homeowner chased a 19-year-old he saw throwing bottles from a pickup, set up a roadblock, ran the truck off the road, broke a window to grab the kid, applied cuffs and called police. Once in a while you read about the real deal, such as the Norfolk, Virginia mechanic who witnessed a hit-and-run that killed a teenage boy. He chased and detained the driver.

Hanging out in international waters

How far out does a person have to sail to avoid U.S. laws against marijuana, gambling, prostitution and underage drinking?—R.R., Miami, Florida

Planning a big weekend? Technically, you can't sail far enough. That's because, while there are international waters, there are no international boats. Each vessel is under the jurisdiction of the country with which it's registered, regardless of its location. The U.S. Coast Guard can board American vessels anywhere in the world if it suspects lawbreaking, and it can do so without a warrant. If you claim your ship flies no flag, the Coast Guard can still board—control of a stateless vessel is assumed by whichever nation stops it. Practically, of course, you stand less chance of being caught if you sail beyond the more heavily patrolled U.S. Customs zone, which ends 24 miles out. The ocean is a big place.

Avoiding jet lag

I will be traveling to Honolulu via Los Angeles, an 18-hour trip. What can I do to arrive in the best possible shape?—C.B., Amsterdam, Netherlands

You're facing serious jet lag. Studies have found that it takes about a day per time zone you cross to recuperate, but you can do it faster with preparation. Beginning two days before you travel, add more water and protein to your diet. Eliminate fatty foods. Continue this regimen during the flight, and avoid alcohol, caffeine and sleeping or motion sickness pills. Wear loose clothing and stretch and walk around periodically. Take a sleep mask, but doze only when the cabin lights dim and the movie has finished. When you arrive, take a two-hour nap. Shower, then set your watch to local time. If it's morning or noon, have a high-protein breakfast or lunch. Order a high-carb dinner to help you sleep. Retire at a reasonable hour and set your alarm to rise early.

Buy me a jet plane

Is it possible for a civilian to buy a ride on a military fighter jet? I think this would make a great Father's Day gift.—M.R., Brooklyn, New York

Come on, don't be a cheapskate—buy the whole jet. You can pick up a decommissioned Soviet MiG these days for as little as $30,000, though the fuel costs might bankrupt you. Defanged fighter jets can be flown in U.S. airspace only for exhibition or pilot proficiency, so rides can't be sold. But there are any number of collectors willing to take a passenger who agrees to split the cost of fuel, which runs a few hundred dollars an hour. For leads, contact the Classic Jet Aircraft Association at classicjets.org. Depending on your budget, you also might get in touch with Space Adventures, which for $20,000 will strap your dad into a MiG-25 at a Moscow military base and take him up 80,000 feet and down again to pull tricks at Mach 2.8 (call 888-857-7223). Many companies and a few museums offer less costly rides in World War II-era trainers such as the T-6 and T-34; you'll find a list at warbirdalley.com. And for $995, Air Combat USA will send your dad up for six simulated dogfights in an Italian-built prop fighter-an experienced pilot handles the takeoff and landing, and your father is equipped with a parachute, a helmet, a flight suit and a few combat tactics. The firm is based in Fullerton, California but has a road show that travels the country. Phone 800-522-7590 or visit aircombat.com.

ONLINE

Brave nude world.

Digital snoop

Years ago I suspected a girlfriend was cheating. Although she denied it, I installed monitoring tools to capture her instant messages and e-mails. I was amazed at how convincing her lies had been. Since then I have monitored other women I've dated, either by shoulder surfing to get their e-mail passwords or by installing software. Anytime I suspect deceit, I obtain the truth. Perhaps this isn't ethical, but it has saved me a lot of time and heartache. I don't want these tools to ruin my integrity as a boyfriend or spoil my ability to trust a good-natured woman. But it's hard to establish that trust when you have seen firsthand how two-faced some people can be. What does the Advisor think?—N.E., Detroit, Michigan

We think the spying is getting you off. When you love a woman as much as you love the technology, maybe she'll be loyal to you.

Porn with a familiar face

I found a collection of porn photos on my boyfriend's computer. I don't mind that he looks at porn, but he put my sister's face on the photos! I'm not sure what to think. What does the Advisor say?—J.C., Portland, Oregon

Look on the bright side—it could have been your mom. It doesn't surprise us that your boyfriend fantasizes about your sister, given that he's attracted to you. But pasting her face onto porn is further than most guys take it. You need to have a talk.

Do not enter, do not pass go

Most adult websites include a disclaimer that says you shouldn't view the site if its content is illegal in your state. How do I find out what's legal? Have people been prosecuted for visiting adult sites?—K.P., Los Angeles, California

Unless you're downloading and sharing child porn, the police won't be knocking on your door. Can we imagine cases where images stored in your browser cache could get you in legal trouble? Yes, but every instance is far-fetched.

The disclaimers are there for the benefit of the adult site, not its visitors. In the unlikely event that an ambitious prosecutor takes a digital porn palace to court for violating local or state obscenity laws, the site figures it can point to the disclaimer and say, "We warned them not to come in." That argument won't take them very far, but it's better than nothing.

What to do with nudes?

What is the protocol when you find nude photos of a female acquaintance online, at a site she apparently created? She's someone I know fairly well and would like to bang. My hours of porn surfing haven't been a waste after all.—J.W., Kansas City, Missouri

Are you sure that its the same woman? We haven't seen the site, but we're guessing it's a fantasy created to make money and not reflective of her personal sluttiness. Rather than being indiscriminate about who she "bangs," you may find her wary, and weary, of your interest. Ask her out, but let her make the first mention of her business. If you come across as another one of her drooling fans, the only way you'll see more of her is with a credit card.

I'm an escort with a website, and having people I know find me online is the biggest risk I take. I went to a new doctor, and the next day I got an e-mail from him through my site asking if we'd met the day before. It was a more honest way to do it, because if he'd asked me out in person I never would have told me I work in the business and he wouldn't have told me he fancies online companions. I would never tell a date what I do, because who I am as an escort is much different from who I would be as a girlfriend. I get paid to always want cock, always have great hair and never reveal my PMS. I wouldn't want to date a guy who is okay with what I do, and I also wouldn't want to live a lie—so dating is not something I do. My guess is that the woman that reader found would prefer to keep her two lives separate.—C.S., Minneapolis, Minnesota

Wouldn't we all.

Throw me a line

I've been surfing chat rooms, looking for a booty call. Is there a way to avoid all the small talk without sounding like a pervert?—T.W., New Orleans, Louisiana

Once you accept your essential pervertedness, you'll be more comfortable being blunt. The FBI agents and guys pretending to be women will appreciate your candor.

Photos of the ex
I've seen sites on which guys post nude photos of their ex-wives. Is that legal? What are the repercussions if the exes find out?—R.S., Randolph, New Jersey

These sites are designed to make you believe that the "ex-wife" in question is being humiliated, which is a turn-on for some guys. In reality, she's a model. We're sure a few former husbands have posted nudes of their exes without permission, but after the lawyers get involved we're guessing they won't do it again—especially men with children.

Can you ask a woman out by e-mail?
Is it acceptable to ask a woman out by e-mail? If she says no, I don't want her to see my disappointment.—F.L., Boston, Massachusetts

It's best to ask in person. If she declines, it's okay to be disappointed.

My horny co-worker
On a new co-worker's computer I came across a chat room she visits while at work. I suspected that if she knew I was in the room, she wouldn't be herself, so I signed in using an alias. During the first session she offered me a blow job and told me she liked to masturbate at work. That's when the administrator of the room revealed that she and I had the same network address, so she knew it was somebody at work. She freaked out and signed off. I e-mailed her later, explaining that I had just been trying to see the real her. Needless to say she seems embarrassed and a little creeped out. Of course I was turned on by her dirty talk and want to make a move. How can I release her sexual side?—C.J., Louisville, Kentucky

It sounds like you already did, but you blew it by being sneaky. How did you happen to be on her computer? After you've both been fired, maybe you can commiserate over a beer.

People often act very differently when they believe they have anonymity. Just because that woman wrote things online doesn't mean she will say or do the same after she signs off. If a guy pursues her in the hope that she will follow through, he may be in for a rude awakening.—S.D, Phoenix, Arizona

Boyfriend is trolling
My boyfriend has posted a profile on a dating site. When I asked him about it, he told me it was completely innocent. He said that because I am

frequently out of town on business, he wants to find "artsy" people to hang out with. His online profile indicates that he's single. When I asked him about that, he said he plans to inform any woman he meets about our relationship "when and if the topic arises." How can I convince him that posting this ad is disrespectful?—M.N., New York, New York

Deranged is more like it. Your boyfriend is reluctant to admit that you exist because otherwise he'd be fishing without a line. He may not be planning to cheat on you, but he doesn't want to miss any opportunity that presents itself. (As Chris Rock says, "A man is basically as faithful as his options.") Unfortunately for your Don Juan, that's not how the game is played. Your boyfriend needs to update his profile or he won't need to update his profile—you know what we're saying?

ORAL

Giant sucking sound.

My girlfriend won't stop sucking

My girlfriend loves oral sex. The problem is that she won't stop, even after I come. I usually have to make up an excuse to get her to quit (my back aches, my leg is asleep, etc.). Do you have any suggestions to bring the festivities to a close without hurting her feelings or lying about it? Things get painful after a while.—G.H., Baltimore, Maryland

If you want a woman to stop sucking your penis (egad—did we just write that?), give her something else to do. Tell her, "I'm so turned on; let's make love," or "Your turn," or "Come up here and kiss me." In the meantime, remember: A few haunted souls can't get blown even once, and right now they hate your guts.

Her blow jobs are "just all right"

My boyfriend and I have been together for a year. We were kidding around and he told me my blow jobs were "just all right." I decided that the only way to prove otherwise was to let him see for himself. I told him to get blow jobs from three women I didn't know and report back to me. Just as I expected, he came back and told me how good I was and how much he appreciates what I do for him. I wanted to let your female readers know that if you trust your man and are secure in your relationship, you should dare him to compare. He'll return if you're better than "all right," and he'll be incredibly grateful.—J.S., Middle Island, New York

You make it sound like your boyfriend was gone for an hour. This is risky business, but you seem cocksure. Now, tell your boyfriend his tongue is "just all right."

She has a ticklish clit

I like to perform cunnilingus on my girlfriend. There is one small problem. Every time I start to touch her or go down on her, she says, "Ooh, my ticklish clit!" and I have to stop. How common is ticklish clit and how can I work around it?—P.B., Oxford, Ohio

Do just that—work around it. Many women don't enjoy stimulation of the clitoris until they're thoroughly aroused, but you can play with it indirectly. Caress, spread and kiss her labia, finger her anus, massage her mons. The wetter she becomes, the less you'll hear about the tickle.

Who farted?

This is a serious question. I was going down on my wife and she let go of a large amount of flatulence. What would be the proper thing for either of us to say or do when that happens? I was grossed out and my wife became angry, saying I had ruined the mood. (She's the one who farted!) What's the etiquette for this situation?—D.L., Buffalo, New York

It's always unpleasant to learn the hard way that your wife's gas doesn't smell like potpourri. We suggest that in the future you both make use of a technique described to Jay Leno by an audience member on The Tonight Show. *She explained that whenever someone in her household felt the need to release, he or she would say, "Safety." This alerted other family members to stand clear. That's an easy courtesy to extend to anyone giving you pleasure.*

The classic blow job

My boyfriend loves blow jobs, but I haven't had much practice. Do you have any tips?—K.L., Mesa, Arizona

Of course. How do you think we got this cushy job? Actually, we often come across great advice in unexpected places. In this case it was a humorous anthology called The Vice Guide to Sex and Drugs and Rock and Roll, *in a chapter by Christi Bradnox, who is one of those goddesses who believe that giving good head is an art form. Here are a few of her suggestions: "(1) Before you head south, prepare the landing pad with your hand. Horse around until he's hard as stone. Assure him that he's going to get some heavy mouth action, but don't let it start until he's ready to crack. Rub through his pants like it's a baby animal about to be born. (2) Your teeth should not exist. Use the same principle you apply when eating a Popsicle with sensitive molars. (3) If he steers the ride (hand hovering over or on your head), ask soft questions. Are you going too hard, soft, slow? You're not looking for a discussion, just a yes or a moan. (4) Your hand should form a tube like a skirt around your mouth, with your thumb and forefinger like a belt that meets your lips. Most of the feeling is in the head of the penis, so don't waste too much time on the shaft. The area should begin to feel like a wet, greased, slow moving internal combustion engine. (5) At some point, lock eyes with him. Remember, he's filming this with his brain and may use it as masturbation fodder for years. You can even jerk him off a bit, which is a nice break for everyone. (6) When he's about to come, increase the speed of your hand and mouth. Let him feel you pulling his orgasm out of him. Make swallowing motions, press your tongue against his shaft and slightly relax your lips. Moan hard and low in anticipation of the best climax you've ever created." There you go. Your boyfriend won't know what hit him.*

As one of those women who view giving head as an art form, I take issue with a few of those suggestions. Your source essentially recommends that a woman make her mouth feel like a pussy. But much of the pleasure a man receives from oral sex lies in the fact that it provides different sensations than intercourse. It's good to swirl your tongue at the apex of the upstroke, but never neglect the shaft. A blow job isn't a blow job if you sink only the tip. Rather than two fingers, use your entire hand and squeeze gently, like a pulse, on the upstroke. See how he reacts if you turn your head to the right on every downstroke. Don't overlook the rest of his body. Caress his belly and the inside of his thighs. Gently run your nails through his pubic hair. Stroke a finger along his perineum. Continue sucking as he comes and you'll prolong his climax. Take your time about disengaging, and give his cock a good-bye kiss. The look on his face will be worth it.—A.M., Tacoma, Washington

Thanks for writing. We love your work.

Don't overlook the importance of eye contact. My wife gives incredible head, and what drives me wild is that she stares into my eyes while doing it. Why is that such a turn-on?—R.T., Richmond, Virginia

As John Updike once noted, oral sex is even more intimate than intercourse because you're fucking your partner's face. Staring into her eyes drives that home. It also tells you that your wife is not ashamed or reluctant to be doing what she's doing—she loves the fact that you're watching. As porn actor Marc Stevens said of co-star Tina Russell: "God, what a cocksucker she was! She'd fuck my eyes with her eyes while she was sucking me."

I love giving my boyfriend blow jobs, and he enjoys getting them. The trouble is, I want him to crave them. Do you have any suggestions for fine-tuning my technique? I've always imagined being so good that he would greet me at the door one day after work, weak with desire, begging me to suck him off.—C.T., Rapid City, South Dakota

The next time you go down on your boyfriend, prop his head on a pillow to make sure he can see what you're doing. Tell him how hot he is, how much you love sucking him and how hard and beautiful he is. Let him know that you're in no hurry. With his erection in your mouth, begin to hum softly. (The warmth of your breath and the vibrations on his cock will drive him crazy with desire.) At that point, we'd be happy as clams, but we're easy. Judy Kuriansky, author of Generation Sex, *offers a description of the classic BJ that had us fidgeting in our seats: "Start licking at the tip, gently. Circle your tongue around the head and then slide the head into your mouth. Create suction and roll your tongue around the head, lingering on the frenulum (the underside of the tip where the ridge meets the shaft). There's no need to bob your head up and down. Slip your mouth over the tip and run your moistened lips up and down the sides of the shaft of the penis (while you caress the head with your hand) and return to slipping the head inside your mouth. Lower your mouth farther down on his erection each time. Or close your lips around the head, licking the frenulum, and grasp the shaft with one or both hands to give him the sensation of being inside you."*

I shared your oral sex tips with my girlfriend but wanted to add one: If a woman starts a blow job with her mouth, she should finish with her mouth. It's not a BJ if she uses her hand.—D.L., Green Bay, Wisconsin

Our rule has always been, "If a woman starts a blow job with her mouth, God bless her."

Can I come in your mouth?

Exactly what percentage of women perform oral sex to climax? I was married two years before I even put my hand on my husband's penis. It was seven years before he succeeded in having me put my mouth on it. This all changed when some women I know at church were talking sex one Sunday after service. When one said she enjoyed having her husband come in her mouth, the rest of us were aghast! We were told that the taste was not objectionable, and if the come was swallowed immediately you hardly knew it was in your mouth. Reluctantly, I let my husband come in my mouth, making him think I was just too slow to get out of the way. The next time we had oral sex he performed on me until I was aroused beyond comprehension. When I went down on him, I had about half of his penis in my mouth and was pumping the shaft with my hand. I knew he was coming so I pumped faster and let him shoot into my mouth. I continued to suck and he started squirming and said I was killing him, but I was determined to finish the job. It was terrific! At last, after ten years, I had given my husband a real blow job. Now we have more fulfilling sex than ever. I did not know how wonderful it could be until my eyes were opened that Sunday morning after church.—T.L., Denver, Colorado

Now, there's a confession you don't hear every day. Have you come in his mouth yet? According to surveys we've seen, nine in ten people engage in oral sex. It's fun. There has been much less research into the number of women who allow men to come in their mouths, but we're working on it. In a poll of college students conducted by Playboy, *about 60 percent of the female respondents said they let their partner do this. Of those, a third said they swallow; a third said "it depends." We like to think it depends on if you ask nicely.*

The games men play

I am happy to give my husband what he says are the best blow jobs of his life. Although I prefer his undivided attention, I don't have a problem with his watching porn while I pleasure him. But the other day he wanted one while he was playing a video game. I told him to finish the game first. When I came back 10 minutes later, he told me he had started another game and no longer wanted a BJ. What gives?—N.T., Dover, Delaware

Your husband has confused his joystick with his joy stick, which is a risky thing to do.

You missed the call with that response. As selfish as it may be, guys love spur-of-the-moment BJs. His wife's offer to come back after he finished the game made it an appointment, and the fantasy evaporated.—S.P., Indianapolis, Indiana

It must be a treat to receive so many blow jobs that you start to categorize them.

He stroked himself when I paused

What does it mean when a guy jacks off after I pause while giving him head?—C.B., Toronto, Ontario

It means he misses your mouth. If he masturbated to orgasm, you may have pulled away just as he was about to come. In that case, his reaction was instinctive. Otherwise, he stroked himself to stay hard. The next time you need to take a break, keep your hands moving. Keep your lips moving as well, by telling him how much you love sucking him.

Lick it good

My new girlfriend wants me to go down on her, but I've never done it before. (None of my previous girlfriends liked getting head.) I'm a little nervous, because I want her to enjoy the experience. Are there any special techniques?—R.N., Honolulu, Hawaii

The simplest way to find out how a woman likes to be licked is to ask her. By doing so you won't reveal anything except your skill as a lover. As porn star Nina Hartley says, "Good pussy eating is a team effort." Here are some general tips: (1) To help her relax, caress the insides of her thighs, talk to her softly, massage the muscles around her vulva. Demonstrating on her video Nina Hartley's Guide to Better Cunnilingus, *Nina gently squeezes and kneads the muscles around her partner's vulva like a baker. These muscles are stronger and more pliant than most people realize—and who thinks to massage them? (2) Forget the movies— porn actors move aside for the camera. Lose your face between her thighs. Lou Paget, author of* How to Give Her Absolute Pleasure, *says, "The men who are best at this resemble glazed doughnuts." (3) On the approach, be sure to coat your tongue and lips with saliva. Don't flick your tongue (another porn move) unless she's already turned on—it's likely to cause dryness and discomfort. (4) If she's on her back, put a pillow under her ass for a better angle or have her put her legs over your shoulders. (5) Gently separate her outer lips with your fingers, for better access. (6) Nina reminds guys that the clitoris is not a doorbell. It's extremely sensitive, so when you caress, kiss, lick, suck and tug on your lover's labia and other parts of her vulva, the clitoris feels the tremors and responds. (Nina claims she once produced an orgasm by tugging on her lover's pubic hairs.) Work slowly, to build tension. Focus on stimulation, not penetration—all of the most sensitive nerves are at the tip of your tongue. Alfred Kinsey found that only 20 percent of women insert anything while masturbating, and most of those just barely. (7) Take a moment to tell her how good she tastes. (8) Try long, broad licks from the bottom of her vulva (often overlooked) to the top. (9) If you find yourself at a loss for your next move, get back to basics: Write the alphabet with your*

tongue, then do it backward. (10) Try kissing her genitals the way you kiss her
lips. Suck her clit the way you suck her tongue. (11) If she says, "That's great" or
"There!" don't speed up. But do keep going.

You left out a crucial piece of information: A man should always shave first.
A day's growth never feels good against labial tissue. Rub your tongue or the
head of your penis along a woman's unshaved leg and you'll see what I
mean.—S.S., Manchester, Connecticut
   We'll take your word for it.

Are there any exercises you can do so your tongue doesn't get sore?—L.S.,
Brooklyn, New York
   We like the Lifesaver technique described by Lou Paget in How to Give Her
Absolute Pleasure. *Hold a Lifesaver in your mouth vertically between your lips*
and teeth. Using tiny motions, dissolve the candy with the tip of your tongue from
the hole out. It takes time, patience and a nimble tongue, which builds stamina.
If you need to take a breather during cunnilingus, hold your tongue against your
upper lip and move your head instead. And there's no rule that says you can't put
the rest of your face to work. If your tongue gets tired, use your nose or chin to put
pressure on her clitoris.

My husband and I have discovered the best position for oral sex. The
woman lies on her back with knees bent. The man lies on his side at a right
angle to her, facing her pussy. His lips and tongue align with her labia,
allowing complete coverage and range of motion. It's not a problem if he
hasn't shaved, since his beard never comes in contact with her delicate tis-
sues. The man doesn't have to worry about a stiff neck or sore knees, and the
woman won't be distracted by her concern that her partner is uncomfortable.—L.M., Hollywood, California
   As luck would have it, that's the same position we get in to watch TV.

Blow jobs and TMJ
After two years of marriage, my wife now refuses to give me blow jobs. She
says it aggravates her TMJ. I knew she had occasional pain and discomfort,
but this is the first time she has mentioned it in relation to sex. Is this for
real?—A.L., Chicago, Illinois

When a woman performs fellatio, she may open her jaw wider than usual and for an extended period of time. That can aggravate temporomandibular joint syndrome, which is damage to the sliding joints that join the lower jaw to the skull. (TMJ syndrome affects four times as many women as men, and most often women in their 30s and 40s.) The detrimental effect of temporomandibular disorders on a couple's sex life has not been given much space in medical literature, but jaw-locking and pain are common concerns. Dentist John Taddey, author of TMJ: The Self-Help Program, *points out that in extreme cases, a hug, a kiss, or even being jostled in bed may cause pain. A woman's feelings about fellatio also can play a role. One specialist recalls a patient who disliked giving blow jobs so much she clenched her teeth before sex. That aggravated her TMJ at least as much as fellatio. But the consultation gave her an out on "doctor's orders." (We assume her partner soon began suffering from stress-related disorders of his own.) If your wife doesn't have such misgivings, physical therapy and jaw exercises can ease her pain in and out of the bedroom. In the meantime, let her know that it's not necessary for her to imitate a suction pump when she gives you a blow job—instead, she can use her tongue, hands and lips to tease you into oblivion. For women who find that fellatio occasionally leaves their jaws sore, take a minute to stretch before-hand. If your partner asks what the hell you're doing, tell him, "You're so big, I'm afraid I might pull something."*

Can vegetarians swallow?

My wife is a vegetarian. She's worried that she might be ingesting meat by-products when she swallows my semen. Can you put her mind at ease?—J.F., Toms River, New Jersey

For your sake, we'd better. Vegetarians don't eat meat because of concerns for the welfare of animals, or because they believe it's healthier. Assure your wife that no living thing suffered in the production of your semen—except you, waiting for your next orgasm. Semen contains protein but no meat, eggs or fish, and it's low-fat. Even vegans, who are stricter about the rules, agree that swallowing is not an issue. We found this at eatveg.com: "Oral sex is vegan even though it may involve putting flesh in your mouth, as it shouldn't involve any cruelty or exploitation, and said flesh is eventually returned to its owner." By the way, many women report that vegetarians' semen tastes better.

Her dirty mouth

I thought I was a clean freak until I met my boyfriend. If I ask him to go down on me, he acts like it's going to make him sick because it's "dirty down there." (Of course, his penis is never dirty when he wants a blow job.) He'll engage in foreplay only when we're in the shower and I've been scrubbed for 15 minutes. This is affecting my ability to climax because he makes me feel dirty with all his complaining. What should I do?—K.J., Chattanooga, Tennessee

Dirty? Is he nuts? We think your pussy is adorable, and you haven't even blown us. In fact, a woman's vagina is more sanitary than her mouth. We don't see much of a future with this guy. Make a clean break—and don't forget to kiss him goodbye.

He gets blown, I get nothing

Whenever I initiate sex with my husband, it turns into a blow job. I don't mind, but when I'm done, he says he's tired and rolls over. If I ask for something in return, he says, "I promise, tomorrow night," but tomorrow never comes. I've resorted to pleasing myself right in front of him. Any suggestions?—G.T., Pittsburgh, Pennsylvania

Quit extending credit. It's like a fire sale—when the door opens, you have to grab what you want. Once you have your husband erect, take charge of his cock and use it for your own pleasure. He'll get his along the way. Tell him you'll blow him anytime he wants, but only if you're sitting on his face. Wake him up with a wet pussy in his mouth. Sit him on the bed, blow him until he's moaning, then shove him on his back and climb aboard. One lick for him, two for you. That's the formula. Tape it to the refrigerator so he won't forget.

How can I deep throat?

I'd love to deep-throat my husband, but I always gag. Any suggestions?—R.C., Cleveland, Ohio

Besides keep trying? We asked a few of the women who have deep-throated us for their advice. They all said it helps to date a guy with a small penis. (Funny.) Keep one hand on the base of your husband's erection at all times to maintain control over the depth of penetration. You also should tell him not to thrust—if he does, party's over. Some women take a slow, deep breath and swallow a little at a time; others find it easier to breathe normally. One girlfriend practiced on a dildo before surprising us. Another said the worst time she had was when she felt queasy from drinking. The more turned on you are, the easier it may be. Coming down on the guy from above might help. Have him lie or sit. If you're kneeling, his erection is going to hit the upper part of your palate, which is more likely to trigger a gag. Violet Blue offers another method in her Ultimate Guide to Fellatio: *"The best position is lying on your back, with your head tilted back and slightly off the edge of a bed or couch. Time your up and down strokes with each breath. Inhale as you draw him in, exhale as you draw him out."*

Yoga love

My girlfriend first sat on my face, then arched her back and gave me head. Does this position have a name?—K.R., Telluride, Colorado

It's a yoga move called the chakra-asucka.

Do women like blow jobs?

Do women enjoy giving oral sex?—M.S., Seattle, Washington

Most women enjoy the reaction they get.

Dipstick mark

I'd like to treat my husband to a blow job that leaves a lipstick mark on his cock. I have found, in practice, that most rouges don't adhere. Any suggestions?—D.B., Phoenix, Arizona

A heavy layer of Red Coromandel Chanel once left a deep impression on us. How about a game of lipstick dipstick, in which you try repeatedly to extend your best mark? Everyone wins when you leave a ring that touches his belly and balls.

Blow party

My friends and I conducted an experiment with our girlfriends and wives. Whenever we requested oral sex, we used the term "blow party" instead of "blow job." What woman wouldn't rather go to a party than a job? What do you think?—G.T., Huntington Beach, California

The revolution starts now. Just don't talk about your blow parties near any cops.

Am I blowing him too much?

I have been sleeping with a friend for the past five years. Sex always starts and ends with my giving him head. Can a woman blow a guy too much? If I cut back, will it change the way he thinks about me? I think I'm spending too much time giving one man so many blow jobs. I guess I wish he appreciated them more.—C.S., Columbus, Ohio

Appreciated them or appreciated you? After five years this isn't a friendship— it's a cheap date. You won't hear complaints from your buddy, because even routine sex is better than nothing. And while we could give you a long list of techniques to shake things up, those would eventually become routine as well. If you want more intimacy, you need to find a more intimate relationship.

Hiccup cure

My wife couldn't get rid of her hiccups, so she said she wanted to deep-throat me to relax her throat. Have you heard of this?—B.T., Indianapolis, Indiana

Until we received your letter, hiccups had no known purpose.

I've deep throated my husband so many times to cure hiccups that now he jumps when I cough. This morning, when I started hiccuping while he was at work, I left him a voice mail: "I, hic, need you, and you're, hic, not here!"—S.B., Salem, Indiana

Making an impression

This girl and I were making out on a couch in a friend's apartment. After we had sucked on each other for a while, I made my move downstairs. A moan and a groan later she asked if I wanted her to kiss my penis. She sucked until I came in her mouth, then she lifted my shirt and spit the semen on my stomach. Next she pulled off one of my socks and used it to wipe up. She turned the sock inside out and threw it on the floor. Thank God I remembered not to put it on the next morning. Have you ever heard of this technique, or was she just fooling with me?—J.F., Mishawaka, Indiana

That's a technique? It sounds more like an audition.

A bite to remember

Soon after my divorce I began dating a stunning redhead. One evening, as we did 69 on her new sofa, I felt a sting in my penis. Her upper denture had caught on the skin of my erection. She got the denture out of her mouth, but we couldn't remove it from my now limp penis. We had to go to the ER, where a doctor used a wire cutter to get it off. I ended up with an inch-long scar and a memorable story for my urologist. The accident turned out to be a blessing in disguise, because from that point on her blow jobs were all toothless, which is a hell of a sensation. With all the people who wear dentures, it's hard to believe we're the only couple who have had this misadventure. Have you heard of this happening to anyone else?—A.J., Ardmore, Pennsylvania

You're the first. Congratulations. We're sorry you had to go through that trauma to discover the joys of the gum job. Joan Elizabeth Lloyd, author of Nice Couples Do, *has collected a number of anecdotes online about toothless sex, including one from a guy who wrote, "It wasn't until my wife had dentures that she was able to perform oral sex beyond a kiss on my penis. She has a small mouth, and oral sex had been too demanding. Now she says it's more sensual for her because she can feel on her gums what she never could with teeth." But one woman wins the prize for dedication. "Because my husband is so good to me, I decided that I would make all his oral sex special," she wrote. "I've had only one cavity since I was a child, but I eventually found a younger dentist who was willing to pull all my teeth without keeping records. Some people might find this perverse, but I believe that when two people truly love each other, sacrifices like teeth are worth any inconvenience." Personally, we prefer our blow jobs with a little danger.*

About a year ago the Advisor received a letter from a woman who planned to get braces. She feared that her orthodontia might hurt her husband when she gave him oral sex. I hope it's not too late to share a story from my early days as a doctor. In the summer of 1949 I was a resident in urology at a large Midwestern hospital. Late one evening, two couples came into the emergency room, one leading the other. The second couple caught my attention. The husband was walking backward, followed by his wife, who was bent over at the waist. The first couple had covered the woman's head and the man's midsection with a towel. We led them to an exam room. You guessed it. The uppermost tip of the husband's foreskin had become wedged in his wife's new braces. She couldn't speak. The man was afraid he'd have to be circumcised. I did a penile block and injected the foreskin with anesthesia. A few careful cuts and he was free. A dental resident removed the skin from the woman's braces while I sutured the fellow's penis. An hour later, he was back in the ER. The couple had gone home and had intercourse, and his stitches broke.—G.G., Scottsdale, Arizona

A few stitches wouldn't have stopped us, either.

ORGASM
What goes around, comes around.

Let's have another

When my girlfriend and I were having sex during a cruise vacation, I had an orgasm and remained inside her mostly erect. Nothing new. But after catching my breath, I again became fully erect and achieved orgasm with ejaculation within a few minutes. This scenario was repeated twice (my girlfriend actually said, "Again?"). Short of taking a cruise every weekend, is there a way to attain this level of sensuality on a regular basis?—C.M., Fort Lauderdale, Florida

You may be a natural. A rare breed of man apparently can have multiple orgasms—each including ejaculation—without training. In 1995 a 35-year-old man contacted Beverly Whipple, a sex researcher at Rutgers University, claiming he could come repeatedly without any recovery period, and he agreed to demonstrate. Whipple and her colleagues monitored the man's heart rate, pupil dilation and ejaculate volume as he masturbated to a video of his favorite porn scenes. He achieved his first orgasm (and ejaculated) in 20 minutes. Two minutes later he came again. According to Whipple, the man reached orgasm and ejaculated four more times in the next 14 minutes without losing his erection. The Advisor occasionally hears from well-rested men who claim two or even three ejaculations without losing their erections. The guy at Rutgers, however, told researchers he comes five to ten times a day and once reached orgasm and ejaculated five times in six minutes. That's a horse you can bet on. One hypothesis is that he and other men produce little or no prolactin, a hormone that appears to control a man's recovery period after climax. In 2003 scientists at the University of Essen in Germany tested this by giving 10 men either synthetic prolactin or cabergoline, a drug that blocks the production of the hormone. They asked each man to masturbate while watching a porn movie. The men who received cabergoline were hornier, had stronger erections and got hard again more quickly after climaxing. If the pill pans out, it could end the world orgasm shortage.

While research continues, there is a natural way to improve your stamina and shorten your refractory period. Whipple says the key is your pubococcygeus

(PC) muscle, which wraps around your anus and the base of your penis. A standard exercise is to clench as if stopping the flow of urine, hold for three seconds and release. You can do sets at stoplights, during boring meetings or while watching TV; no one will be the wiser unless you grunt. The goal, Whipple says, is to build up to about 150 reps a day. She suggests men track their progress by placing a tissue on their erection and lifting their penis up and down. Eventually you should be able to lift a hand towel, then a bath towel. Women can test their strength by inserting two fingers into their vagina, spreading them into a V and trying to close them by clenching. In studies, people with stronger PC muscles report more control, sensitivity and desire, as well as stronger orgasms. Men also become better at delaying orgasm or even stopping ejaculation, allowing them to have "dry" climaxes and keep going.

My husband, who is 56, can climax three or four times with no downtime. He didn't suspect he was different until he visited prostitutes as a young man in the Navy. He would covertly ejaculate in his hand, then wipe it on the sheets. That way he could get off five or six times for the price of one. My husband says that after cabergoline arrives, "I won't have anything special going for me except you." That earned him an afternooner or two or three, depending on how you count.—H.H., Los Angeles, California

Your husband has another rare talent—he undressed you with a single line.

Unusual reactions

Whenever I'm making love and about to climax, I begin to laugh. The more intense the orgasm, the louder I laugh. My reaction makes it difficult to keep partners. No matter how hard I try to explain, they think I'm laughing at them. I've tried everything I know to keep quiet, including pinching myself and stuffing socks in my mouth. I am now seeing a woman I'm crazy about, but I'm hesitant to make love to her. What should I do?—N.N., Sacramento, California

We can understand that your lovers would question your situation, but many people report spontaneous laughter, yawning, sneezing, crying or sighing during orgasm—reactions consistent with the release of tension. Because your laughter is persistent, you may suffer from gelous seizures, which are triggered by the wave of pleasurable impulses that spreads through your nervous system during climax. (A related condition is gelasmus, *or hysterical laughter.) Neurologists typically diagnose the condition after a brain scan and control it with prescription drugs. If you don't expect your current relationship to lead into the bedroom immediately, hold off on sex until you can see a doctor and have the last laugh.*

After I climax, I always sneeze four to six times. Why?—B.D., Miami, Florida

Arousal causes the mucous membranes in the nose to expand, which has been known to induce sneezing in people whose nasal passages are chronically swollen. A decade ago, the Journal of the American Medical Association *reported the case of a 60-year-old man who said he sneezed four to five times about a minute after orgasm. He found relief with a prescription nasal spray. There may be other factors involved. Research has shown that the vagus nerve, which controls involuntary actions such as breathing and swallowing, may also carry signals for sneezing, yawning and orgasm. As one scientist has noted, a sneeze could be described as a respiratory orgasm.*

My girlfriend says that she feels numb, usually in her hands, after she has an orgasm. Is this normal?—C.T., State College, Pennsylvania

We initially wondered if this might be caused by the blood rushing to your girlfriend's genitals. But after reading your letter and our response, a physician wrote: "This numbing is caused not by diversion of blood but by hyperventilation, which is well known to be associated with sexual activity and orgasms. In fact, hyperventilation can cause carpopedal spasm (numbness and tingling in the fingers and toes) and circumoral paresthesia (numbness and tingling around the lips). These are caused by overbreathing, blowing off too much CO_2 and altering your acid-base balance. Early in one of my own relationships, my girlfriend noted that her fingers and toes felt numb after sex. I asked if her lips also felt numb. She said they did but that she had attributed it to the vigorous blow jobs she gives me. Another time she fainted after orgasm. Being a multi-orgasmic woman may carry unexpected medical risks and dating one requires vigilance and preparation."

Four-points orgasm

Have you heard of the four-points orgasm? It requires a partner with ample breasts. Just before she climaxes, the woman squeezes her tits together. That's a signal for the man to place his thumb on her clitoris and to suck both of her nipples. He then power strokes and hangs on for dear life. What do you think?—S.M., Philadelphia, Pennsylvania

Keeps you busy, doesn't she?

The orgasmatron

Supposedly a doctor somewhere is testing a device that can be implanted in your back to give you orgasms. Can that possibly be true? Where do I sign up?—L.T., Las Vegas, Nevada

You're thinking of Stuart Meloy, an anesthesiologist in Winston-Salem, North Carolina who may someday be remembered as Dr. Orgasmatron. A few years ago a patient he was treating for chronic pain began moaning with pleasure when he directed electrical impulses to her spine. She told him, "You need to teach my husband how to do that." Meloy has since patented his orgasm stimulator and has recruited 10 women who had trouble climaxing to test it. (He says there's no reason it wouldn't have the same effect on men.) The FDA has approved the device to treat pain, so Meloy is confident enough to offer it off-label for sexual healing. For $3,000 he will insert an electrode that can remain near your spine for up to 10 days before it must be removed to prevent infection. A nine-volt battery powers it. Looking for something more durable? Meloy will implant a permanent electrode under your skin and hand you a remote control for $17,000, which covers the cost of surgery and equipment. He notes that the device doesn't create instant orgasms but instead "launches the events that lead to orgasm. It's not subtle." If you have cash to burn, there's more information at nasfonline.com.

Showing off for grandma

When I was in high school my family and I visited my grandmother one Sunday afternoon. While everyone talked in the living room, I fell asleep on the floor. When I awoke I discovered I'd had a wet dream. Are the mental images during a wet dream so realistic that they alone cause an orgasm, or does there have to be physical stimulation as well? I hate to think my poor grandmother was watching me hump the floor. Please ease my mind.—R.G., Indianapolis, Indiana

Your grandmother? What about the rest of your kin? Rest easy. If you had been acting out your dream, someone would have woken you, especially if the cat was in danger. We reach climax more quickly during sleep than when we're awake. What likely happened is that the muscle convulsions during climax woke you. To the outsider it looked, at most, like you were sleeping deeply and then jerked yourself awake. You don't need physical stimulation or even an erection to have a wet dream. You also can reach orgasm without ejaculating—you just might not realize it without the sticky mess as evidence. That same lack of physical evidence is one reason wet dreams among women are underreported. Alfred Kinsey found that while men had sleep orgasms most often in their teens, women had them most often in their 40s.

Guys faking

Recently *Playboy* quoted a college sex advice columnist who said, "All a guy has to do is grunt, give a body shudder or throw on a porn-star face and he can fool his partner." Her point was that men don't have to work as hard as women to fake an orgasm. That's true for the most part, but there is a sure way to tell if a guy is coming. As one of my girlfriends and I were having sex, she asked, "Ever heard of Lucky Pierre?" Before I could respond, she slid a lubed finger up my ass. As I ejaculated she nibbled my ear in time with the contractions in my sphincter. There was no way that I could have faked that. Anybody care to validate this?—A.A., Santa Ana, California

We'd love to. What's her number?

Sexual records

If *Guinness* doesn't archive sexual records, is it possible that *Playboy* does? In certain positions, my boyfriend and I have direct penis-to-G-spot connection. By lifting my hips slightly, he can give me orgasm after orgasm. I once counted 25 in three hours. This can be physically and emotionally draining, but if there is a record to be broken, we would be willing to give it a try.— S.D., Miami, Florida

Your experience is unusual but far from a record. Sex researchers have documented a woman having 134 orgasms in an hour, and that was in a laboratory. Guinness currently tracks records such as the most valuable postmortem penis (Napoleon's, $3,800), the heaviest pair of breasts (12 pounds, four ounces) and the most breasts (10) but ignores individual sexual achievements. That may be because it's tough for erotic overachievers to meet the burden of proof. For example, the book requires that each attempt be verified by two independent witnesses, preferably a respected local doctor, lawyer, politician or cop. Rather than pursuing 2.25 orgasms a minute, see how long your lover can make you not come (e.g., three hours of teasing and foreplay). Given how easily you climax, that would be a truer test of endurance.

Five minutes to liftoff

In her book *Five Minutes to Orgasm*, D. Claire Hutchins writes that "most women can achieve orgasm in three to five minutes while masturbating. And this is starting cold, before fantasy or stimulation begins." It takes me at least 15 minutes to come, and then only with intense concentration. Are her numbers real?—W.S., Appleton, Wisconsin

Hutchins took her figures from a survey conducted by Alfred Kinsey in the 1950s of about 1,900 women who said they had masturbated at least once. Seventy percent of the women reported that they climaxed within five minutes. However, it's not clear that each "started cold," and later research in a sex lab found the average closer to 20 minutes. (The fastest orgasm took 15 seconds, but many women needed an hour or more.) We asked Betty Dodson, author of Sex for One, *what she thought of the race to climax. "What's the goddamn hurry?" she said. "The longer we spend getting there, the more pleasurable the orgasms will be. When I'm working with a woman who is learning to come, I may have her masturbate for two hours." In other words, coming fast isn't a skill, but coming slow can be.*

A reader asked about my book. In your response you quoted Betty Dodson, who said, "The longer we spend getting there, the more pleasurable the orgasms will be." I disagree. Women have been brainwashed to feel thrilled about having any orgasm at all. The ideal is to delay orgasm only as long as lovemaking continues to be fun. Prolonged thrusting can be tiresome for the man and painful for the woman. Relying on vibrators and oral sex may inhibit a couple's enjoyment—both require a lot of work for the guy, and his erection isn't involved. The fact is that couples who have been together for years are not going to have a splendidly romantic encounter every time—yet orgasm should be the reward of every lovemaking experience. My book suggests that women take responsibility for their own climaxes. They can do that by assuming the superior position (missionary is probably the worst position for bringing a woman to climax), masturbating during intercourse and fantasizing. Five minutes or 50—as long as both partners are enjoying the sex, it's fast enough.—D. Claire Hutchins, Grand Prairie, Texas

Thanks for your response. Guys appreciate any help we can get.

Hutchins writes that "missionary is probably the worst position for bringing a woman to orgasm." I can come only in missionary. Is there something wrong with me?—G.F., Williamstown, New Jersey

Nothing at all. There's one thing that can bring you to orgasm in any position: your partner's finger (or your own). It may seem like cheating to finger your clit during intercourse, but the penis is a team player.

The doctor is in

My grandmother confided to me that some women used to have to go to a doctor to have orgasms. Could that be true?—R.D., Santa Barbara, California

From the fifth century B.C. until the 1920s, many women sought out treatment for "hysteria," a vaguely defined illness thought to arise from a lack of sexual intercourse. Before the invention of the vibrator, treatment consisted of a physician fingering or massaging his patient until she climaxed. In 1653, a doctor described how, with the help of a midwife, he massaged a patient's genitalia "with one finger inside, using oil of lilies, musk root, crocus or something similar." The technique proved most effective on widows and nuns. In her book The Technology of Orgasm, *Rachel Maines notes that few doctors relished treating hysteria—they found it time-consuming and tedious. Some preferred to prescribe horseback riding, long train rides or high-pressure water massages. More often than not, the condition proved to be chronic.*

Female ejaculation

When I climax, I sometimes squirt a clear liquid. My husband and I separated recently, and during that time, some bimbo told him I was peeing on him. Now we're trying to work things out, but he refuses to bring me to orgasm. He won't listen to anything I say, but he devours your every word. Can you help?—F.A., Modesto, California

Sure. It's not pee. During arousal or orgasm, some women release a fluid has been found to be chemically distinct from urine. In many cases a woman who ejaculates does so after her G-spot is stimulated, leading researchers to suggest that the fluid originates from the same tissue that becomes the prostate gland in men. Female ejaculation is accepted as a matter of course in some cultures. The Batoro of Uganda, for example, teach unmarried women the custom of kachapati, *or "spraying the walls." It's also common in erotica—apparently men fancy the idea they can make a woman so excited that she gushes (or at least spurts). Your husband should consider himself lucky.*

Headaches during sex

My new girlfriend is the wildest lover I've ever had, but every time we have sex, I get a headache as I climax. Is this something to be concerned about?—N.M., Albuquerque, New Mexico

Most likely, no. Sex headaches are so common that pain specialists have divided them into three categories: (1) "Dull" headaches intensify as you become more aroused and peak during climax. The pain usually occurs at the back of the head and is likely caused by muscle tension. (2) "Explosive" headaches consist of a throbbing pain at climax, generally on both sides of the head. These are the most common benign sexual headaches, but no one is sure what causes them. They may be hereditary. One doctor treated four sisters who suffered from climax headaches but had never mentioned it to one another. (3) The rare "postural" headache occurs during climax at the back of the neck and head and could indicate a spinal fluid leak, which is bad news. In fact, there is an off chance that any type of sex headache could be the result of an aneurysm or tumor, which is why it is always wise to see a doctor. In most cases, treatment is as simple as gentler fucking or massage as foreplay, or drugs used to treat migraines. Harvard neurologist Donald Johns says sex headaches seem to occur most often among people in their 40s and during stressful encounters—say, during an affair or with a crazy new lover. They also occur more often in men, by a 3-to-1 ratio. Presex headaches, another challenge altogether, occur more often in women, by a 20-million-to-1 ratio.

Sex can also ease the pain. When I wake up with a headache, I ask my husband to make love to me. The pain is gone within minutes.—J.B., Springfield, Illinois

You just gave "I have a headache, dear" a wonderful new meaning. In a study conducted at Southern Illinois University, 24 of 53 women who had sex while suffering from a migraine found that it relieved the pain; only one said her headache got worse. Other research suggests that vaginal stimulation increases a woman's pain threshold. One scientist hypothesized that when the vagina is stimulated the body responds as it does during childbirth—by releasing painkillers.

Orgasm reflex

An article about Pavlov's dogs gave me an idea. If I masturbated to the same song every day, would my pussy be programmed to have an instant orgasm? I decided to experiment. I chose *Got Till It's Gone*, Janet Jackson's duet with the rapper Q-Tip. It's four minutes long (which seemed like enough time to consistently reach orgasm), and the beat picks up speed. Each day at 6:35 p.m., I put *The Velvet Rope* into my CD player, pressed track four and fell onto my bed with legs spread. I usually began moaning three minutes into the song, when Q-Tip raps "Why you wanna go and do that?" I always climaxed before the song ended. After three months, I stopped the routine, then waited to see how I would react when I heard the song at random. A week later, I was a passenger in a friend's car when a guy driving a Mustang convertible pulled up next to us at a red light. His radio was blaring, and my song suddenly flooded through the open window and headed straight for my pussy. My ass tightened, my breath quickened and my thighs burned with anticipation. I tossed my head back and felt my panties getting wet. I didn't actually climax (I was too shy to wiggle around much with my friend sitting there), but I was extremely turned on. A few days later, the song played over the loudspeakers at my health club. I pedaled furiously on my stationary bike and had an intense orgasm. My instructor praised me for my hard work. Advisor, what do you think of my little experiment?—S.R., Los Angeles, California

What a sweet story. You and your hand have your own song. Now it's time to rejoin the world of irregular pleasure. Masturbate at different times, in different positions, to Bach, Benny, Miles, Garth or silence. Come in a minute, five minutes, 30 minutes. Climax once, twice, seven times. Heck, you can even invite a friend over and use his hand.

How can I come more slowly?

When you read about a guy who has a problem with premature ejaculation, what does that mean exactly? How soon is too soon?—K.L., Miami, Florida

PE occurs when a man consistently ejaculates before or shortly after penetration following minimal foreplay. That's a common clinical definition, but it has never satisfied anyone. Guys want numbers. So in 2004 a team led by psychologist Stanley Althof of Case Western Reserve University gave stopwatches to the partners of 1,587 men, including 207 who had been diagnosed with PE. After tabulating the results, the researchers found that the men who suffered from rapid ejaculation had an average "intravaginal ejaculatory latency time" of 1.8 minutes, compared with an average of 7.3 minutes among the other men. Althof notes that PE is a lifelong problem in two-thirds of cases; the other third are "acquired," meaning the condition shows up later. Anxiety over ejaculating too quickly can contribute to the problem; in trials of a drug called dapoxetine, men given placebos had double the stamina. Traditionally PE has been treated with squeeze or start-stop techniques, antidepressants that stifle arousal (dapoxetine is similar to Prozac but doesn't stay in the body long enough to be effective for depression) or numbing creams or condoms. It is often frustrating for both partners, not only because of the bad sex but because the man's shame or frustration can bring an abrupt end to the intimacy. Althof says teaching men to avoid such a response is an important part of treatment. In rare cases PE can be a symptom of illnesses such as diabetes or multiple sclerosis, so there is added concern when it appears later in life after years or decades of control. As we mentioned, the two most common non-drug treatments have been the penile squeeze (the woman squeezes her partner's erection as he nears climax to help him focus) and the start-stop tech-nique championed by Dr. Helen Singer Kaplan in PE: How to Overcome Premature Ejaculation. *(The woman gives the man a hand job until he is near climax; when his arousal wanes a bit, she repeats the exercise.)*

I also suffer from premature ejaculation, so I went for a consultation at Boston Medical Group. The doctors told me that PE is often caused by an oversensitive head of the penis. To treat it they prescribe a combination of drugs that are injected into the penis. The drugs keep your dick hard regard-less of ejaculation, so you can continue lovemaking for about an hour. They say this gets you used to the sensation of having sex for longer periods and desensitizes the head so it will toughen up. (They compare it to your feet get-ting calloused when you walk barefoot.) BMG claims that after doing its pro-gram for a few months your mind and body will be trained to go without the medication and your PE will be cured. It sounds reasonable, and they are doctors, but I'm having trouble finding any independent verification of BMG's claims or success rate. I'd like to fix this problem, but the treatment costs $1,000, and I don't want to blow my wad if it's junk science.—T.H., Dallas, Texas

We can't tell you much about Boston Medical Group beyond that it doesn't have an office in Boston and its doctors aren't eager to discuss their kooky methods with journalists. The American Urological Association has just updated its guide-lines for the treatment of premature ejaculation, and nowhere does it mention sticking a needle into your dick.

Stand by your man

What does it mean when a woman can have the biggest orgasm of her life simply by standing next to a certain man? This has happened to me three times—the first was 10 years ago, and the most recent was last year. My girlfriend and I waited for the guy to see if it would happen again, and it did—twice. The man is Willie Nelson. Is this normal? I don't want to wreck his marriage or mine. But I would be a cheap date.—M.J., Newark, New Jersey

God works in mysterious ways.

Get back

My husband and I recently found that I have an orgasm when he scratches a certain spot on my lower back. Is this normal?—J.R., Prince George, Virginia

It's unusual but not unheard of. Beverly Whipple, who for years studied the nature of orgasms at her physiology lab at Rutgers University, documented women climaxing from clitoral, G-spot, cervical and breast stimulation—as well as those who could lie still and fantasize to climax. She has also heard anecdotal reports of women who came while having just about every part of their bodies massaged, including the neck and the big toe. This is less surprising in light of research by Whipple and others that shows some nerves take a direct path from the genitals to the brain while bypassing the spinal cord.

Stoned sex

I enjoy having sex (and my husband enjoys my enjoying sex) when I'm high on marijuana. My sensations are heightened, and I can focus intensely. Sex without pot varies from standard to great, but if I'm high, it's guaranteed to be fantastic. I don't get high often—maybe once a month—but I would like to cut back or stop. Is there a way to get that feeling of focus and heightened sensitivity without an illegal drug?—C.A., Toledo, Ohio

Having sex in a public place does it for us, but that's also illegal. Partaking once a month hardly seems excessive, and a lot of anecdotal evidence suggests that low to moderate intoxication can enhance sex. (Smoke too much and you'll be alone with your thoughts.) In Woman: An Intimate Geography, *science writer Natalie Angier notes that, unlike booze, weed "distracts the intellect without dampening the body's network of impulse relays." Many of the 150 experienced smokers Charles Tart surveyed for his 1971 book,* On Being Stoned, *felt they were better lovers when high, especially if their partner had also smoked, because the* marijuana brought on "feelings of tremendously enhanced contact, of being more sensitive, gentle, giving." In other words it slowed things down, which always makes for better sex. (Guys also typically report they have more control.) However, Tart noted that a quarter of respondents said weed didn't make them better in bed because it made them focus too much on their own pleasure. The real benefit of marijuana before sex may be that it helps some women achieve orgasm. Writing of her own experience, Angier says that marijuana "can be a sexual mentor and a sublime electrician, bringing the lights of Broadway to women who have spent years in frigid darkness. All the women in my immediate family learned how to climax by smoking grass. Yet I have never seen anorgasmia on the list for the medical use of marijuana." She later told High Times: "It definitely has something to do with the way in which marijuana releases the inhibitory mechanisms in the neocortex. That's why I say it's better for people who can't get there in the first place because they just don't know how mentally. Though women who can orgasm might continue to like marijuana for sex for the relaxing potential too."

Viagra for women

Why isn't there Viagra for women?—D.G., Cincinnati, Ohio

Because women are . . . complicated. Or at least more complicated than an erection. Early trials with women found that Viagra works as advertised—it increases blood flow to the genitals—but even when the lab instruments showed that female subjects were physically turned on, the women reported not feeling horny. This disconnect between physical and psychological arousal is a chasm that testosterone, Viagra and other pharmaceuticals apparently can't bridge, except perhaps as placebos. A 2003 survey of 853 women led by John Bancroft of the Kinsey Institute concluded that the best indicators of sexual dysfunction in women are emotional factors, such as the strength of their relationship. (Only 8 percent of the women reported an impaired physical response as the primary source of their problem.) A psychiatrist cited in Meika Loe's The Rise of Viagra illustrates this point with a New Yorker cartoon in which one woman says to another, "I was on hormone replacement for two years before I realized what I really needed was Steve replacement."

Orgasmic exercise

While working out at a gym I discovered not one, but two orgasmic pieces of equipment. Both are abdominal machines. One has you strap yourself into a seat and lift your legs into a crunch. With the other you lie on your back with your knees bent and lift your upper body into a crunch. I couldn't believe the intense feelings. The more reps I did, the closer I came to climaxing. My face turned red, my pussy was buzzing and I was so embarrassed that I left the room. How can I duplicate that intensity during sex with my boyfriend?—Y.L., Long Beach, California

You're the reason that gyms ask members to wipe down the machines. Why not enjoy yourself? Everyone turns red while they work out, and even if you scream, "Oh, God!" just follow it up with "Solid reps!" It shouldn't be difficult to take these exercises home. Improvise as your boyfriend lies on his stomach and fingers and licks you, or have intercourse as he stands next to the bed. You're both going to have killer abs.

PAYING FOR IT

For the love of money.

Strip club rules

At the age of 59, after the end of a 25-year marriage, I went to my first gentlemen's club. While I was drinking my cola (no alcohol allowed), a lovely
woman asked if I wanted a dance. She explained that a table dance is where
she dances nude while I sit and watch, and a lap dance is where she moves
around in my lap with shorts and halter top on. We agreed on a table dance.
She told me her name and there was lots of eye contact. It was incredibly
erotic. Later I enjoyed a lap dance with another girl. She gently put my hands
down to my sides, and I had to pretend I was paralyzed from the neck down
to keep them there. I found the experience frustrating, to put it mildly. My
real frustration is that I don't understand the rules. Sometimes the girl onstage
practically put her breasts in my face. Am I allowed to touch, with my face or
hands? I assumed not. In the lap dance, she put her cheek to mine and
caressed my face. Am I allowed to touch her? Again, I assumed not. Are the
rules legal or just conventions? After my table dance, I patted the girl's butt,
which didn't seem to upset anyone.—C.W., Manhattan Beach, California

Generally the rule is look but don't touch, though some clubs are more lax than
others. Local laws may dictate how much contact is allowed. In his lively, cross-
country guide to strip clubs, Live Nude Girls, *J.P. Danko explains the etiquette*
this way: "Any casual contact that would be appropriate if you just met a woman
in a regular bar is also appropriate in a strip club. Appropriate contact includes
a casual touching of a dancer's arm, shoulder or hand as well as a light hug or
peck on the cheek. Contact with any other portion of the dancer's anatomy is
absolutely inappropriate unless initiated by the dancer herself. This includes
resting a hand on a dancer's knee." Gropers ruin the atmosphere by putting
dancers on the defensive. Danko makes another point: If you want to enjoy your-
self at a gentlemen's club, leave your illusions at home. The dancers aren't there to
meet men, which means you'll be judged on two things: your politeness and your
spending habits. Tip appropriately, smile and enjoy yourself.

J. P. Danko says to leave your illusions at home. But don't exotic dancers sometimes connect with customers, or is it always just business?—R.G., Albuquerque, New Mexico

A dancer may find you attractive, but she's not looking for a date. We keep our head at strip clubs by pretending the women are very attractive used-car dealers.

The chances of hooking up with a dancer are slim, but I dated a few before meeting one who became my wife, so it can happen. The only advice I can offer is to be nice to the dancers you meet, spend some money on them and don't treat them like sex objects. Keep in mind that in most cases your jealousy will shut down the relationship. My wife quit dancing after we met— she said she suddenly felt strange when other guys touched her—but many women don't.—F.B., Chicago, Illinois

Not treating a stripper like a sex object is more than most guys can manage.

During eight years as a dancer I dated customers at every club I worked in. I also met my husband on the job. He said he wanted to eat me like a Christmas turkey dinner. He was such a dork that he stood out.—A.T., Washington, D.C.

The fact that your husband scored at a strip club with that line shatters everything in which we have ever believed.

Scent of a woman

This past weekend a group of friends and I went to Cancún. One evening we stumbled into a strip club and found that the dancers there smelled exactly like the strippers back in the States. In fact, the women at clubs in Nevada and California all seem to wear the same perfume. It's a scent I've never smelled on a woman I've dated. Is there a secret combination of oils and pheromones that strippers use to separate men from their money?—T.F., San Luis Obispo, California

It's no secret—it's baby lotion. Jennifer Axen and Leigh Phillips, authors of The Stripper's Guide to Looking Great Naked, *explain that dancers often mix their favorite scent with lotion to get better coverage and help the perfume last longer. It's known as the angel-devil mix because the smell is both familiar and sexy.*

Paying the rent

My boyfriend and I have lived together for almost a year. We rented a nice apartment in a trendy area in L.A. The rent is steep for us, but we enjoy entertaining and this place is perfect for it. My boyfriend works as a bartender, and I work part-time at a boutique in the afternoon and dance at a strip club (with his blessing) in the evening. All is well, except our expenses have grown faster than our wages. We started to pay our rent a week late, then two weeks late, and the last time we were a month late. Last weekend the landlord asked me to meet him at a coffee shop. He said he was considering taking us to court if we were late again. Then he made a proposal: Sleep with him twice a month and he wouldn't charge us rent. My boyfriend couldn't know about this, of course. I'll use the extra money to buy groceries, pay down our credit card debt and/or stash it in a secret account. I know this is crazy, but the more I think about it, the more I am tempted. It beats worrying about our finances all the time. Please advise.—C.B., Los Angeles, California

Have you ever noticed that each year, when you receive a new lease, the landlord has raised the rent? Twice a month now, and soon it will be weekly. Then perhaps it becomes twice a week, because it would be such a shame if your boyfriend found out. Regardless, it seems doubtful he wouldn't find out. He's going to be curious about where the rent money is coming from and why the landlord—who doesn't sound like the most discreet guy—makes those eyes at you. Rather than risk your relationship, we would accept the inevitable here and find an apartment that fits your budget.

Secret agent man

I'm preparing to hire a dominatrix for a role-playing session: captured secret agent. She seems legit and has an excellent website. I've never done anything like this before. How should I expect it to start and end? Should I enter with only the cash I need, and no ID or car keys?—M.I., Washington, D.C.

You seem to have control issues. The dominatrix isn't going to hold you upside down to shake out change, and she won't steal your car. It's a business transaction. You describe what you want, she describes what you get, you agree on a price and soon you're happily incapacitated. Try to hold out for a few minutes before you give up the mission, okay?

Be prepared

Recently I visited a strip club. An attractive dancer asked if I would like a lap dance. Before the dance was over, I experienced a powerful orgasm. The dancer climbed off my lap, smiled and kissed my cheek. I felt guilty. Is this a common experience? Is there any reason to feel like I did?—M.S., Bronx, New York

None. That's what's supposed to happen. Your story reminds us of a memoir published by the sex magazine Black Sheets. *While looking back on a lifetime as a lap-dance customer, Steve Omlid wrote: "The first thing I learned was that wearing a condom is a smart idea." There you have it.*

Tips for tricks

I am planning a trip to Nevada and would like to visit a brothel. How much should I expect to pay? Would I do better to hire an escort?—M.R., Cleveland, Ohio

We don't have much experience in this area, so we called a friend who hires an average of three escorts a month and also has made several trips to Nevada brothels. (He claims his hobby has done wonders for his love life, since he no longer worries about getting laid and has more confidence when meeting women.) Our buddy says the brothel experience is "like visiting a bar, except you know you're going to get fucked." Once you arrive, greet the madam, have a drink, watch the game and meet the women on your own time. Expect to pay at least $200 to $400 an hour for the sex. You'll get a better deal hiring an escort in any major city, but you risk arrest and perhaps disease. (Legal prostitutes are tested regularly.) Our friend pays about $300 an hour for women he rates as eights or nines. He finds them online; sites such as TheEroticReview.com allow you to search for "providers" by location, hair color, race, breast size, piercings and other criteria, then read or post reviews. One tip: Put your cash in an envelope, leave it on the dresser and never discuss it. One further note: Our friend is single.

What's the best way to prepare for a encounter with an escort?—L.J., San Antonio, Texas

Take a shower. While compiling her anthology Paying for It, *Greta Christina asked the prostitutes and dominatrices who contributed what they expect from customers. "Most sex workers don't give a damn about your weight, age, race, physical shape or ability," she writes, "but they do care if you smell bad."*

Hookers and the law

Since prostitution is illegal everywhere except for a few counties in Nevada, how can escort services advertise in newspapers, magazines and the Yellow Pages? It seems they would be easy pickings for the vice squad. Also, let's say a guy were to call for an appointment. How would he ask, without risking arrest, whether the woman is willing to have sex?—S.M., Chicago, Illinois

No need to ask; they know what you're after. The services walk a fine legal line, so caution is the watchword. The official deceit is that they hire out women for companionship, not sex. If mutual attraction leads to a hand job, blow job or intercourse, good for you. The police occasionally make arrests; in one case, the escort service owner's defense was that she led clients to believe they were getting "full service" but told the girls to provide only a strip show. (The jury didn't buy it.) If you're a clod and ask the booker or the escort outright if you can pay for sex, the conversation will end abruptly.

A friend told me that if you want to make sure a prostitute isn't a police officer, you just have to ask her if she's a cop. She has to answer truthfully because it's illegal for the police to entrap you. He said hookers can ask potential johns the same question but that it has to be phrased a certain way. You can't simply ask, "Are you a cop?" Any truth to this?—M.D., Aurora, Illinois

None. It's an old hooker's tale. Undercover cops can lie about their identity; otherwise, they'd rarely be able to make arrests, and in some situations they'd find themselves in danger. The belief stems from a misunderstanding about what constitutes entrapment. Legally, a police officer can't lead you to commit a crime that you would not have otherwise committed. But if you're arrested for soliciting a decoy, you'll have a tough time arguing that you were suckered. For entrapment to be considered, the policewoman would ostensibly have had to cajole and somehow convince you—the choirboy who had no intention of doing anything illegal—to give her cash for sex. Another fallacy is that money has to change hands, or that clothes have to be removed.

Let's say I pay a woman to let me suck her toes. Can I get into trouble with the law?— M.L., East Chicago, Illinois

As long as she removes only her socks, we'd call it a massage. It would help your defense if you didn't climax.

I'm dating a prostitute

A friend introduced me to a woman who works as an escort. I used her services several times and we developed a nonpaying sexual relationship and friendship. I am falling hard for her, and she has expressed the same feelings for me. My question is, in a relationship like this, will she expect fidelity?—E.S., Los Angeles, California

Why wouldn't she?

Do you still have to pay?

If you hire an escort whom you don't find attractive, and you send her away without doing anything but saying hello, do you still have to pay her?—J.H., West Liberty, West Virginia

We've heard of customers offering a third of the fee, gas money or nothing. But that was in the days before the Internet. Today many services post photos of their contractors online, which makes it difficult to claim you didn't know what to expect. If the escort is not as described or doesn't resemble her photo, stop her at the door before she has a chance to get comfortable.

On the prowl

I want to spoil my husband but am not sure how to go about it. Pink lacy panties, ass fucking, role playing, strip joints—they're all getting old. What I have in mind is getting a five-star hotel room on the Vegas Strip and hiring three call girls to be there for us. I don't want sloppy women; I want servants who will wait on my husband from the moment we arrive. I want them to pour him drinks, bathe him, massage him and so on. I'll slip out and come back later so we can all fuck. How much would a night like that cost—$10,000? That may be a lot to spend on sex, but material items can be overrated, and experiences are forever. Can you help me put this together?—S.R., Las Vegas, Nevada

Let's see: Five-star suite: $1,000. Champagne and room service for five: $500. Ten-pack of condoms: $13.99. Trio of escorts for a four-hour shift: $5,000. Coordinating three concubines and wife for "spontaneous" spa treatment and orgy: expensive, complicated and likely disappointing. Although prostitution is legal only in certain Nevada counties outside of Las Vegas, finding escorts online for a party is easy. But locating three strangers who are instantly comfortable with you, your husband and one another will be difficult. Your best bet would be to *hire one experienced escort and ask her to bring two friends. The problem there is that you're not choosing them, she is, and there's no guarantee you'll find them attractive. That's one reason the call girls we asked didn't like the idea of hiring three women, especially for your first time. Having four women in the room puts a lot of pressure on your husband to perform, and most men want their wife involved from the beginning. (Three women giving him a bath is hot, but three women giving him a bath while his wife supervises is hotter.) Based on their experiences with couples, our sources suggest you experiment with a threesome. If that works, then try adding a fourth.*

Co-ed strip clubs

Do you know of any strip clubs that have female and male dancers on the same stage? I enjoy going to clubs, but my husband thought it would be nice for me to have a male dancer to look at.—C.F., Chicago, Illinois

Your husband is a considerate voyeur, but tits and balls are not a combination many guys will pay to see (except perhaps on the same person, which is a discussion for another time). The closest thing you'll find are clubs such as the Masters in Myrtle Beach, the Sugar Shack in Lake Geneva, Wisconsin, Olympic Gardens in Las Vegas, PT's Showclub in Denver or Cleopatra's Viewpoint in Portland, each of which have female and male dancers performing in adjacent rooms or on separate floors.

Cut to the chase

I'd like to ask some girls I know to blow me for $50. How would you approach this? I don't want a relationship, just head. Is it illegal to ask a chick to blow you for money?—D.K., Chicago, Illinois

Generally, it's considered rude to offer a woman $50 to blow you. Technically, it's also illegal, but it seems unlikely that asking people you know would get you arrested for solicitation. If you spend $50 buying a woman wine at dinner and she then blows you, that's okay. A relationship will cost you $50 many times over.

PENIS

The long and short of it.

Are erections larger under a full moon?

My wife told me that my erection appears larger on nights with a full moon. I didn't believe her, so she measured me every night for two months. And, sure enough, on nights just before, during and after a full moon, I was half an inch longer. Have you heard of this before? Does it have anything to do with the moon's gravitational pull?—R.J., New York, New York

That's a new one. Does your pubic hair get thicker, too? We don't doubt your penis grew, but the only moon that has any influence on it is your wife's ass. You both expected it to be larger in the moonlight, which influenced how aroused you became when she prepared you and took measurements. That could easily account for that half inch. Under controlled conditions, there would be no difference. The moon does not move the blood or water in your body as it does the tides, and its gravitational pull is a function of its distance from the earth, not its phase. Nevertheless, your wife should continue to stroke and examine your erection regularly.

Does size matter?

One night about a month ago my new girlfriend and I got to talking about her previous partners. She told me her first lover had a huge penis but that the sex had been painful. My penis is 6.5 inches erect, and she has told me I'm a perfect fit. She also says I'm the first guy to get her off every time. The problem is, I can't stand the thought of her having been with someone so much bigger than I am. She has no clue this bothers me, but I once went soft inside her thinking about it. I keep wondering if she ever thinks her old boyfriend could "fit" her better now. She says I'm the best she's ever had, but she also says that size does matter. Help!—J.B., Atlanta, Georgia

If you want to stay hard during sex and you're not bisexual, don't think about penises. You have a Goldilocks cock—not too small, not too big, but just right. That's a good place to be. Your penis will "fit" with a wider variety of women, most of whom are content with large enough. Only the first few inches of the vagina have nerve endings, and a woman's pleasure during intercourse comes as much from your penis girth (which helps stimulate her clitoris indirectly as you thrust) as length. While an extra-large penis might feel great to some women, just as many will find it uncomfortable. Besides, the vagina isn't a gaping cavern. Its walls stretch and tightly grasp whatever is inserted—nature doesn't discriminate. With your large-enough erection, you'll also enjoy things that big guys miss, such as being deep-throated. We mention all this because your girlfriend is trying to tell you something: She likes your cock because it's attached to you.

My entire life I have been coping with the size of my penis. It's not the problem you'd think. I'm endowed to the tune of 10 inches. This has always been a terrible inconvenience, especially when I try to conceal my penis under clothes, and I dread climbing out of a pool. It also cramps my sex life. Several lovers have said sex is uncomfortable or painful, which makes me feel brutish. (I usually have to spend half an hour massaging their abdomens afterward.) Some women have refused to have sex with me after I've taken off my pants. My current girlfriend is five feet tall and weighs 88 pounds. It is almost impossible for us to make love. I would like men who consider themselves inadequate to know that there is nothing glorious about being huge.—C.A., Virginia Beach, Virginia

You're not the first guy with this problem. In the 17th century, a French doctor recommended that the well-endowed man wear a doughnut-shaped piece of cork at the base of his penis to keep him from bumping his partner's cervix. Given the present-day shortage of cork doughnuts, you may have to experiment instead with different positions. Your girlfriend may enjoy femoral lovemaking, in which she climbs on top of you and rubs her labia along your well-lubed erection. The woman-on-top position also allows her to control the depth of penetration. If necessary, place pillows under her knees to elevate her. Or use pillows to raise her hips as she lies on her back, which allows your penis to follow the curve of her vagina. In some positions, you can place the tip of your erection into the space below the cervix known as the posterior fornix. Some couples report that this allows several more inches of penetration.

A bump in the night

In an attempt to stimulate the G-spots of his lovers, a friend inserted a six-millimeter plastic bead under the skin of his penis. He used a sharp toothpick to make the opening, then let the wound heal (it took about a week). Have you ever heard of this? Does it work?—L.S., Loretto, Pennsylvania

A bead won't do anything except make your penis swell from infection. And after all that effort, your partner might think it's a wart. Penile inserts are most common in southeast Asia, where tribesmen have traditionally implanted bells, stones, jewels, ivory, gold, pearls, balls and shells in their shafts or gland. According to a book called The Penis Inserts of Southeast Asia *(really), some objects are the size of a small chicken egg. "As many as a dozen might be inserted," the authors note. "Kings might remove one of theirs to bestow it on a person deserving great honor." In India, where inserts may have originated, prostitutes sold gold, silver and bronze bells to teenagers to sew into the skin of their penises to impress lovers. Japanese mobsters insert beads out of machismo—each represents a year spent in prison. One mobster's ex-lover said she could feel his 13 "pearls" but that they didn't make the sex any better. In fact, she described the bumps as "hokey." If that sort of feedback turns you on, at least hire an experienced piercer to do the job right.*

Molding your penis

I'd like to mold a dildo for my girlfriend from my own penis. Can you suggest ways to do it? Is there a kit I can buy?—D.S., Orlando, Florida

We wanted to cast our penis, but the cement truck never arrived. Yes, there are kits. Typically, you fill what looks like a Big Gulp cup with alginate, slide in your cock and balls and remain aroused for about five minutes. Once the alginate has hardened, carefully remove your frightened member, pour wax or rubber into the hole, let it stiffen for about 24 hours and—presto—a backup unit, complete with veins. Here are a few places that sell molding kits (you may want to order extra alginate, as most guys don't get it right the first time): (1) The life sculptors at Artmolds.com offer a standard kit for $50. (2) CastingWilly.com has varieties such as a version with a handle for $85, or a $395 bronze casting. (3) CloneYourBone.com sells $30 wax molds that come with wicks so you can make candles. And who can't use penis soap-on-a-rope? Buy Match Your Snatch at the same time and save 10 bucks. (4) For $80, CreateAMate.com provides an alginate kit with three chances to make an impression.

Do black men have larger penises?

I am an African American man in an interracial marriage. Before I married, I dated women of various races, and almost all shared a belief that black men have extraordinary genitalia. At first I took this as flattery, but as I got older, I started to wonder if it could be considered racist. The problem is, some of my black friends seem to believe it too. Am I being too sensitive about this? Is there any truth to this belief?—G.B., Atlanta, Georgia

There haven't been any comprehensive studies to determine if erection size differs among races, mainly because it doesn't matter, or as scientists will tell you, it has "little physiological consequence." Alfred Kinsey asked 2,376 whites and 59 blacks to measure their penises and mail him the results; the average self-reported erection, regardless of race, measured about six inches. The belief that all black men have large penises dates back to at least the 15th century. It was later spread by anthropologists who drew broad conclusions based on their discovery of single well-endowed tribesmen. This particular myth reflects the stereotype that all black men are sexual beasts. Not that other races haven't tried to claim the penis prize for their own. One "sexologist" who measured the penises of a sample of men of various nationalities found that the longest white, English penis extended at least two inches beyond the longest African, German, French, Danish, American or Swedish variety. The researcher was, of course, a white Englishman.

Illegal boners

A friend claims that having an erection in public is illegal in some states. If so, how is it enforced? What's the penalty?—M.V., San Diego, California

Control problems? Steer clear of Indiana and Tennessee. In Indiana, appearing in a public place in a "discernibly turgid state" is a misdemeanor punishable by as long as a year in jail and up to a $5,000 fine. In Tennessee, your bulge could lead to a $500 fine, though the state exempts boners that appear in restrooms, locker rooms, doctor's offices, college art classes and nudist camps. Even in states that don't specifically ban erections, police officers may make arrests. Bob Morton of the Naturist Action Committee notes that many statutes distinguish between nude, which is sometimes legal, and lewd, which is always illegal. He says cops reason that if a guy is visibly aroused, something lewd must be going on, so they bust him. Morton also notes the difference between turgid and well endowed but flaccid, and that certainly some men have been falsely accused. These laws typically are designed to intimidate customers at strip clubs and to prosecute gay men who cruise for sex.

Answering a tough question

What do you say when a guy asks if his penis is too small? It seems like a no-win situation. If you say it's huge, he won't believe you. If you say it's small, he'll be hurt. Should you tell him, "Yes, but your tongue makes up for it"?

And guys, this isn't a good thing to bring up when you're basking in the after-glow. It ruins the moment, believe me.—A.L., St. John, New Brunswick

You're right. You can't win. Say, "It feels wonderful to me."

Enlarging your penis

I am 35 years old and my erect penis measures about five-and-a-half inches. I've always been insecure about my size, and lately have seen a lot of ads for penis-enlargement surgery. Do you recommend it?—G.S., New York, New York

This is one of the most common questions asked of the Advisor, and we're always amazed at what some men are willing to risk to add a measly inch to their normal-sized, functioning penises. Thousands of men have had globs of fat injected into their dicks or ligaments sliced to create the illusion of greater length, and certainly some have been satisfied with the results. But when things go wrong during cosmetic penis enlargements, they really go wrong, which makes us wonder about anyone who would recommend or perform the surgery. In 1994 a surgeon in Miami was convicted of manslaughter after a patient bled to death following cosmetic surgery that included a penis enlargement. More recently, Dr. Melvyn Rosenstein, who claims to be "the world's leading authority on penile surgery," had his license suspended after a judge ruled he was negligent and incompetent. More than 40 of his former patients claim that he botched their surgeries so badly that they suffer from symptoms including intense pain, scarring, deformities, loss of feeling, decreased sexual function, and a decrease in size. If Dr. Rosenstein was the world's leading authority, how confident does that make you about the other guys?

I dropped $400 on Enzyte, a product that claims it can increase the size of a man's penis by an average of 24 percent. It goes so far as to instruct the user to discontinue use if he gets too big for his lover's vagina. I used a full dose for about three months and saw no change. How can this company advertise such great results? Doesn't the government regulate claims like these?—T.R., Seattle, Washington

Unless a company says its over-the-counter product prevents or cures disease, the FDA doesn't investigate. As a result, you see a lot of bullshit about herbal mixtures that allegedly can add as much as four inches to your length. Save your money. Dr. Stephen Barrett, vice president of the National Council Against Health Fraud and editor of Quackwatch.com, says all penis-enlargement pills should be regarded as fakes. In fact, he has yet to find a mail-order health product that lives up to its claims, and he's been searching for 25 years. Many readers have asked the Advisor *about Longitude, a big-dick pill containing zinc, yohimbe, oyster meat, oat straw, cayenne, pumpkin seed, licorice root, boron, ginseng and other ingredients. In 2002 Arizona law enforcement and U.S. Customs officials seized $30 million worth of homes, offices, luxury cars, jewelry, bank accounts and cash from the three principals of the company (two guys and one guy's mother) that marketed Longitude over the Internet, on the* Howard Stern Show *and in men's magazines such as* Maxim *and* Penthouse. *Enzyte is smarter about the pitch; it refuses to offer a money-back guarantee (which is what got the makers of Longitude in trouble), never promises that changes will be permanent and notes that the product "doesn't work for everyone." The only evidence it presents is a survey of 100 customers, nearly all satisfied. Dr. Barrett says not to put too much value in testimonials, which are often solicited with cash or free products.*

Are you saying there is no hope for small guys like me to increase their size?—H.M., West Bloomfield, Michigan

There's no method to increase the size of your cock outside of surgery, and even that will increase your length only when flaccid. The good news is that you're probably not as small as you think. Most men measure four to six inches when hard. Only two percent have erections longer than 7.2 inches.

I guess you've never heard of jelqing. It works, but it's a pain to set aside 30 minutes six days a week to do it. I jelqed for a couple of months. The increase was especially noticeable in the flaccid state, with the most pronounced growth near the head. One must jelq regularly to keep the gain, and there is potential for serious injury if you're overzealous.—M.N., Walters, Oklahoma

Your experience with this risky and unproven method, which involves "milking" your penis regularly for months, is unusual. Why not spend that three hours a week on something productive, like volunteering at a homeless shelter, or therapy?

Your attitude toward penis enlargement is uninformed. I used moist heat, massage and stretching daily for two years to go from six to seven inches. In the flaccid state I now have a nice bulge. The boost to my confidence, not to mention the satisfaction of the ladies, is immeasurable.—H.M., Stockton, California

We can measure it. If it's tied to your penis size, it's still low.

Curving penis

During the past few weeks, my erections have started to curve to the left. Is this something to be concerned about?—S.R., Wheeling, West Virginia

Maybe it's the girl next door. You're likely suffering from Peyronie's disease, named after the French physician who first diagnosed it in 1743. In many cases it appears after an injury to the penis causes scarring or fibrosis. A common analogy is to imagine a long balloon being inflated with a piece of tape on its side. Some erections have a slight natural curve; Peyronie's is distinguished by sudden, unexpected bending down, up or to either side (depending on where the scar tissue forms; you may feel it as a ridge or knot). Most of the time the condition runs its course without treatment, but it can take months or years and may be painful initially. Urologists have battled Peyronie's with vitamin E, Potaba steroid therapy, corticosteroids, radiation, ultrasound and surgery, among other treatments. Visit a urologist, but give the condition time to correct itself before agreeing to anything as drastic as surgery.

Check your balls

One of my balls is larger than the other. I'm hoping it's not a sign of cancer. Is there a self-exam that I can do like the ones women perform on their breasts?—R.K., Burlington, Vermont

One testicle is almost always larger than another—no worries there. Eight out of 10 times the left ball hangs lower. What's not normal are hard, painless lumps. Testicular cancer is relatively common among men under the age of 35, so it's prudent to check yourself once a month after a warm shower. Gently roll each testicle between the fingers and thumb of each hand. Don't be confused by the soft, tube-like structure behind each testicle—that's the epididymis, which carries sperm. And free-floating lumps in the scrotum are not cancer. See a doctor if you feel anything out of the ordinary, if one of your testicles swells or decreases in size, if you feel a heaviness in your scrotum or a dull ache in your abdomen or groin, if you have pain or discomfort in your balls or scrotum or if your breasts are enlarged or tender.

The penis-foot connection

Is it true that the bigger a man's feet, the bigger his penis?—H.T., Mesa, Arizona

Urologists at St. Mary's Hospital and University College in London gently stretched and measured the flaccid penises of 104 patients, average age 54, but

found no correlation to shoe size. Greek researchers at the Naval and Veterans Hospital of Athens had more success correlating the flaccid size of 52 men between the ages of 19 and 38 with the length of the men's index fingers. We know of several body parts that correspond with the length of a man's penis, but they all belong to women.

Is circumcision necessary?

What happens if one parent opposes the circumcision of a newborn son and the other parent insists on it? My wife and I have been discussing this as we try to have a child, but I can't convince her that circumcision is an unnecessary and painful procedure. Who does the doctor listen to? If my son decides he wants to have it done when he's older, fine, but no infant should be forced to endure it.—S.G., Calgary, Alberta

We would want to hear your wife's reasons for wanting this procedure, because we can't think of any good ones. If a physician knows there is a strong disagreement between the parents over whether to circumcise an infant, he would be foolhardy to perform the surgery. Point out to your wife that you are not alone in believing circumcision is unnecessary—rates in the U.S. have fallen from 80 percent to 90 percent in the early 1970s to about 60 percent today, in part because more parents are being educated. The American Academy of Pediatrics doesn't recommend it, and scientists who have taken a closer look at the prepuce have found that it contains a huge number of nerves. In fact, the nerve endings of the foreskin have been compared to those in the fingertips and lips. To remove either of those organs from an infant would be considered barbaric. Most men in the world aren't circumcised; the surgery only became popular in the U.S. because 19th century doctors thought its removal would discourage masturbation, which they believed led to disease. When that justification fell from favor, doctors argued that circumcision improves hygiene. There is evidence that circumcised infants have fewer urinary tract infections and that circumcision may help prevent the transmission of HIV. But these risks can be addressed by less radical means, such as regular washing and condoms.

Penis piercings

I had my nipples pierced last year and now would like to get my penis done. I've settled on a Prince Albert, which, as you know, is a ring that enters the opening of the urethra and exits in the center of the V formed by the glans on the underside of the penis. I figure I can't go wrong with a permanent G-spot tickler and added stimulation for the most sensitive part of my cock. Is there anything I should know before I have it done?—T.R., Reno, Nevada

Having someone punch a hole through your penis takes a special sort of faith. Readers tell us that besides the physical sensations, the best thing about having your penis pierced is walking around knowing you have a pierced penis. The Prince Albert is the most common penile piercing, and should be the least painful. You'll bleed for anywhere from one to four days, particularly at night when you have involuntary erections. It takes about eight weeks for the wound to heal and as long as 10 months before you can remove the jewelry. You can attempt intercourse after the first few weeks, but proceed cautiously and keep everything sparkly clean. (Even healed piercings can create tiny tears in the skin that allow STDs a foothold.) Use plenty of lube on the inside and outside of a condom with an extraroomy head to cover the jewelry. Oral sex presents its own challenges: Penis jewelry has been known to chip teeth. So don't rush her. The PA can stimulate the G-spot during doggy style, but if she prefers other positions you might consider an apadravya, or vertical bar through the glans. Some men also pierce their frenums, coronas and/or scrotums. One step at a time.

Will my penis piercing set off airport metal detectors?—H.J., St. Louis, Missouri

Piercings rarely set off alarms—when they do, it's usually because your jewelry is concentrated in one area or the rings are of a particularly heavy gauge. Handheld wands, however, may pick them up, which could create a scene straight out of This is Spinal Tap. *What gets you in trouble typically isn't the piercings but the baggage you're carrying. About five years ago Turkish authorities stopped a British dancer who had triggered an airport alarm, and a search revealed a total of six metal rings in her nipples and genitals. She also had three kilos of heroin strapped to her chest. More recently, a woman posting to the online Cock and Ball Torture Forum related how she had asked her husband/slave to pick her up at the airport. He was delayed not because of his thick nipple and penis piercings, which had never been a problem, but because of two small padlocks his wife used to tightly bind his balls whenever the couple were apart. Let that be a lesson.*

Tanning while nude

Whenever I tan nude at the salon, I feel the need to cover my penis. Is my package in any danger from the ultraviolet rays if I don't cover it?—B.G., Evansville, Indiana

They won't boil your sperm, if that's what you mean. Because your penis and testicles haven't been dangling in sunlight, they'll be more sensitive. Ease them into the rotation.

Me and my big dick

I often travel to Europe, where it doesn't seem to be a problem to mention to women that I'm well hung. But here in the U.S. I can get the strangest looks. I believe in being up front about this because so many women have told me they enjoy my ample size. If women can wear low-cut blouses and short skirts to advertise their goods, why can't I mention my endowment?—M.S., Prescott, Arizona

You don't know anything more interesting to talk about?

Your response was perfect. I talked to some of my girlfriends about this, and the majority of well-endowed guys we know are jerks. One guy I dated called his penis "the weapon." Has there ever been a study relating a man's penis size to his personality?—M.B., Glendale, Arizona

No, just as there has never been a study of breast size and personality.

Boxers or briefs?

Is it better for your balls if you wear boxers or briefs?—M.S., Portland, Oregon

There's no difference, at least according to a study reported in the Journal of Urology. *The scrotum is generally a few degrees cooler than the rest of the body because sperm like it that way. The idea is that wearing briefs raises the temperature and limits production, which can be good or bad, depending on your desire to be a father. One experiment in the 1960s attempted to raise scrotal temperature using an insulated jockstrap and a lightbulb. But it wasn't until the mid-1990s, when two urologists at the State University of New York at Stony Brook took careful measurements of 97 patients, that we had any real insight into the matter. They found the average boxer ball temperature to be 97.9 degrees and the average brief ball temperature to be 97.7, leading to the conclusion that "the hyperthermic effect of briefs has been exaggerated." More recently another State University of New York urologist found that sitting with the knees together to support a laptop caused the scrotal temperature of his 29 volunteers to rise by about one degree, even before the computer was turned on. Long-term, he said, this could cause fertility problems. The only previous research on this topic was a 2002 letter to the*

Lancet *in which a physician described a patient whose laptop got so hot it burned his penis through his pants and underwear.*

Penis transplants

Has there ever been a successful penis transplant?—C.D., Seattle, Washington

Are you in search of one or looking to donate? What might have been the world's first transplant took place in 2003 at the Nil Ratan Sircar Medical College Hospital in Calcutta, India. Doctors transplanted the penis of a one-year-old who had been born with two to a seven-month-old born without one. As John Wayne Bobbitt can attest, it's more common to have your own penis reattached. We'll keep this brief, but here are two cases of note: (1) German doctors twice reattached the penis of a psychiatric patient who cut it off in incidents 10 years apart; (2) in Milwaukee in 1992 a man who lost his organ in a lawn mower accident had it sewn beneath the skin of his forearm (with the head protruding) for a month to keep it alive while his perineum healed. The surgeons who performed this amazing operation concluded that "in penile amputation, replantation remains the treatment of choice." God forbid.

That lawn mower incident sounds like bullshit. I bet he got Bobbittized by his wife and needed a story to tell the doctors. I thought the Advisor, if anyone, would be more skeptical.—G.C., Dallas, Texas

There was grass in the wound. That's all the evidence we need.

Will a fish bite my penis?

I have never gone skinny-dipping because I'm afraid a fish will bite my penis. Do you know if something like that has ever happened?—A.E., Loveland, Colorado

As long you don't swim in a jungle river near a dam, you'll be okay. That's because the fish most likely to take a chance like that is the speckled piranha or one of its toothed cousins, and they gather near dams. They aren't aiming for your privates but for whatever flesh they can find to defend their young. Dr. Vidal Haddad Jr. of the Botucatu School of Medicine in Sao Paulo, an expert on fish attacks, knows of only one study that even mentions penis bites (published in 1972), and he hasn't heard of any incidents in his own research. There is a well-documented case of a tiny catfish, known as a candiru, jumping into a man's urethra as he stood thigh-deep in the Amazon to urinate. He needed surgery to remove it.

While skinny-dipping in the Severn River near Annapolis, Maryland I was stung by a jellyfish on the most sensitive square inch of my body. I set a record for the one-armed dog paddle to shore. The pain and swelling eventually subsided, but I still have a faint red mark the size of a dime on the head of my penis. Fish attacks may be rare, but there is good reason not to swim nude at night in strange waters.—C.M., Richmond, Virginia

While researching attacks on the penis, we found the case of a farmer in Brazil who was stung through his pants by a scorpion. You two should have a beer.

Penis tattoos

I plan to get a tattoo on the shaft of my cock and perhaps the head. My girlfriend has agreed to keep me hard, but any other advice you can offer would be appreciated.—V.J., Ashland, Wisconsin

We have never placed anything sharper than a woman's teeth near our penis, so we asked for counsel from Gerry Beckerman of Ozark Ink Tattoo in Ava, Missouri (and formerly of Phoenix and Fort Lauderdale), who has done a number of penis tattoos during his three decades in the business. He says you don't need to be erect to have it done; the skin simply needs to be pulled taut. It's usually stretched by the artist, an assistant or a girlfriend or wife. "The tattooing isn't that painful, but it's still a sobering experience for most guys," he says. "I just did the penis of a friend who wanted 'Mary' in Old English script on his shaft and a tribal design on his scrotum. Mary pulled the skin as I worked. The skin of the shaft is thin, so it may scar unless you hire an experienced artist. The underside is less forgiving than the top. The scrotum is another matter. It's like tattooing a basketball." You can draw just about anything on a penis, Beckerman says, though most men keep it simple. "I've done more than one fly or smiley face on the head," he says. "But I also turned one guy's shaft into a barber pole." Other designs at the body-modification site bmezine.com include stars, an eyeball, ladybugs, butterflies, an elaborate dragon whose wings and tail extend up the guy's abdomen, an entirely green or black shaft and/or head, hot-rod flames, hula dancers, roses, a fish, webbing, scorpions, a dagger, Satan and labels that read "USDA Inspected" and "Warning: Choking Hazard."

PORN

It's all in the lighting.

How can I break in?

I am a 50-year-old retired professional who would like to act in porn. I'm six feet tall, 200 pounds, with brown hair and blue eyes, and I've lasted more than seven hours. What do I need to do?—T.E., Oklahoma City, Oklahoma

You don't want to work in porn; you want to have sex with porn babes. In all likelihood, you don't have what it takes to be a professional fucker. Build and penis size have nothing to do with whether you would be cast. All that matters is whether you can get hard and come on cue with a woman you don't necessarily find attractive, under hot lights, in front of an impatient crew. Once you're erect, you must remain hard for hours as you're repositioned to create the illusion of spontaneous sex. You have to get hard again after lunch and potty breaks. You'll spend much of your time absentmindedly stroking yourself. The pay sucks—maybe a few hundred dollars for a shoot that includes two or three pop shots. You need to live in southern California. And there's no way you'll get an audition unless (1) you know a director or producer who will take a chance on casting you, since he'll be out a good sum if you can't perform, or (2) you know a woman who's supermodel gorgeous and who wants to become a hard-core star but insists she won't fuck anyone but you. If you can attract someone like that, you don't need help getting laid. You also could make your own videos, which might work as an introduction. But you'll have to find the women by yourself.

My wife and I were watching a talk show that featured a couple who had launched a sex site. They set up a camera in their bedroom and transmitted live images to the Internet. Surfers pay by credit card to watch the couple have sex. They claimed to gross around $30,000 a month. Is this easy to set up? What software do you need? Is it legal?—S.W., Louisville, Kentucky

Check out ifriends.com. You supply a webcam, the site provides the software and you earn 50 percent of revenues from pay-per-view and private sessions. It's much more difficult to launch an independent site. The market is saturated, and it takes a substantial investment to attract enough surfers to churn a profit. We can't get into the legalities (they vary from county to county) but you'll find guid-ance at the Adult Webmaster Resource Center at ynot.com. It includes information on software, hardware, billing, suppliers, commerce, hosts, designers, advertising and promotion.

I have this great idea for a porn film

I've toyed with the idea of writing a porn movie. Where should I send my screenplay? Are the sex scenes scripted, or is that left to the actors and director?—D.S., Oakland Gardens, New York

We could provide a list of production houses, but unless you're giving the stuff away, it's a waste of your time and theirs. Most porn directors write their own scripts. Even if someone purchased your 35 pages of dialogue, you'd earn only a few hundred dollars. Plots, when they exist, are usually inspired by convenience—a director considers which locations, sets, props and actors he can get on the cheap, then weaves a story around them. The sex isn't scripted unless there's some plot point, such as a good girl refusing anal sex. Plus, the director is going to film his fantasies, not yours.

Land of the free

My wife and I enjoy watching adult videos, but stores in this area don't sell or rent them. I e-mailed two websites and both said they don't ship to Alabama. We thought about getting a satellite dish, but our state is one that doesn't allow hard-core channels. How can we get movies without having to travel out of state?—J.L., Montgomery, Alabama

While most high-profile sites refuse to ship porn to Alabama or other sexually repressive states for fear of prosecution, hundreds of smaller operations will take the chance to have you as a customer. They don't advertise this fact, for obvious reasons, so the only way to know for sure is to submit an order. If you get an e-mail saying it's been canceled, continue your search. If you prefer to return the evidence, a number of sites offer seven-day porn rentals for about $5 each.

3-D porn

Is there such a thing as 3-D porn?—G.H., Pueblo, Colorado

Sure. Open your eyes during sex. Porn shot in 3D, like porn that's not shot in 3D, is mostly disappointing. You have a few options. The 1992 3D video Princess Orgasma and the Magic Bed *is still available. It comes with a pair of Pulfrich*

glasses (one lens is darker than the other, and the image viewed through the darker lens reaches the brain slightly later). Vidmax-3d.com sells 16 collections of sex scenes shot in the mid-Nineties with alternate field stereography. (The two best are Bedroom Cries *and* Boudoir Babes.*) To view the effect, slide one of the $50 videos into your VCR, then plug a pair of $125 shutter glasses into the player's output jack. Outrageous Films released the first and apparently only 3D porn DVD,* Erotek Dimensions, *in 2001, but it's now hard to find and also requires shutter glasses. Two dreadful hard-core films shot in the mid-1970s for anaglyphic (red-blue) lenses,* The Lollipop Girls in Hard Candy *and* Disco Dolls in Hot Skin, *are popular on the midnight movie circuit. Finally, if you happen to attend the annual National Stereoscopic Association convention,* Adult Video News *editor and 3D photographer Mark Kernes sometimes presents a midnight show of eye-popping hard-core shots taken on porn sets. Some images also appear as slide shows on the DVD versions of* Unreal *and* Chloe Cums First. *No glasses necessary—just stare hard.*

Where's my fluffer?!

Do fluffers actually exist? They are the women who supposedly get a porn actor hard before the scene?—R.R., Washington, D.C.

The position has never been common, mostly because budget-minded directors aren't willing to pay for sex they can't get on film. One former porn actor recalls using a fluffer only once in his long career—his co-star didn't want to mess up her makeup. The most notable recent use of the position was during the filming of two World's Largest Gang Bang *videos in which porn actresses set new standards for continuous acts of sexual intercourse. We've long been fascinated by the idea, so we experimented with a sex trick by the same name: Your partner does all she can to keep you hard without benefit of intercourse and without exciting you so much that you lose your cool. You act nonchalant, trying not to give anything away, all the time thinking like a jaded movie stud. The object is to come without her suspecting you were close. Play fluffer for her and everyone's a winner.*

How big is the industry?

I've read that commercial sex in all its forms is the fourth-largest industry in the U.S. That includes videos, magazines, websites, topless bars, prostitution, phone sex, fetish services, etc. Do you know of any statistics to back this up?—C.H., Van Nuys, California

It's fourth behind food, shelter and clothing. We've seen estimates of $10 billion, $11 billion, $13 billion, $14 billion and $20 billion, excluding prostitution. Because most adult businesses are privately held and don't have to release financial data to stockholders, you're left with extrapolations from sales. For example, the Video Software Dealers Association estimates that Americans spend $8.4 billion each year to rent videos and DVDs. It guesses that porn rentals make up three percent to five percent of that total, or $253 million to $422 million. A survey of adults-only stores by Adult Video News *found they earn a total of $970 million annually from sales and rentals. A VSDA survey of 90 stores that carry mainstream and adult titles found that porn accounts for an average of 16 percent of their gross. Using that figure, AVN pegs the total hard-core video and DVD market at $4 billion, not including mail order. Forbes calls that number "wildly inflated" and points out that even if each of the 13,000 porn titles released annually sold 2,000 copies at $20 apiece—all generous assumptions—the total would be just $520 million. The magazine estimates the annual gross from adult movies, websites, pay-per-view and magazines at $2.6 billion to $3.9 billion. So, who knows? We'll start saving our receipts.*

Great porn

Can you suggest any adult films that won't be a waste of time? I prefer erotica to pornography.—M.F., Annapolis, Maryland

Is a movie erotic if it turns you on but pornographic if it turns someone else on? We consider just about everything erotic on some level, so it's hard to come up with a surefire list. But we can point you in the right direction. We asked Richard Freeman, who edits a monthly newsletter about porn films called Batteries Not Included *($3 from 513 North Central Ave., Fairborn, Ohio 45324), for films that seem to have wide appeal. He suggests, in no particular order,* Chameleons: Not the Sequel, The Opening of Misty Beethoven, Face Dance, New Wave Hookers, Justine: Nothing to Hide 2, American Babylon, Neon Nights, Unnatural Phenomenon, 800 Fantasy Lane *and* Latex. *"These ten may not be the best ever made," he says, "but I can watch any of them and feel I've found my sexual center." We know what we're doing this weekend—how about you?*

Is the porn made in other countries any better than what's coming out of Los Angeles?—P.L., Tallahassee, Florida

Some is better, although mostly it's familiar. European porn tends to have more plot, fewer boob jobs and nary a condom in sight. Sample a few titles from Private, *which films primarily in Budapest (our favorite director: Pierre Woodman). Or pick up a copy of International Porn, a sampler of European and Asian porn compiled by Tom Weisser of Video Search of Miami (vsom.com or 888-279-9773). A quick rundown: The Japanese are best known for an era of soft-core films that ended in 1988; it wasn't until 1994 that directors could legally show genitalia. German porn is the most perverse ("If a director shows a dildo, it will be as big as someone's leg," Weisser says). The Italians are obsessed with interracial and anal sex. The French have the most beautiful actresses, which may explain the many lesbian scenes. Get it while it's hot. European porn has become more homogeneous of late: The same 30 women show up in films made all over the continent.*

I'm a woman who loves watching porn. But some things get on my nerves: (1) Orgy scenes in which the guys give each other "Dude, we're so lucky!" looks and exchange high fives. Is that necessary? Concentrate on what you're doing! (2) Female performers whose fake orgasmic shrieks sound like the Emergency Alert System. (3) A guy who walks up to a girl who is already busy with two penises and taps her on the head with his cock. Wait your turn! (4) Hearing the disembodied voice of the director say, "Honey, lift your leg a little so he can get his fingers deeper into your asshole." Hello, postproduction? (5) Squeamish female performers who dodge the money shot so it flies onto some rented couch. (6) Directors who don't hire a backup stud to step in when their lead can't get it up. I don't enjoy watching my sex life with my ex played out on video.—C.M., Los Angeles, California

Porn and condoms
Who decides whether a porn star wears a condom? Every now and then you see a film in which every guy isn't wearing one. I know it's not because of the female stars, as I've seen the same women perform with and without them. Can you explain?—S.G., Calgary, Alberta

Given the choice, only a few performers (about one in six, according to the Adult Industry Medical Health Care Foundation) insist on protection—those who don't get hazard pay and more work. The performers who work bare comfort themselves with the idea that they're having sex within a relatively small group and that monthly HIV testing is mandatory. This despite two scares in recent years that involved multiple HIV infections. Plus, there are other risks. AIM has seen an increasing number of cases of gonorrhea and chlamydia. The next time you watch sex performers work without a net, appreciate the risks they're taking for your arousal.

If the shoe fits

Why do so many of the women in porn movies wear shoes, even during the sex scenes?—N.G., Minneapolis, Minnesota

Heels make the performer's legs seem longer, lift her buttocks and give her a wobble when she walks, which makes her appear vulnerable. Plus, would you walk around barefoot on a porn set?

What is bukkake?

Two women in my office were discussing bukkake. I asked what it meant. They laughed and said it's sexy and that I'd like it. That's all I could get out of them. I thought I could get an explanation from you.—J.C., Buffalo, New York

Bukkake is a form of pornography in which a group of men ejaculates onto one woman. Where the hell do you work?

The money shot

Why do porn films always include an annoying close-up of the guy's face as he strains and groans before orgasm?—R.C., Dallas, Texas

Because porn is fantasy. Sex scenes are filmed as a series of starts and stops, not in one glorious fuckfest. The finale is typically done the same way: The action stops, everyone gets into position, and the actor strokes himself to climax. No cameraman in his right mind would pan to the actor's face and miss the money shot, so the director will later have the actor fake his come face for the two-second transition. A few years ago, Joani Blank made a video, Faces of Ecstasy, *in which she recorded the faces of a dozen men and women as they climaxed. One challenge was getting the subjects to keep their eyes open as they came. "It's so much hotter that way," Blank says, which suggests that readers of this book should give it a try. It may also be fun to use that digital camera to take photos of each other making the faces you think you make at climax and, later, the ones that actually appear.*

Is that for real?

Are any of the "reality" porn sites such as *Bang Bus* and *M.I.L.F. Hunter* real? Although I'm sure there are women out there who would get into a van and, after half an hour of coaxing, have sex with a stranger for $100, I can't believe any would do it while being filmed.—J.R., Richland, Washington

There's no pulling the Kleenex over your eyes. Yes, they are fake. The women are actors who apply for the job, then improvise their dialogue. Frankly we're surprised by their talent: Many are almost convincing as random women who accept an invitation from three drooling strangers—one of whom is peering through a camcorder—to climb into a van with tinted windows. Producers for these types of sites typically recruit swingers, strippers and the underemployed and pay upwards of $700 for an hour of coy conversation and sex. In a 2004 report, WPLG-TV in Miami revealed that "the women [of Bang Bus] are actually paid performers, and the incidents are all set up in advance." Stop the presses! The station even took a videotape to the police to see if any laws had been broken, but the cops said none had. WPLG, you are officially no fun.

Celebrity porn

While appearing on *The Tonight Show* to promote the latest Bond film, Halle Berry talked about doing a bedroom scene with Pierce Brosnan. She said that their genitalia had been covered by something, but she was cut off by applause and laughter. Did NBC bleep her? What did she mean to say? Do all actors cover their privates during shower or sex scenes so their genitals don't touch? I can't believe it's easy to avoid a natural reaction to the opposite sex.—J.L., Washington, D.C.

We think Halle meant to say plywood. Under normal circumstances, it might be difficult to avoid a stiffie or tingly moment during an intimate embrace. But filming is not a normal circumstance. The actors are in a confined space with hot lights and surrounded by crew members. Nearly all of their movements have been mapped out. That's not to say it doesn't happen. Many people suspect that Carre Otis and Mickey Rourke completed the circuit during their climactic scene in Wild Orchid. *Others believe the same thing about Jane March and Tony Leung in* The Lover, *and there's no doubt Donald Sutherland went down on Julie Christie in* Don't Look Now. *Other films that have raised questions:* Tattoo, Color of Night *and* Boxcar Bertha. *For screen shots, see MrSkin.com or Scoopy.net.*

I've read stories online about celebrities who appeared in porn early in their careers. Is that true? If they exist, where can I find them?—T.M., San Antonio, Texas

The creator of MrSkin.com, Jim McBride, suggests that everyone calm down and think about this for a minute. "With all the celebrity hounds such as the National Enquirer *and* Inside Edition, *don't you think we'd have heard by now if some Hollywood star did a porno?" he asks. There are loops that feature women who resemble celebrities. The female lead in a Forties smoker is said to be Marilyn Monroe, but it's actually look-alike Arline Hunter, whose stock pin-up shots were used for an early* Playboy *centerfold. Joan Crawford supposedly made a stag in the early Twenties called* The Casting Couch; *one story has it an MGM lawyer watched the film and concluded it wasn't her, another that Louie Mayer destroyed as many copies as he could find. A biography of J. Edgar Hoover alleges that the FBI director threatened to circulate a stag film starring a "well-known female singer" unless she toned down her support for the Black Panthers. That might be a reference to a sixties loop that features a woman whose nose resembles Barbra Streisand's. (She says it's not her, but the film is grainy, so people will always see what they want to see.) Sylvester Stallone and Madonna made their screen debuts in bad soft-core movies, a few hard-core stars such as Traci Lords and Kobe Tai have landed mainstream roles, and Pam Anderson, Rob Lowe, Jayne Kennedy and Paris Hilton have been reluctant home video stars. Video Search of Miami (vsom.com or 888-279-9773) offers a sampler of "celebrity porn" for $20 that includes the "woman with a big nose" loop and a scene featuring a performer who resembles Linda Blair. Prepare to be disappointed.*

POSITIONS

Assembly required.

How many are there?

How many sex positions are there? My girlfriend and I found a site online that claims to have more than 500. We would like to try one new position every day, and I figure that could keep us going until next summer. Then we could start over.—R.T., Hartford, Connecticut

That figure comes from the Indian scholar Yashodhara, who centuries ago wrote commentary on the Kama Sutra. *He said there are precisely 529 positions, but he used some creative accounting. For example, here's his description of the* dhenuka, *which translates as "congress of the cow": "In the same way can be carried out the congress of a dog, the congress of a goat, the congress of a deer, the forcible mounting of an ass, the congress of a cat, the jump of a tiger, the pressing of an elephant, the rubbing of a bear, the mounting of a horse. And in all these cases the characteristics of these different animals should be manifested by acting or producing sounds like them." So, if your partner barks one day and whinnies the next, you've completed two positions—or you need to move off the farm.*

For the guys

What is the best position for men?—T.S., Omaha, Nebraska

Given the importance of visual stimulation in male sexuality, the best position would have to allow the man to see his partner's reactions. A guy loves to know he's the reason she's moaning, groaning, sighing, grabbing and begging for more. That eliminates the reverse cowgirl, also known as woman on top facing away. Next, comfort. Missionary position can be one of the most uncomfortable. To maintain the best angle and allow his partner to breathe, the man must rest his weight on his palms or elbows. Over time, that takes a toll. It also doesn't give him easy access to her clitoris. Doggie style is fun, and you may get to stand. But she's facing the other way and you can't see her breasts unless you crane your neck. We can't overlook the spoon position, though the angle can be tough there, too. In our view, that leaves the cowgirl as a favorite. It's comfortable for the guy because he's on his back with a great view and the woman can control the depth and positioning of his thrusts. It also leaves the guy's hands free to roam.

My wife and I prefer a variation on the missionary position. She lies on her back and bends her knees so they're touching my shoulders. After a few ball-slapping thrusts, I lower her right leg and place my left outside of it. I turn my body to a one o'clock position, resting my weight on my left knee and on my right shoulder and chest. My left hand is now free to massage her temples, and she loves it when I put my fingers in her mouth. (She likes to have something to suck on.) I can caress and fondle her breasts or—and this is what she begs for—reach between her legs. I slide my right hand under her ass and lift it slightly for better thrusting. The best thing about this position is that I'm close enough to hear every groan and whisper. The position is comfortable, so it allows us to talk and fondle each other following orgasm. We do this until I fall out of her, and if the sex was really good, we start over. I'm sure this isn't anything truly inventive, but it works for us.—D.A., Pittsburgh, Pennsylvania

Your positioning is creative, but of course you're not the first. You'll be interested to know that, according to anthropologist Edgar Gregersen, the Nambikwara Indians of South America preferred rear entry and "a position not recorded elsewhere as a standard form of intercourse. The woman lays on her back, with the man on top facing her, his right leg between her legs and his left leg outside them."

My wife and I have a position we call the Magnificent Screw: Once the man is inside the woman, she squeezes her vaginal muscles and slides up and down on his erection. She doesn't go far enough to stimulate his head (very important—the guy won't last long if she consistently hits his sweet spot) or so far that his cock comes out of her body. The formula my wife uses is 8 to 10 shallow thrusts to one deep one. She then slowly rotates so that she's facing my feet, before repeating the process. She continues to rotate as long as either of us can stand it. I also play with her clitoris and anus to stimulate her, and I have wonderful alternating views of her beautiful breasts and her astounding ass.—T.W., Philadelphia, Pennsylvania

The A-attack
A buddy who spent some time in Japan mentioned the A-attack as something he had done there. He winked at me like I should know what he was talking about, so I said, "Yeah, that's a great one." Can you tell me what it is?—F.W., San Francisco, California

If you visit a Japanese bathhouse and ask your "health girl" for an A-attack, she will stimulate your anus with a vibrator or finger while masturbating you with her free hand. You can also turn the tables and "attack" her. A variation is the A-attack pearl, in which the hostess inserts a string of pearls into her client's anus and then, while blowing him, pulls the string out pearl by pearl. These and other sexual delicacies are described in Japan's Sex Trade, *a guide by Peter Constantine. In* daisharin asobi *(the "big wheel game"), a "soap lady" lies on top of the man, then slowly rotates her body so he can lick and touch the parts that cross his face. Variations are* daisharin, *in which the partners rotate in opposite directions, and* tokei asobi, *in which the woman fellates the man while crawling clockwise around his body. If you're lucky, she'll take an hour to do it rather than a minute.*

The tall and short of it

My girlfriend is five feet tall and I'm 6'3", so it makes it difficult to 69. Do you have any suggestions as to how we could pull this off?—B.T., Baltimore, Maryland

We take it she's not interested, or you wouldn't have written. Most couples of disparate height find that, with minor adjustments, every position works. That's because, as a 5'4" lover once told the 6'5" Advisor, "We're all the same size in bed." Ralph Keyes concluded the same after interviewing hundreds of tall and short Americans for his book The Height of Your Life. *"As is apparent in any room full of seated bodies, height variation above the hips isn't nearly as great as that below," Keyes noted. "With rare exceptions, the only real difference in sex between couples whose height isn't matched and those whose is is that their toes don't touch when they make love lying down."*

Worker's position

What is the worker's position?—K.A., Oakland, California

We've heard it described as any position in which you're being screwed. Actually, according to Brenda Venus, author of Seduction Secrets for Women, *it's similar to making spoons. Instead of both partners curling together on their sides, only the man does while the woman lies on her back. She lifts the leg closest to her partner and places it over his pelvis. Lying on his side, he puts his top leg between her legs, then slides inside her. If the coordinates are right, he should be able to kiss and suck on one of her breasts as he thrusts. Venus says it's called the worker's position because it allows you to rest after a long day.*

Chuukese hammer

Recently there has been an influx of immigrants here from the island nation of Chuuk. We've heard references to a position called the Chuukese hammer, but when we ask for details, our new friends just respond with big smiles. Can you help?—L.Y., Agana, Guam

The Chuukese hammer (also known as wechewechen chuuk, *which translates as "Trukese striking") requires the man to sit with his legs spread. The woman kneels facing him and scoots forward so her partner can slide the head of his penis just inside her labia. He then grasps his erection and moves it up and down (the "hammer") to stimulate her clitoris. As the couple reaches climax, the man draws the woman closer and slides inside her. To signal the height of her arousal the woman may place her finger in the man's ear. The Chuukese hammer reminds us of an American-made trick called the builder's grip. During intercourse, the man occasionally pauses, wraps his hand around the base of his penis, withdraws and gently "hammers" his erection against his partner's clitoris. Just make sure her fingers are out of the way.*

Have you ever heard of a variation of the Chuukese hammer called *gichigich*? It was invented by the Yapese.—R.R., Berkeley, California

Who hasn't? Gichigich is essentially the same position. The woman sits on the man's lap, facing him, and her inserts his erection between her outer labia. He then moves the head of his penis up and down and sideways, varying the speed and the direction. Eventually, this stimulation makes the woman "frenzied, weak and helpless," writes anthropologist Edgar Gregersen, working from field notes recorded near the turn of the century. "The woman experiences one orgasm after another and involuntarily urinates a little after each orgasm (the sensation for the man is that he is on fire)." The position is supposedly practiced only by single men and women; married Yapese fear it could leave them unable to work the next day.

RELATIONSHIPS

It takes two to tangle.

What are you thinking?

What does it mean when a woman asks, "What are you thinking?"—W.G., Bowling Green, Ohio

She's looking for a pulse—some acknowledgment and reassurance that the relationship is humming along. The question usually confuses guys. They figure if the relationship isn't working, one person will leave. They think, Does she want me to catalog my current random musings on baseball, tits and blow jobs? That will only piss her off. But if you respond with those old standbys "nothing" or "you," that doesn't satisfy her either. Men need to recognize that the exchange of seemingly mundane details is how women establish intimacy with their best female friends. She's approaching you in the same way. Deborah Tannen, a linguistics professor at Georgetown who wrote the best-seller You Just Don't Understand: Women and Men in Conversation, *says the best way to deal with this is for couples to acknowledge what's going on. The man should get in the habit of bringing up topics for discussion. The woman needs to reassure herself that, absent other signs the relationship is suffering, his silence doesn't mean he's unhappy. Linda Vaden-Goad, a social psychologist at Western Connecticut State University who has studied how couples use silence, says even if men are willing to share their thoughts, they are more comfortable with action than analysis. "Disclosure makes them feel vulnerable, and they're supposed to be strong," she says, "though some men in our studies admitted to using silence as a strategy to maintain power because it keeps their partner guessing." Which is interesting but not something we want to talk about.*

We're dating, but are we friends?

I have tried in vain to explain to my girlfriend that we are not friends, just as a parent is not his child's friend. While elements of friendship might be present in these relationships, calling each other friends isn't accurate. I believe my view is logical, while others are using their emotions. They see not being "friends" as horrible, while I view it as it should be: something better and deeper. Either I'm not explaining myself well enough, or I'm wrong. Help!—K.P., Lancaster, Ohio

Are you expecting to get laid anytime soon, Mr. Spock? We see your point, but you're belaboring it. Lovers, as well as children and their parents, are more than friends. But a relationship that isn't built on the combination of loyalty, respect and empathy commonly described as friendship isn't going anywhere. While you and your girlfriend aren't just friends, you also aren't just lovers.

Keeping it real

My girlfriend found one of my adult videos in the VCR and she hit the ceiling. Since then, we've split over a different issue, so the truth can be told· A man can hang a given woman just so many times before it becomes a bore. The precise number of times depends on several factors, including her attractiveness, the degree of variation in the sex and the guy's age and sex drive. (As I've gotten older, fewer women appeal to me sexually, and I grow tired of those sooner.) Whatever the reason, eventually it happens: You'd rather masturbate to a photo of a 23-year-old with perfect breasts than have sex with your 50-year-old wife after she's had your kids. Unfair as hell, but true.—P.M., Oakland, California

Yeah, but what's the wife thinking? Most aging moms would love to spend their sexual energy on a 20-year-old. So why doesn't every married slug leave his or her spouse at the first sign of wrinkles? Your equation is flawed. We've never been naively romantic about relationships—they're hard work—but you overlooked love, or even affection. For most older-and-wiser guys, that plays a huge role in who they choose to "bang." The sight of a 23-year-old babe still turns them on, but they have enough invested in their significant other that it works better as fantasy. Having sex with a stranger every week or month or year comes with its own sort of boredom.

He won't call me his girlfriend

I'm 26 and the guy I've been seeing for three months is 28. Although we spend three or four nights a week together, he won't call me his girlfriend. I asked him about it, and he said he wants to "take it slow." (It did take him three weeks to sleep with me.) I've since heard him describe me as "my girl," and he doesn't correct members of his family when they call me his girlfriend. He treats me like his girlfriend—should I be content with that?—K.G., Redlands, California

Your boyfriend is tongue-tied because he's hoping that someone better will come along. Until that happens, you'll do.

While it might be true that he's just waiting for someone better, it's also possible that he refuses to label the relationship because he is dealing with intimacy or commitment issues. Perhaps she should evaluate why she wants this label, and they can come up with something that meets both of their needs.—J.S., Tucson, Arizona

You mean like fuck buddies? Rebounders? Someday-maybes? You may be correct about his issues, but he should work them out on his own time rather than wasting hers. Labels may be confining, but after three months "girlfriend" threatens no man.

Breaking up is hard to do

I'm trying to break up with my girlfriend. I no longer feel any passion for her, and I want to date other women. (I'm only 21.) She calls me her one true love and tells me that if I loved her I would try to work things out. Whenever I talk about breaking up, she cries and pleads. How can I leave without making it seem as if it's her fault?—J.T., Reno, Nevada

It's always difficult to dump someone and have them be happy about it. If your girlfriend believes you are her one true love, you have no choice but to disappoint her, because that person doesn't exist.

Should I go, or should I fight?

I have a girlfriend who is everything to me; she is my life. Three weeks ago she told me there was another guy and that she isn't sure who she loves more. Should I leave or fight for what I think is mine?—J.P., Los Angeles, California

If your girlfriend is your life, you need to get a hobby. She's already made her decision—she chose not to choose—and that's your signal to back away. While it's possible to love more than one person, it's difficult to coordinate.

Mending a broken heart

How do you mend a broken heart?—P.J., San Francisco, California

How about this: Think about your former lover constantly. (You've tried to forget her, and that hasn't worked.) We just read a study of 110 men and women who were asked by University of Virginia psychologists to bring to mind a past

love. While one group spent eight minutes pining, the other group tried to suppress the memories. Afterward, the fingers of each participant were checked for sweat—a sign that their emotions had been working overtime. Those who had tried to suppress their memories were much more stressed. The research suggests that focusing on a recently lost love—thinking about her, writing about her, talking about her—may make the affair lose its luster more quickly. You'll also inspire your friends to fix you up with someone new, since you'll be boring them to tears.

Let's be friends

Why is it that when women want to end a relationship, they say they want to be friends when they actually want nothing to do with you? In most situations, I would like to be friends.—S.Y., Boulder, Colorado

They're being polite. It's difficult to maintain a friendship after a serious relationship, largely because most people don't have the energy for the charade. What usually happens is that the dumper feels guilty. It's not that she dislikes you. If you win the lottery, she'll be happy for you. If you become famous, she'll boast about how she dated you (or trash you to Jerry Springer). Meanwhile, the dumpee is thinking, This is just a phase before we get back together. That's why most post-breakup friendships are shams. The Advisor hereby calls for a worldwide ban on any couple saying they are going to be friends after a relationship dissolves. Get it over with, already. You may be friends someday, after you both find new lovers. But not now.

The fine print

What do you think of this? "On this day, I do wish and desire of my own free will to become the mistress of [man's name] for a period of seven years. During this period, I shall be given the support of the man to bear his children. We shall agree upon support and accommodation fees to assist the mistress with living costs and expenses. Her duties shall be to escort the man when called and to engage in intimate activities such as dating, romance and sex. She shall be treated with respect and also treat the man with respect. The man shall date and romance her and engage in sexual activities that satisfy both of them. During this time the mistress and the man shall be allowed to date and engage in activities with other partners as often as they desire."—H.G., San Jose, California

Only a fool would show that contract to a woman, because she might sign it.

Love is a process

Last night I was with the girl I've been dating for about two months. (I'm 21, and this is the first girlfriend I've had.) I told her I loved her. She replied that she "really likes me." This was like a kick to my chest. I couldn't sleep the rest of the night thinking about it. I feel like breaking up with her, even though I know I wouldn't find anyone better for a long time. What do you think?—M.P., Cambridge, Massachusetts

She did you a favor. You're not in love, not after eight weeks. You haven't seen this woman at her worst, and there's too much lust and emotion involved to accurately gauge how you feel for the long term. Love is a process, not a revelation. If you're hoping for a relationship rather than just a romance, tell your girlfriend that you didn't mean to scare the shit out of her, if that's what you did. Whatever it's called, at this point all you know for certain is that you enjoy being with her.

The Advisor says "love is a process, not a revelation." You are so wrong. I met my husband when we were both 17 and knew from the first moment that we were soul mates. We've been married for 14 years and have two children. How can you deny love at first sight?—T.R., Dallas, Texas

We're glad things worked out.

How can I ask her to lose weight?

My girlfriend, whom I love deeply, has been slowly gaining weight in her thighs and butt. We kid about it, but how do I tell her that maybe she should start losing weight? I don't want to hurt her feelings.—J.A., Newark, New Jersey

There are a few rules in life that should not be broken. Never wear a belt with suspenders. Never pass on a blind curve. And never, ever tell a woman she's fat, even if you're "just kidding." If you do, it won't matter whether she's thin or fat, because you won't have sex with her again. If she asks, you will say she's beautiful and that you wouldn't change a thing. If you're concerned about her weight, lead by example.

What you should know about women

Cheryl Lavin, who writes a relationship column in the *Chicago Tribune*, has been asking her female readers to suggest things that guys should know about women. I thought I would share my favorite responses, in the hope they might educate your male readers: (1) We'll stop faking it when you stop asking us. (2) Don't compare our breasts with Pam Anderson's, especially since you have a shot at ours. (3) Don't count our shoes and we won't count your *Playboy*s. (4) We are not nags, it's just that you never do it the first time. (5) If it itches, wash it. (6) Only the worst kind of a pig stares at other women when he's with us. We look at other men, but we do it discreetly.—G.T., Arlington Heights, Illinois

We read Lavin's columns, too, but we marked different items—namely, the more reasonable suggestions provided by men. Here is a sampling: (1) If you think you're fat, you probably are. (2) Don't rub the lamp if you don't want the genie to come out. (3) It is in neither your best interest nor ours to take any quiz together. (4) If something we said can be interpreted two ways, and one of the ways makes you sad or angry, we meant it the other way. (5) Our relationship is never going to be like it was the first two months we were dating. (6) We notice other women because we are men and we are alive.

Wild women

I broke up with a woman who was the most amazing lover I've ever had. Unfortunately, she was a head trip. She had been abused by her mother, abandoned by her father, sexually assaulted by her stepmother and raped by two men in her teens, plus she is addicted to alcohol, cocaine and painkillers. She is bipolar and has panic disorder. But she wanted sex daily—oral, anal, bondage, spanking, role playing, exhibitionism (she worked as an exotic dancer), dominance and submission. Because she is bisexual, she had a habit of bringing her girlfriends home for me to screw while she licked my asshole or organized a tag-team blow job. She also had the uncanny ability to get gorgeous strangers in bars, malls and restaurants to show me their tits. Does a woman have to be completely fucked in the head to be such a godsend?—P.J., Arlington, Virginia

There are plenty of well-adjusted women who love crazy sex. They're just harder to find.

A reader asked if it's possible to find a woman who is wild in bed but not wild in general—a situation that makes someone fun to sleep with but a nightmare to date. Many women (and men) suffer from borderline personality disorder. I read up on the topic and discovered that women who have BPD are often sexually aggressive or display impulsive behavior such as substance abuse, excessive spending, reckless driving, suicide attempts, etc. People with the disorder have a crippling fear of abandonment, which may have resulted from being abused as children. The first hint a guy gets is usually when his new girlfriend loves him beyond description one minute and hates him more than anyone she knows the next. Whatever the perceived trouble may be, it's his fault. There's even a book on BPD called *I Hate You, Don't Leave Me.* Unfortunately, the disorder is difficult to treat, but sometimes drugs and intense therapy can help. I loved a woman who had BPD, and she almost destroyed me.—A.S., Los Angeles, California

BPD affects an estimated 2 percent of the population, and 75 percent of its victims are women. A relationship with a BPD sufferer usually begins as an intense, impulsive, romantic affair before disintegrating into an anxious and sometimes frightening drama. (Many people compare their relationships with BPD sufferers to walking on eggshells.) Some people who accept a diagnosis of BPD avoid relationships, resigning themselves to going it alone.

Invite to a wedding

My ex-girlfriend asked me, "If you got an invitation, would you come to my wedding?" We dated for seven years and we've been apart for 18 months. Should I go?—J.T., Philadelphia, Pennsylvania

Do you want to go?

Back to the fold

One of my friends says he never goes back to his old girlfriends because the same problems would come up. Another friend says he frequently dates his exes because people mature and that makes for better relationships. Who's right?—E.S., Richmond, Virginia

It depends on the guy. We only date other people's exes, but we'll sleep with anyone.

I'm in love with a friend

I told a friend I would like to have a romantic relationship with her. She said that she found me attractive and liked to spend time with me but wanted to just be friends. She said that she would understand if I didn't want to see her anymore. I decided to keep things the way they are. I'm hoping she will change her mind. Is there any chance of this happening?—D.B., Detroit, Michigan

It's possible but not probable. It's difficult to maintain a friendship when you want more than a person can give.

My girlfriend won't have sex

My girlfriend and I have been dating for seven months. Two months ago I moved 200 miles to start a four-year graduate program. She told me she would not follow me unless we were engaged. Now she doesn't want to have sex again until we're married. She says she has feelings of guilt related to her faith. I have a problem with going from an active sex life to none at all, but I love her and want to make it work. Should I agree to her wishes and spend the next four years masturbating, or should we discuss an alternative?—J.B., Des Moines, Iowa

What alternative? Even if you were having sex, four years is a long time to maintain a long-distance relationship, and you don't know her well enough to make a decision about marriage.

On the rebound

After we broke up, my ex-boyfriend and I remained friends. We did everything together, even had sex. It was like we'd never split up. But then he found a new girlfriend and stopped calling. We haven't spoken in three months. I think he hates me. Should I try to reconcile or let him go?—P.C., Tuscaloosa, Alabama

You already know the answer. Being the rebound relationship is always tough, especially when you're also the ex.

I've been seeing this guy for a month. He and his girlfriend of 12 years broke up two months before we met. We have spent almost every night together. The sex is great and so is his personality, but he doesn't seem to believe in foreplay. I love giving oral, but it's not much fun when I know he won't reciprocate. Maybe he doesn't like my cookie. I have a large clit, and my lips aren't the cute tucked-away kind. Or maybe he doesn't like oral. I am a clean girl and have even tried bathing right before the action starts. Maybe his ex didn't like it and that ruined him. How can I turn this around? I told him I love to be eaten out and that I'm more likely to come that way, but no progress yet.—K.G., San Bernardino, California

Some guys are reluctant to lick for any number of lame reasons. But our guess—this will be hard to confirm since your boyfriend probably won't admit it, because to do so would threaten the low-obligation sex that's currently soothing his psychic pain—is that he finds going down on you too intimate. He's not over her yet, not after two months.

Girlfriend has almost moved in

My girlfriend lives with her parents but spends 28 days of the month at my place. I have no problem with that, but whenever I ask her to help with the bills, she gets angry. She says I make her feel like an intruder. What should I do?—M.B., Little Rock, Arkansas

Ask her to move in—it's only two more days a month. That may be the source of her hostility. But be careful. If you can't get together on the bills, it doesn't speak well for your future together. Money is the root of all evil arguments.

The lingering ex

I ran into my ex and her new boyfriend at a restaurant. She began to flirt with me as if he wasn't there and even asked me out for the next day. But when I showed up at the bar she'd suggested, she had her boyfriend with her. She again flirted and this time asked me to lunch. I called in the morning to confirm and she said she couldn't make it. What's my next move?—J.T., Orlando, Florida

You don't have one. Your ex is playing you for cheap thrills or to make her boyfriend jealous—probably both.

Say I'm out with a new girlfriend and her ex shows up and tries to win her back, and I have to have a talk with him to set things straight. What is the best thing to say to make him go away and stay away?—S.T., Atlanta, Georgia

What is this, Wild Kingdom? *To him you're a nobody, a big mistake, so anything you say will sound as if it's coming from Charlie Brown's teacher. It's a bad situation; step back until your girlfriend can convince her ex that it's over. It becomes your problem only if she needs to convince herself.*

My fiancée left me after four months, saying that God was calling her closer to him. She called to say she wants me back, but I'm happy with my new girlfriend. Should I tell her about the call?—B.S., St. Louis, Missouri

What call?

Why won't my boyfriend get rid of videos of him and his ex making love? They had a bad breakup, and he says he hates her. We even made new videos of us making love, but that hasn't changed his mind.—E.R., San Antonio, Texas

The question is, why do they bother you? They're mementos. She's not coming back. Just make sure your videos are better lit.

Your advice to the woman who was upset about her boyfriend keeping sex videos of him and his ex is way off the mark. Why shouldn't a woman be upset with the idea of her boyfriend sitting down with a bowl of popcorn and a tub of lube to "reminisce"? No man needs videos to remember sex. His refusal to consider his girlfriend's feelings shows his attachment to the past. If he isn't ready to let go, he isn't ready to film a sequel.—E.P., Kent, Ohio

We'll stick with our response. First, every guy knows not to masturbate while eating popcorn—it makes the fast-forward button too slippery. Second, while no man needs a video to remember sex, it sure helps. Finally, the letter wasn't about sex videos as much as it was about a desire for control. We've seen this before. Like a good boy, a guy destroys his videos. His girlfriend then demands that the photos go, then the letters, then the gifts. But you can't have a guy's past—only his present and, if you're lucky, his future.

My girlfriend and I have been together off and on for three years. Six months ago, while we were broken up, another of her exes stayed at her place. As she slept, he videotaped her with one hand while masturbating with the other. She found out about it but continues to hang out with the guy. Months later, after we were back together, she told me what had happened. I was outraged and told her I couldn't trust him around her any longer. She said I couldn't tell her who to be friends with. I love this girl, but she refuses to see that this guy is a psycho who violated her. We've broken up again over this. What do you think?—B.W., Portland, Oregon

Sounds as if they're meant for each other. Don't be surprised if tapes exist in which your ex-girlfriend isn't asleep.

How to fix a long-distance relationship

I realize most long-distance relationships fizzle, but my girlfriend and I were okay for two years before we recently began hitting a few rocks. Any suggestions how I can improve things?—P.L., Fort Walton Beach, Florida

Move.

She's afraid of being hurt

I was dating this girl for six weeks. One day, out of the blue, she called it off. I found out that she left because she was afraid of getting hurt. How can I convince her that I won't hurt her?—E.S., Las Cruces, New Mexico

You can't make that promise. Every relationship of any value carries this risk.

Will she come back to me?

Several months ago my fiancée came home from work and told me her feelings about me had changed. I moved out, hoping it would blow over. A week later, she started dating her boss. Two weeks after that, she moved in with him. I went to a psychologist, who told me that, based on the statistical evidence, the odds are 80 percent to 90 percent that my fiancée will return. At the suggestion of the psychologist, I went to a psychiatrist, who told me that she wholeheartedly expects my fiancée to return. Now I'm confused and more depressed. Should I expect her to come back, or should I go with my feeling that she's gone for good?—D.R., Miami, Florida

Go with your gut. Even if your ex comes back, she destroyed your trust. That was probably a fatal blow to the relationship. As for these counselors, they can't know what your ex is thinking. Ask a friend to recommend a professional with a spine. You need help managing your grief, not a shoulder to cry on—and not false hope.

Am I engaged to a control freak?

My fiancée has been married before, but I have not. She complained that her first husband devoted too much time to interests she didn't share or that weren't couples-oriented. I've been a blues-metal bass player for years; she says not only does this activity leave her on the sidelines, but there's too great a chance I'll meet women at gigs and cheat on her. Now that I've left the band, she's upped the ante, raising a fuss whenever I leave a disc in the CD player by a band she doesn't like. She used to tell me that my musical ability turned her on. Is there more to this than issues of musical taste and male neglect? I'm beginning to think I'm engaged to a control freak.—J.R., Chicago, Illinois

Beginning to think? Your first mistake was quitting the band. Will they take you back? It seems harsh to break off an engagement over music—or a subscription to Playboy *or whatever your manly appetites may be—but we always tell guys to proceed with caution, because this stuff is a warning shot over the bow. There will always be something else she doesn't like—you just may not hear about it until after the rings are exchanged. If you two have any hope of a successful marriage, your fiancée needs to realize that she can't change you and shouldn't try. In other words, she has to love the entire album, not just the singles. Frankly, working this out in counseling may be a challenge; it sounds like she still has issues from her first marriage. If you marry her now, you'll also get her ex-husband.*

I had a similar experience. I stupidly let my wife drive away my friends, dispose of my guitars, tell me what type of beer to drink and limit me to an allowance of $10 a week. She had me convinced that if I made "just one more little sacrifice" she would be happy. After I'd given up everything enjoyable in my life, including sex, she began complaining that I used too much toilet paper, shampoo and deodorant. I came to my senses one night while lying awake worrying that she would find my secret stash of toiletries. We divorced, and I've never been happier.—K.C., Great Mills, Maryland

Welcome back. You sound like a good guy to have on a camping trip.

When are we together?

At what point do two people become a couple? I say it's the first time they're expected to attend an event as a unit.—R.P., Bloomington, Indiana

We say it's when they've both seen each other on the john.

She says she can't date me

My best friend's sister says she can't date me because I'm close to her brother. Should this be a problem, and if so, how can I get her to see past it?—C.P., Fort Collins, Colorado

The bigger problem is she's not interested.

Young love

Could you give me some insight into this situation? My older brother is 18, and his girlfriend is 16. She is his first girlfriend. At some point she dumped him. He was a mess, crying and everything. Then they got back together, and he was like a lost puppy following her around. Everything he did had to be with her or he wouldn't do it. Now they're taking a "break," and he's a mess again. What's the best way to handle this?— N.C., Jackson, Michigan

Your brother isn't himself at the moment, mostly because he's on drugs. Specifically, he has a cocktail of hormones rushing through him that he has never

dealt with before, and it's making him temporarily insane. The Beatles sang about this: "I'm in love for the first time. / Don't you know it's gonna last? / It's a love that lasts forever. / It's a love that had no past." In other words, because your brother has no experience with relationships, he has given the first one more weight than it deserves. Even Hef went through this phase, as he describes in his Little Black Book: *"I projected everything that I was interested in onto Betty [his first serious crush], everything I had observed in my life, all the dreams I had extracted from the movies, all of this onto her. She couldn't possibly have lived up to that. It was an illusion." Your brother will come around. Be there to help him when the permanent breakup comes and he needs to be distracted. Watch and learn and work on your own independence so you don't become a lost puppy. This may sound heavy, but store it away: You'll have more fulfilling relationships if you can accept the fact that no one else can make you content. You accomplish that alone.*

Twenty years later I am still having dreams about my first love. She broke up with me, and I reacted badly. Eventually I recovered and am now happily married. But every few months she shows up in my dreams, in which I usually apologize to her. I wake up feeling bad. Then I feel worse because I wonder why the hell I'm still anxious about someone I knew in high school. Can you provide any insight?—L.T., Miami, Florida

Paging Dr. Freud! As many people have found, your first love lingers as a symbol of the perfect relationship. At the time, your brain was flush with the chemicals that accompany romance, but the relationship didn't last long enough for them to wear off. You also didn't live with her, so you saw each other only in prepared moments. Twenty years later she is truly a ghost—the 17-year-old girl you dated no longer exists (nor, for that matter, does the 17-year-old boy who loved her). The next time you have one of these unsettling dreams, recognize that your mind is putting into a familiar form the anxiety we all have about being rejected. We all have regrets about our behavior, but it's difficult to regret being young. If you knew then what you know now, you would have been dating older women.

As a psychology professor at California State University who since 1993 has studied lost loves and their effect on relationships, I feel you may have underestimated the power of his teenage attraction. In a survey I conducted of more than 1,000 people who had rekindled relationships after at least five years of separation, two thirds had reunited with loves they'd lost when they were 17 years old or younger. More than 70 percent stayed together after reuniting. In a more recent survey of 1,300 adults who never tried to reunite with a lost love, 30 percent said they would like to and 18 percent said they would leave their spouse if their lost love showed up. In general, men express much stronger emotions about these relationships than women. I would advise anyone who wants to see a lost love again for "closure" or to "catch up" to be careful. What seems innocent can destroy even a strong marriage. This is not a fantasy, as an affair with a relative stranger or even a co-worker may be; it is a love that was interrupted. When I first started my research, 30 percent of the respondents who reconnected with a lost love said the reunion led them to cheat on their spouse. Because the Internet makes it so much easier not only to find lost loves but for those initial contacts to develop in a seemingly casual way, that figure is now closer to 80 percent. There's more information as well as a message board at lostlovers.com.—Nancy Kalish, Sacramento, California

Thanks for writing. We've lost and found a few loves, though it's never the same the second time around because both people have changed. If she hasn't, we're suspicious.

The Advisor takes a stand

What's your position on withholding sex as a means of gaining power in a relationship?—M.L., Springfield, Ohio

Uh . . . we're against it. If a person believes refusing sex is the only way to assert power, the relationship is out of balance in other ways. You also sacrifice your own pleasure.

How many is too many?

I can't get over the fact that my girlfriend has had more lovers than I have. She is my first lover and is five years younger than I am. When I ask her for details, she refuses to say anything. That fuels my paranoia. I wish she would just tell me how far she went with the three guys I know about. If that would ease my mind, shouldn't she tell me everything?—J.C., Chicago, Illinois

Your inexperience shows here, because unless you're recruiting virgins for sacrifice, the number of notches on a woman's bedpost has nothing to do with the future or strength of her current relationship. Someday your girlfriend may provide her history, but she's a smart woman who recognizes that you're already judging her. We're often asked, usually by men, "How many is too many before I should get upset?" and find the question frustrating and ridiculous. We've never had any desire to know more than a woman volunteers; she's not a used car. We find it more useful to quiz a partner about the best and worst behavior of her exes so we can refine our moves. We don't have an easy solution to rid you of this insecurity. We suspect that as you mature and get more experience it will be less of an issue. You are worthy of being with this woman, and she wants to be with you. Don't let the saps she left behind sabotage what you have.

You implied that J.C.'s concern is because of his insecurity or immaturity. Wrong! He has a right to know; the quantity and quality of her partners say something about his girlfriend's character and commitment. (Six is reasonable; 60 suggests a pattern.)—P.N., Montreal, Quebec

A pattern of what? Meeting people? A better indicator of a woman's character is how she treats waiters.

I've read that the average straight guy has 12 sex partners in his life, while the average woman has three. How is that possible? Even if there is a small percentage of women who have hundreds of partners, that still raises the average of the average woman.—E.M., Columbus, Ohio

Social scientists encounter this discrepancy frequently when they ask men and women how many partners they've had in their lifetimes. However, it all but disappears when researchers narrow the focus to the previous year. In other words, our memories can be imprecise. Two researchers addressed this issue in the Journal of Sex Research. *After asking 1,800 college students how many sexual partners they'd had and how they arrived at that number, they concluded that men and women generally use different calculation strategies. Sexually promiscuous people usually don't keep a running tally, so when they're asked to come up with one, they take their best guess. Women tend to produce as accurate a count as possible, but they also underestimate. Men tend to make rough guesses, which skew upward. Cultural factors also play a role. Men may subconsciously exaggerate to appear macho, while women may understate to avoid being judged as promiscuous. There's also the hooker factor. Researchers have estimated that about 65,000 Americans prostitute themselves full-time, and that each has an average of 694 clients per year. Added to existing data, these figures more or less eliminate the discrepancy.*

The surveys about how many partners people have had in their lifetime never break it down by age. That is, a 24-year-old who has had 10 lovers is vastly different from a 50-year-old with 10. I have a female friend who estimates that most guys in their mid-20s have slept with 80 to 90 women. That seems high. I'm 36 and have been with 65 women. Is that above average? I had a 25-year-old girlfriend who had slept with 75 guys.—N.F., Austin, Texas

Those numbers are robust. In one study of 3,126 adults, about 10 percent of the respondents reported having had at least 21 lovers since age 18. That held true regardless of age, with the exception of 18- to 24-year-olds, who just need more time. The median was six partners for men and two for women, meaning that half the respondents had more and half had less. At the extreme, one man claimed 1,016 partners and one woman said she'd been with 1,009. (What's more amazing—their promiscuity or that they were both so precise?) In 1982 we surveyed 100,000 readers and asked them tally their lovers. The median for men was 16; the median for women was eight. Which goes to show that reading Playboy *gets you laid more often—or at least it did in the 1970s.*

Shrieking banshees

When I married I picked a woman who didn't want children, and we've had a great 20 years. But her two sisters decided to start families when they were in their 40s. In the space of four years they have procreated a combined total of nine times. Now I'm stuck with these self-centered moms who feel their undisciplined brats are welcome at any event. When we were invited to a princess birthday party, I went to a ball game instead, and my sister-in-law blew a gasket. After working a 50-hour week, why should I drive three hours to spend a weekend with a pack of shrieking, sugar-intoxicated banshees? Am I being an ogre? My wife isn't angry, but her sister is really pissed.—J.C., Buffalo, New York

Next time say you have to work. But you also need to lighten up about this. You can't ditch every family gathering, and it doesn't pay to irritate a sister-in-law (they can do a lot of damage). Some of this is your attitude going in. If you arrive thinking you'll be miserable, it becomes a self-fulfilling prophecy. Enjoy the fact that they aren't your kids.

SEMEN

The stuff of life.

Funky spunk

My husband wants me to swallow and I can't stand the taste. I've read that pineapple juice helps prevent funky spunk. Exactly how much should a man consume, and how often, to alter the taste of his semen? And how soon should I expect to notice a change?—M.L., Virginia Beach, Virginia

Adam Carolla of Loveline *has a great take on this. He says, "If a guy drinks 400 gallons of pineapple juice, his semen will taste like semen with a little bit of pineapple juice in it." Nevertheless, many female readers insist that, in their experience, fruit juices work when consumed in large enough quantities at least a day before. But that could have more to do with the guy's being well hydrated, which may dilute what's commonly described as a bleachy, salty or bitter taste. Some women have told us they are happier swallowing when their partner eats less junk food and red meat. One recipe posted outside the* Playboy *test bedrooms calls for three stalks of celery (diced), two capsicums (minced), two bananas (sliced), half a cup of orange juice and half a cup of sweet sherry, but no pineapple. The brewmaster wrote, "Mix the ingredients and have the guy eat it for breakfast. He also should avoid dairy products, onions, garlic and fish for the day." Good advice before any date. The only way to settle this is a series of blind taste tests, which are being arranged as we speak.*

My husband and I tried a recipe from the newsletter *Batteries Not Included*. In a juicer, we blend a stalk of celery and a third of a fresh pineapple. My husband drinks six ounces of the mixture every day. The celery and pineapple contain high concentrations of aspartic acid and the amino acid phenylalanine, the same ingredients used in sugar substitutes. What do you think?—G.A., Chicago, Illinois

Your recipe may not work for everyone, but it will prevent outbreaks of scurvy.

All my past lovers have told me that my semen is bitter or salty. But my current girlfriend says it doesn't taste like anything. Could it be that some women are more aware of the taste than others? After all, some people like broccoli and some don't.—R.W., Colorado Springs, Colorado

Perhaps. Researchers have documented differences in the sense of taste. In one study, scientists asked test subjects to place a bitter synthetic chemical on their tongues. A quarter of the people tasted nothing. Half said it tasted bitter. A quarter found it so bitter they retched. The last group are "supertasters"—men and women who have a large number of taste buds (as many as 1,100 per square centimeter of tongue). For a supertaster, frosting tastes too sweet, coffee is too bitter and alcohol too sharp. Supertasters don't like the feel of oil or fat on their tongues, and they dislike salty or spicy foods. Women are more likely to be supertasters—about 35 percent of Caucasian women fall into the category, compared with ten percent of white men.

Stopping the flow

As I'm about to come, my wife presses gently but firmly on the area between my balls and anus. She keeps the pressure on throughout my orgasm. This not only makes my climax feel a hundred times more intense, but she can control the rate of my ejaculation to the point where nothing comes out—very handy for cutting back on the mess. If your lady doesn't like to swallow, she can follow through with the blow job without worrying about a surprise. It's also been my experience that my recovery time is cut in half when we use this technique. My question is, does the constant pressure or the prevention of the semen from leaving pose any long-term health risks?—G.T., Rome, Georgia

The technique you describe, whereby pressure is applied to the perineum, is well-known to premature ejaculators. Some Hindu sects such as Tantrism believe that if a man climaxes without ejaculation, the semen will be drawn up the spinal cord to the brain, where it fuels superhuman powers (note to Stan Lee: Retrograde Ejaculation Man!). In reality the semen is drawn into the bladder, where it's expelled the next time you take a piss. But she doesn't have to know that.

Getting out a semen stain

What is the best way to remove a semen stain?—T.R., San Diego, California

Assuming the stain isn't a memento from some unforgettable quickie, warm water should do the trick. Semen consists of water, seminal plasma, spermatozoa and trace amounts of more than 30 other elements, but nothing that soaking or washing can't remove. Treat the stain within a few days for best results. If you prefer dry cleaning and care to be discreet, the technical term for bodily secretions is albumin (your cleaner has seen it all before). Should the ejaculate miss your garment and plop on the office floor, the Carpet and Rug Institute provides semen removal instructions at its website (carpet-rug.com) that begin: "Blot with a dry, white absorbent cloth or white paper towels. Gently scrape up semisolids with a rounded spoon. Break up solids and vacuum." You can take it from there.

Yellow semen

Sometimes when I ejaculate, my semen comes out either yellow or partly clear. At other times it contains gelatinous lumps. Should I be concerned?—C.B., Falls Church, Virginia

Semen may appear white, gray, yellow or silver, and it can be watery or thick. It also will vary from guy to guy and ejaculation to ejaculation. If you haven't had sex in a while, it may appear more yellow than usual, and certain medications also might change its color. If it has brown or red streaks, that's blood. Typically it indicates that you broke a vessel or have a minor infection. In rare cases it points to something more serious, such as prostate cancer, but you don't need to be concerned unless you see blood in every ejaculation for weeks at a time, or if you feel pain. The gelatin-like lumps you mentioned may be globules of protein and enzymes that form naturally in the prostate gland. They could indicate a mild infection, or simply that you haven't ejaculated in a while.

He's gonna blow!

An article in *Playboy* stated that the most semen recorded in one ejaculation was 2.23 teaspoons. Are you sure you didn't mean tablespoons? The last time I gave my boyfriend a hand job, he came in gushes. How would I measure his load to give him the new record? Would he win a prize?—P.H., Pittsburgh, Pennsylvania

You sound like the prize. The 2.23 teaspoons was produced by the power hitter in a fertility study of 1,300 men. The typical ejaculate measured about half a teaspoon. Until someone with a lab coat and an advanced degree agrees to measure your boyfriend's spunk, his talents must remain the stuff of legend.

I have a technique for increasing volume and distance. Here it is: (1) Whatever method you use to come, make sure it's consistent. Don't surprise your penis. (2) Keep all the promises you make to your body. For example, at the moment you feel yourself about to come during a blow job, don't pull your penis away. Come all over her face, because your penis thinks that's what you're going to do. If you don't, your body will consider you a promise breaker. (3) Use your imagination. It's easier for me to have a forceful orgasm if I have a fresh fantasy in mind. I don't have a large penis, but I'll match my ejaculations—for volume, intensity and distance—against any porn stud.— M.A., Troy, New Jersey

Your methods may provide more force, but not more volume. The only reliable way to increase the volume of your ejaculation is to hold off from having sex or masturbating for a few days. Penis size has nothing to do with how much semen you produce. And you won't have a second chance to work on your technique if you come on a woman's face without her okay.

Is my fiancée rejecting my sperm?

My fiancée and I are trying to have a child. When I ejaculate inside her and pull out, my semen spills out a few moments later. We've tried crossing her legs or holding them straight up in the air, but she still hasn't become pregnant. Could it be that my sperm doesn't react well with her body?—W.A., Philadelphia, Pennsylvania

Not at all. Backflow is normal. You are shooting hundreds of millions of sperm into the back of her vagina, but only the strongest will make it through her cervix. The oldest and weakest sperm tend to be those first out of the hatch, so they end up at the bottom of the pool of semen and are sent back. There are various notions about why men produce so much sperm in each ejaculate, but basically the little buggers are fragile, difficult to make and must complete a difficult and lengthy journey. The woman has so many defenses that trim down the number of invaders that it takes hundreds of millions of sacrifices to get just a few hundred sperm to within striking distance of the egg.

How much do sperm donors make?

What's the going rate for donating sperm?—M.H., Los Angeles, California

The standard rate is $75 a pop, and the chance to reread your favorite articles in Playboy. *But it's not easy money. At California Cryobank, based in Los Angeles, donor applicants go through an elaborate screening process. First, you must be 19 to 39 years old and college-educated. Second, you must meet the same public health standards as a blood donor, have a physical exam and answer* *numerous questions about your medical and genetic history. Third, your sperm must be able to survive being frozen and thawed. After all that, fewer than 2 percent of applicants qualify. (Technically they're paid for their time, not the sperm.) Each contributes to the bank two or three times per week for one to two years. A single woman or couple browses a catalog that lists the donors based on general characteristics such as educational level and race, selects one, then receives his samples until she becomes pregnant. If he chooses, a donor can allow the children he helps create to contact him after they turn 18.*

Does semen cause weight loss?

A friend sent me an article he found online that reads: "The secret to keeping pounds off may lie in the chemical makeup of semen. A 12-month study of 200 women showed that those who performed fellatio to completion (swallowing) gained an average of 48 percent less weight than those who did not. 'We are focusing on an alkaline substance found in semen,' said Ingrid Fleischer, a professor of science and medicine at the University of Hamburg. 'By itself, it has no effect on burning calories, but when mixed with other elements in semen, the results are staggering.'" A group of us are debating whether this could be true.—R.K., Duluth, Minnesota

Don't believe everything you read on the Internet. But pray she does.

Is semen still potent after freezing?

Let's say I collect my semen and freeze it. If my girlfriend inserts the frozen cube into her vagina, could she get pregnant?—J.H., Montgomery, Alabama

Are you being deployed? It's more likely you'll forget about the thing and get a surprise in your next drink. To preserve sperm, banks freeze it in liquid nitrogen at 196 degrees below zero. They also add a solution to prevent ice crystals from forming inside the spermatozoa.

Does swallowing affect a fetus?

I love oral sex. But now that I'm pregnant, I fear that swallowing semen will affect my fetus. A friend told me not to worry because semen is just protein. Is semen harmful in this situation?—R.T., Philadelphia, Pennsylvania

Not at all. It may even be beneficial. Research suggests that exposure to semen through intercourse (and possibly oral sex) prevents preeclampsia, a dangerous form of high blood pressure that can occur late in pregnancy. The semen can't

come from just anyone—it has to belong to the father, and exposure has to be repeated over months. Prolonged contact with the father's antigens apparently boosts the mother's immune system. That may be why one study found that first-time moms who become pregnant within the initial four months of a sexual relationship are at greater risk of preeclampsia.

What's causing this chin pimple?

I've been married about a year, and I blow my husband nearly every day. But I developed a pimple on the center of my chin that wouldn't go away. It finally cleared up when he went on a trip for a few days. Could blow jobs be giving me acne?—J.C., Bloomingdale, Indiana

You could get us in a lot of trouble with millions of teenage boys. We suspect that the pimple is caused by the excess saliva created during these regular blow jobs, for which we know of no solution that doesn't compromise the integrity of the BJ. If this were anything more serious, such as an allergic reaction to your husband's semen, your lips and tongue would probably swell. According to Dr. Jonathan Bernstein of the University of Cincinnati College of Medicine, who has studied semen allergies, the most serious involve burning, itching, blisters, congestion, shortness of breath, dizziness, nausea, diarrhea and loss of consciousness. It's possible, he says, that some women are reacting not to semen but to foods or drugs passed through their partner's body. Some women have also had immunotherapy with proteins isolated from their lover's seminal plasma. Another solution, less popular, is to change partners, although even that doesn't always work.

SEX TOYS

Let's get buzzed.

Choosing a vibrator

Can you recommend a good vibrator?—G.B., Phoenix, Arizona

Besides the washing machine? Every woman (and man) is different, so we can tell you only what sells well at shops such as Babeland (800-658-9119 or babeland.com). We've written about the top three before: the workhorse Hitachi Magic Wand, the classic Rabbit Habit and the discreet Pocket Rocket. Innovative products include a vibrator charged by the sun; the Petal Ring, which is designed to stimulate both partners at the same time; a vibe you can attach to your laptop's USB port; and the Audi-Oh Butterfly, which vibrates to sounds such as voices or music. In general, vibrators are becoming smaller and more powerful, largely because many now run on watch batteries. The trendiest new toys are vibrating objets d'art sold by the London boutique Myla (myla.com). Japanese ceramic artist Mari-Ruth Oda created Pebble ($190) and furniture designer Tom Dixon created Bone ($380).

Sex toys at the airport

Is it safe to carry sex toys through airport security?—M.T., San Francisco, California

Sure. But avoid delays and in-flight temptations by transporting the toys in your checked luggage. Certain toys, such as handcuffs or strap-on dildos, might raise suspicions, especially if you wear them. And take a lesson from the passenger who caused a bomb scare in Springfield, Massachusetts. Police evacuated the city's train station after Amtrak personnel reported an unusual sound coming from a checked suitcase. It turned out to be a vibrator that kicked on after being jostled. Our advice: Remove the batteries.

Vibrating panties

Nothing irritates me more than when someone's cell phone rings in the middle of a meeting, or in a restaurant. So I bought one with a vibrating device. That's when the lightbulb went on over my head. I bought a beat-up cell for ten bucks, set up an account for it and ran home. I hooked up the signal receiver to a pair of vibrating eggs that my girlfriend places in her vagina. The whole thing is powered by a small battery pack that tucks neatly in the small of her back. She tells me she forgets she's wearing it, but that may be because she has started wearing it all the time. I call her whenever the mood strikes, perhaps while she's sitting at her desk, or talking to her girlfriends at the watercooler, or briefing her boss. I let it ring once, as a tease, or three times, to make a point, or for 15 minutes, to drive her nuts. She can't answer the phone, so she's at my mercy. My favorite trick is to call her ground line, ask her some insipid question to lull her into a long answer, then dial her "privates" number. The change in her tone of voice is priceless. Now she goes limp at the sound of any phone ringing. I'd still like to get a remote vibrator, something that can be activated quickly at a party, from my pocket, without pulling the phone out every time. Maybe I could build it, but I don't know enough about electronics. Does anyone make this sort of product?—V.K., Ottawa, Ontario

If you build it, she will come. There are remote-controlled panties and vibrating eggs, but the reviews we've heard haven't been enthusiastic. Because the panties are one-size-fits-all, their strategically placed nub often shifts out of position. The woman could keep it snug with tight pants, but then she may not need any vibration to get off. The setup is usually too noisy for anywhere but the dance floor, and it won't have the range you expect. Plus, each pair costs about $100. Still game? Order through reputable outlets such as the Xandria Collection (xandria.com or 800-242-2823). We'd tell you more, but someone just paged our testicles.

Cyberskin

I have seen catalogs that offer sex toys made of cyberskin. Supposedly it feels like the real thing. I've read elsewhere that it's hard to keep clean, that bits of it can break off and that it should be cleaned with talc, which has been linked to cervical cancer. What do you know about it?—M.C., Boston, Massachusetts

The sex toy store Good Vibrations (goodvibes.com or 800-289-8483) sent us a dildo and a fake vagina (positioned at the end of a 10-inch cylinder called the Fleshlight) so we could handle the stuff ourselves. We found it to be soft, pliable and clammy. It also easily picked up smudges, was difficult to clean and looked like bits could flake off. Yet we can understand the appeal—every guy who stopped by our office stuck his finger inside, then examined his digit as if he felt it should be wet.

Good Vibrations recommends using cornstarch rather than talc to preserve the surface of the toys, and to rinse it off before penetration. However, cyberskin becomes stickier after being washed, which attracts more grunge. You could slide condoms over the toys before you use them, but that certainly doesn't help the fantasy. Despite these drawbacks, the Fleshlight sells well enough, and you also can find butt plugs and even fake mouths that are made of cyberskin. The question is, does anyone buy them a second time?

I thought that your response was too negative and might discourage people from enjoying these wonderfully textured toys. My husband and I have found that as long as the cyberskin is wiped down with a cleaner such as Safe Suds, dried well and dusted with cornstarch every time the toy is used, it stays in great shape. As for the "clamminess" you found so disconcerting, a touch of lube makes that go away.—V.T., Phoenix, Arizona

Am I just her vibrator holder?

My wife has taken to calling me her "vibrator holder." I think she may be kidding, but I can't tell. Should I be offended?—P.M., Milwaukee, Wisconsin

That depends on when you're holding it. If your wife considers you a vibrator attachment, that's a problem. If you can touch her vibrator only when it's unplugged, you're in trouble. If you're in the next room cleaning her vibrator while she fucks the neighbor, call a professional. However, if she's saying in a slightly awkward way that her vibrator feels best under your control, you're ahead of the game. Ask for specifics: Would she prefer a holder or a handler? As Joani Blank points out in Good Vibrations: The Complete Guide to Vibrators, *it's difficult for even the most diligent lover to please a woman with a vibrator as well as she can herself. That's why some women enjoy having their partners hold the vibrator still while they move against it. Or they take the reins as they near orgasm to ensure optimum pleasure. Since vibrators are unisex, perhaps your wife could demonstrate her holding and handling techniques on your body. There's nothing more wonderful than two vibrator holders in love.*

Can't see, can't move

My girlfriend lets me tie her to the bedpost but only if she is blindfolded. Is she ashamed, or is there something extra-erotic about this?—R.P., Reno, Nevada

This is supersize erotic. Gather a sexy tool kit that includes feathers, velvet gloves, massage oil, her favorite vibrator (plus a new one to surprise her), dildos in three sizes, a book or CD of erotic stories, ice, a hand warmer, chocolate (to reward her), a small butt plug and extra lube. And take your sweet time.

The best sex toy ever

I'm 19 and my girlfriend is 18. Before we have sex for the first time, should I get some sort of lube? Which do you recommend?—G.G., Indianapolis, Indiana

You're already thinking like a great lover. Many guys are threatened by lube—the world's most underrated sex toy—because they feel inadequate if they can't get their partners sufficiently wet. But many factors affect how much a woman lubricates, including her menstrual cycle, pregnancy, diet, dehydration, exercise and stress levels. What you need (and what most drugstores carry) are water-based lubes such as Astroglide, ForPlay, ID and Wet. Some people prefer silicone-based lubes such as Eros or Wet Platinum, which stay slick longer and don't get sticky. However, they don't clean up as easily. (One company sells a substance you can use to "degrease" after sex with silicone lube.) Never use vegetable oil, Vaseline, cooking oil, baby oil, lotion or moisturizer. These substances break down latex condoms and are difficult to wash out. Plus, they don't stay wet.

Fair warning

My vibrator has this warning: "Do not use on unexplained calf or abdominal pain." Why is that?—F.F., Las Vegas, Nevada

Because that unexplained pain could be from a blood clot, and shaking it loose might send it toward the heart or brain. The notice appears on most vibrators and massagers sold in the U.S., courtesy of Underwriters Laboratories, which tests products and advises companies on consumer warnings. You'll see other vibrators labeled "for novelty purposes only," which means they don't claim to do anything but entertain you. When you read as many vibrator instruction manuals as we do, you stumble across some peculiar admonishments. Wahl Corp., for example, makes massagers that are sold by sex-toy stores as vibrators. The Wahl family would prefer that their products not touch unauthorized body parts, so it warns customers, "Do not use massager on genital areas." A spokesman says the company is concerned any time electric appliances are placed near moisture but admits the warning is included for moral reasons. The Wahls don't approve! That makes it even naughtier. The Advisor now uses Wahl massagers for all his personal pleasure needs.

Ring around the cock

While stroking me during foreplay, my girlfriend slid a large rubber band over my cock and behind my balls. After a few more strokes and licks, she had given me the biggest, hardest erection of my life, and it seemed to last forever. My girlfriend loves this trick because it prolongs her pleasure. I am curious as to what it's called and why it works. Are there any side effects?—J.A., Austin, Texas

Your girlfriend improvised a cock ring. It works by restricting blood flow from the penis, which can heighten sensation and provide staying power. But a ring may cause serious damage if worn for more than half an hour (don't fall asleep with it on). Avoid using metal or latex rings, which can only be put on or taken off when you're flaccid. If the metal ring starts to pinch after you're hard, you can either wait for your erection to subside (ice might help) or visit the emergency room. Latex rings are safer because you can snip them off, although that means placing a sharp point perilously close to your penis. But we prefer leather rings that fasten with snaps or Velcro. The deluxe models have straps that separate the testicles or stretch each ball downward, if that's your thing, and/or D-rings to which your lover can attach a leash. Rough, rough.

Glass dildos

One of my girlfriends owns an expensive glass dildo she says is made of the same material as the Pyrex bowls in her kitchen. She raves about it and even offered to lend it to me. I'm afraid it will break. Have you ever heard of these toys?—M.D., Orlando, Florida

They were introduced by two guys in Florida—Steve Ritchie was a yacht captain and Dave Reynard owns an answering service. The partners had already patented two sex toys, the Aqua Vulva and the Whip Lite, when Reynard and a girlfriend discovered the illicit pleasures of a glass martini mixer. The men realized that inserting a glass stick into orifices wasn't safe for the masses, so they investigated making dildos from borosilicate glass, better known as Pyrex or, in this case, Boronex. The advantage of borosilicate glass over rubber or latex, they say, is that you can drop it in hot water for a few minutes and it will stay warm for 10 to 15 minutes of sex play. Glass also feels smoother and, because it's nonporous, requires only a few drops of lube. Finally, it's easy to clean. Each toy is handmade, which accounts for the higher prices (most cost between $100 and $200). Get info online at asstroknots.com, or phone 800-292-9173 for a catalog. If *you invest in a glass dildo, keep in mind that it's not the best toy for sex in the driveway. But you won't have any problems in bed.*

Please advise your readers of a potential hazard with dildos made of borosilicate glass. I learned the hard way that kitchenware made from this material can explode if it has even a hairline crack.—V.E., Los Angeles, California

That's unlikely to happen with a dildo unless you expose it to extreme changes in temperature, which is not recommended or practical. While toy companies advertise that the products retain heat and cold, most people find that room temperature works best. (The glass will feel cool because of higher body heat.) Lately the number of sites selling inexpensive glass toys has risen, in part because of a crackdown on bong shops, which has led to a glut of unemployed glass-bong craftsmen. John Sanchez of the Original Glass Dildo Company suggests that anyone considering a glass dildo keep it simple. While most guys order 12-inchers with all the trimmings because they think that's what their partners want, most women buy clear, smooth eight-inchers. Sanchez suggests going to 10 so you have a few inches to hold on to.

THE SINGLE LIFE

Looking for love.

Where to find single women

I have lived in Silicon Valley for the past 10 years. I'm 40, never married, no children, average height and in great shape. I'm interested in art and music and participate in all kinds of sports. I can cook, iron and take care of myself. The *San Jose Mercury News* recently published data that showed Silicon Valley having among the worst ratios of eligible men to women in the country, including some parts of Alaska. The region is filled with single male engineers. The women I meet don't feel the need to keep a date (two have canceled on me in just the past week), because they sense it's no big deal; they can go to any party and be outnumbered three to one by guys. I've decided the best thing to do is move. Can you find me a list of cities that have the best ratios of women to single men?—W.T., Palo Alto, California

You cook? You iron? Find another town, man, and now. The women are waiting. In the meantime, look on the bright side: You don't live in the absolute worst place to meet women. That would be Jacksonville, North Carolina, home to two Marine bases. (If any single females are planning moves to Jacksonville or Silicon Valley, consider the lament of one woman who lives in the latter: "There are lots of guys, but they're all the same guy.") To send you in the right direction, we hired the market research firm Claritas to identify the cities with the most available women. It's an inexact science. The standard census data on unmarried, separated, divorced and widowed females include anyone aged 15 or older, which includes teenagers and retirees alike. The figures also can't be divided more precisely by age, though we did cross-reference the data against local populations of all women aged 18 to 40. Finally, the figures don't account for prisons, nursing homes, lesbians, serious boyfriends or the Playboy Mansion. For you stats majors, here's more detail (the rest of you can jump to the list below): We first ranked each of the country's 318 metropolitan statistical areas (MSA) by its percentage of excess single women of all ages—that is, he compared the number of single women to the number of single men and determined what percentage of the single females would still be available if everyone paired up. Second, we weighted the results by ranking each MSA by its number of excess women, single or married, aged 18 to 40. We further weighted the rankings by the percentage of each MSA's total population made up of women aged 18 to 40. Finally, we added the three rankings together. Thus, an MSA that ranked 2nd in the first list, 15th in the second list and 10th in the third list ranked 27th overall.

ALL CITIES:

 1. *Hattiesburg, Mississippi*
 2. *Jackson, Mississippi*
 3. *Jackson, Tennessee*
 4. *Bloomington-Normal, Illinois*
 5. *Waterloo-Cedar Falls, Iowa*
 6. *Monroe, Louisiana*
 7. *Rocky Mount, North Carolina*
 8. *Muncie, Indiana*
 9. *Springfield, Massachusetts*
 10. *Greenville, North Carolina*
 11. *Des Moines, Iowa*
 12. *Lexington, Kentucky*
 13. *Florence, South Carolina*
 14. *Laredo, Texas*
 15. *Richmond-Petersburg, Virginia*
 16. *Birmingham, Alabama*
 17. *Lynchburg, Virginia*
 18. *LaCrosse, Wisconsin*
 19. *Tallahassee, Florida*
 20. *Athens, Georgia*

MIDSIZE METRO *(500,000 to 1 million):*

 9. *Springfield, Massachusetts*
 15. *Richmond-Petersburg, Virginia*
 16. *Birmingham, Alabama*
 26. *Baton Rouge, Louisiana*
 27. *Little Rock, Arkansas*
 29. *Toledo, Ohio*

MAJOR METRO (1 million plus):
24. *New York*
28. *Memphis*
32. *Greensboro/Winston-Salem*
47. *Louisville*
49. *Raleigh-Durham/Chapel Hill*
52. *Nashville*
57. *Indianapolis*

Support the troops

I thought you'd like to know about my organization, Operation Take One for the Country. I created it to encourage single women to hang out at bars and clubs frequented by single servicemen, especially those about to go into harm's way. We aren't arranging charity sex or suggesting that women pursue dangerous behavior in the name of patriotism. We're just saying they should give single servicemen a chance; they're worth knowing.—K.M., Tequesta, Florida

Having a woman say "I want you" is more fun than hearing it from Uncle Sam.

America has a long tradition of this sort of behavior. According to *No Magic Bullet: A Social History of Venereal Disease in the United States Since 1880*, during World War II doctors and social workers frequently commented that the professional prostitute had given way to the patriotic prostitute, or charity girl. One social worker wrote, "Girls idealize the soldier, and many feel that nothing is wrong when done for him. One girl said she had never sold herself to a civilian but felt she was doing her bit when she had been with eight soldiers in a night." These women were also known as amateur girls, khaki-wackies, victory girls and good-time Charlottes.—J.S., Los Angeles, California

Why didn't they mention this in history class? We would have gotten better grades.

Is there any way to be taller?

One thing that limits the number of beautiful, intelligent, sexy women I can date is my height. It's intimidating to be the shortest guy around, and because I'm 5'5", that's usually the case in almost every bar or club. Are there any viable solutions to growing taller once you've reached your 20s? I've seen suggestions on the Internet that range from doing stretching exercises for months to injecting human growth hormone to visiting an endocrinologist.—A.K., Washington, D.C.

Besides lifts in your shoes or radical surgery, there's nothing to be done. The growth plates have fused in nearly every person by the age of 20. We suggest you accept your height as one of your many unique qualities and spend your energy on something more productive, such as learning 100 good short-guy jokes. You should know, as a matter of routine, some of the shorter men who did more for the world than the 10 tallest guys you know: Mozart, Beethoven, Gandhi, Churchill, Hitchcock (Napoleon, at 5'7", was closer to today's average of 5'8"). There are drastic measures you can take if you're completely nuts. Years ago we wrote about a guy who was two inches shorter than the height requirement to become a Detroit cop. He slept in traction for several months but managed only to add an inch and a half. In 2000 a 4'9" British teenager hoping to grow tall enough to be a flight attendant had doctors break both her femurs. She spent four weeks in traction and gained five inches, one inch shy of the requirement. The point is, you could go through all that, be released from the hospital in pain and in debt, and then fall in love with a woman who's 6'1". Taller guys, you should realize, have their own complaints—they tower over most women, slam their heads on unfamiliar doorways, can't hear what's being said at parties and look awkward dancing.

Writing an effective personal ad

Do you have any suggestions for writing a personal ad? I don't want to spend a lot of money and not get any responses.—N.T., New York, New York

A well-written personal ad will prevent you from being swamped with inappropriate responses, which can be nearly as annoying as not getting any. Describe the traits that make you stand out in a crowd. Realize that every guy in the personals is affectionate and sensual and enjoys intelligent conversation. They're also fit, handsome, look younger than their age, love sunsets and have a refined sense of humor and superior listening skills. Dig a little deeper. Instead of "going to the movies" as a pastime, say that you "love comedies and Westerns" (if that's true, of course—don't set yourself up for a fall). Instead of "dry sense of humor," say that you "can't wait for Larry Sanders to interview Spinal Tap." Read other personals and mark those that stand out. What they'll have in common are details that together form an enticing, well-rounded grab for attention. Whatever else you do, don't use negative words such as lonely*: How much fun can a lonely guy be? And don't include "scanning the personals" among your hobbies.*

I put an ad in an alternative weekly to meet some new people, and every guy I have had lunch with so far has been a creep—about half are married and just looking for quick sex. Can you help?—H.T., Atlanta, Georgia

Personal ads attract mostly misfits and cheaters, so it becomes a numbers game. Keep at it and you'll get better at screening prospects. For the big picture, pick up a copy of My 1000 Americans *by Rochelle Morton. (Guys should read it as a primer on how not to act.) Morton placed an ad and shared a meal with every third guy who responded to it. She managed to meet several dozen nice guys, but mostly her book is a catalog of creeps. The most memorable was a married guy who brought along his four-year-old daughter. When he went to the rest room, the girl said her daddy wanted Morton to touch his pee-pee. When the guy returned, the girl blurted, "I said it, Daddy," while he feigned ignorance. Morton says that if she had to do it again, she would be more specific in her ad and initial conversations about what kind of guy she hoped to meet. "If you go into the process with low expectations, you won't be disappointed," she writes. "And you might hit the jackpot."*

"Personal ads attract mostly misfits and cheaters"? That's a gross exaggeration based solely on Rochelle Morton's disappointing experiences. When I started responding to ads after my marriage ended, I was surprised by the number of young divorced women who were searching for companionship. I didn't meet a single creep, misfit or cheater. When I placed an ad, I had seven responses within hours. I stopped at number three, and we married two years later. Ads work if you know what you want.—J.D., Mount Vernon, Virginia

The lesson of Morton's experience is to be specific. She used the phrase "fun times" in her ad, which most guys took as code for casual sex. That and her "delete-delete-meet" selection process (to ensure a random sample) may explain the high number of misfits.

She's gorgeous, but her breasts are too small

This woman and I have been on three dates, and the sparks aren't exactly flying. I wonder if I would be more interested if she had larger breasts. That thought upsets me. I mean, how shallow can you get? How would I feel if she said to me, "I'm sorry, I'm not interested in you because your penis is too small"?—D.S., Minneapolis, Minnesota

Don't blame the breasts. We received a letter from a reader who insisted he broke up with his girlfriend because her forehead was too big, as if that were the reason. If this woman had blown you away with her charm and personality, her breasts would have been the perfect size.

Libido overload

I am an adult-film producer having trouble finding a girlfriend. I'd like to meet a woman who is not in the industry, because I would get jealous if my girlfriend had sex with another guy, even on camera. I know that sounds hypocritical. I've been with nearly 100 women, all of them one-night stands. Sometimes it's difficult for me to enjoy sex or stay hard because I look at porn and interview models for 100 to 120 hours a week. You know how it is when you come home and see something that reminds you of work and you get annoyed? That's my situation. Any advice?—C.T., Philadelphia, Pennsylvania

You're suffering from libido overload. Porn is fun, but an overdose can make unscripted sex with an actual human being seem disappointing. Producer Adam Glasser, a.k.a. Seymore Butts, had similar problems meeting women, which Showtime documented during the first season of Family Business. *Most of the women he met through online dating sites found his work interesting but not enamoring. (Glasser eventually began dating one of his ex-assistants, who became a performer.) There are women who won't have a problem with your job, but it may take some effort to find them. It may also be wise to be discreet ("I work in video production") until you have a chance to make an impression. One thing is certain: You won't meet anyone outside the business if you're immersed in it 17 hours a day. You also won't be very interesting at dinner. Stop working on weekends and find a hobby that doesn't involve genitalia.*

Dating models

Do you have any strategies for picking up models? I don't want any of your usual coy or sarcastic bullshit, either. I need some practical advice.—G.T., New York, New York

You're making this difficult. We pick up models the same way we approach any beautiful woman—by introducing ourselves. But there are some rules. First, don't compliment her on her beauty. She hears that all day, along with dimwitted

pickup lines. It's also painfully obvious, the equivalent of informing a tall person, "You're tall." Her beauty is nothing she has any control over, so it's hard to take as a compliment. Instead, comment on something she chose, such as her shoes, which are usually the last thing a guy notices. It sounds corny but it works. If you happen to know something about shoes, all the better. Or comment on her jewelry, such as a ring. Don't be overbearing, which translates as desperate, but also don't look uninterested in some weird attempt to be mysterious. Make eye contact; let her take you in. Many guys have trouble with this, because uncommon beauty can be intimidating, and you look like you aren't listening or lack confidence. It almost goes without saying that you should be well dressed and well groomed. Being handsome is a plus, but if that's not an option, try to be rich. If you can, catch her when she doesn't have her war paint on—you may find her vastly more approachable. If you land a date, keep the physical stuff to a minimum initially, but make it clear that you like her. One of the great fears among models is that they're being set up as a trophy fuck. Ask for her e-mail address rather than a phone number, which allows you to show your hipness but also gives her some space. But then don't bombard her with bullshit messages like some cyberstalker. By the way, this advice applies to any woman you find attractive, not just the ones who appear in magazines.

What are the odds that a guy will date a supermodel?—G.P., Canton, Ohio

We'd settle for a regular model. Gregory Baer tackles this question in his book Life: The Odds. *Assuming that the top 25 supermodels date five American guys a year and that the average guy spends 10 years searching, your odds are 88,000 to one. You improve your chances dramatically—to about 10 to one—if you're in New York City or Paris and are an actor, musician, athlete, photographer, producer, director or male model. Using supermarket tabloids, Baer tracked the dating patterns of 44 supermodels and found that these groups constitute 82 percent of supermodel boyfriends. The other 18 percent are nearly all lawyers, doctors or other wealthy individuals.*

Tripped up

The other night at the bar, two of my friends pointed out a gorgeous woman. After she and I made eye contact, off I went, plowing through the crowd to introduce myself. As I approached, I put my latest pickup strategy into action: I pretended to trip, fell to the floor in front of her, then feigned embarrassment and let her feel sorry for me as I scrambled to my feet. It worked like a charm. The problem is my friends and I often go to the same bar, so before long my "falling for you" move will be well known. Can you suggest any techniques?—T.L.,Roanoke, Virginia

Wow, that's desperate. Granted, your method makes an impression. As a general rule, however, "klutz" should never be the first thought to cross a woman's mind when meeting you. Women are more impressed by confidence than cons.

He likes "older" women

I'm 18 years old and attracted to older women, like 30. Is this normal?—T.D., Omaha, Nebraska

First, never tell a 30-year-old you consider her an older woman. Second, act now: When you hit 30, you'll be fantasizing about 18-year-olds.

Surprise package

Recently I met an amazing Asian woman at a bar. For the next few weeks we saw each other almost every day. The extent of our physical contact was my fondling her breasts and her giving me head. One day, after it started to get intense, she shut down and asked me to leave. She called me later to tell me she "wasn't a real girl." She said she hadn't told me sooner or in person because she feared my reaction. I know most guys would walk away, but I'm crazy about her. (She acts, talks and dresses like a woman, so it's hard for me to think of her otherwise.) I'm not gay, but I'm in love with a man. What the hell should I do? If it were only physical, it would be an easy decision.—M.K., Indianapolis, Indiana

Love is a mysterious thing. Gender can be too. Since you don't have an immediate urge to flee, continue the conversation. If labels are a concern, you're bisexual.

The smell of success

I had a blind date that went so well, we ended up having sex. But when I went down on her, I was bothered to discover that she had perfumed her pubic area. This woman has many of the qualities I look for in a potential spouse, but the fact that she was ready to go to bed with a stranger has me wondering. Am I being a prude, or do I have a legitimate concern?—R.H., Prunedale, California

We love a woman who is prepared for any circumstance, although who's to say she doesn't perfume herself all the time? Regardless, you were no longer a stranger when she went to bed with you.

He wrote to ask if he's a prude, but he is actually a hypocrite. He too was ready and willing to go to bed on the first date.—B.A., Fairview, Oregon

Some guys are never happy. I bet if she had refused sex, he would have asked how to get a blind date into bed. Besides, most women do not spray perfume on their genitals, as that would taste nasty for the guy. Instead, they dot it above the kissable zone.—A.M., Monrovia, California

I wonder what his date thought when she learned he had washed his balls.— P.Y., Metairie, Louisiana

For her sake we hope he did.

Are some guys hopeless?

A few months ago you published a letter from a guy who couldn't get a date. Another reader said the guy's problem must be his choice of ladies. That's not it. Having listened to hundreds of women over the years, I've concluded that there are simply men nobody wants. Women call these guys jerks, creeps, nerds, losers, dorks, dweebs, etc. If it's not his lack of money, he is either too short or losing his hair. The world's zeros need to leave women alone. The Advisor has pioneered other social issues—pioneer this one. Your female readers will thank you.—R.S., Garland, Texas

We've heard from thousands of women over the years, and we don't share your cynical view of their outlooks or motivations. Many say that short, bald guys are better companions, and more attentive in bed. Besides, if there weren't any jerks, creeps, nerds, losers, dorks or dweebs, we wouldn't look so good by comparison. Let's keep them circulating.

So the Advisor believes that "many" women prefer short, bald guys? As a short, fat, bald guy, I can say you're dead wrong. Women are as shallow as men when it comes to dating. Their rules are more numerous than those used by men— but no deeper. Both sexes are driven by evolutionary biology: Good-looking

= healthy = good mate. Admit it: Losers exist. I know. I'm one of them—and you have no idea how it hurts to write that.—V.P., Knoxville, Tennessee

Tommy Lee Jones had a line in the movie Jackson County Jail *that applies here. He said, "I'll play what's dealt." You can't be taller, and you can't get your hair back, but you can lose weight—and the chip on your shoulder. We know some hefty guys who do okay, but they possess rare charm. Without that, you have to work harder. Most guys talk their way into women's lives rather than leading with their perfect chins. Social skills don't come naturally for everyone, but awkward and shy people still manage to reproduce. A major obstacle for many men is their belief that having a girlfriend or spouse will solve larger problems. If you're searching for a savior, you'll judge every woman who crosses your path solely on whether she can change your life. That puts incredible pressure on the encounters, and it changes how you are perceived.*

The reader who claimed that "losers, creeps and dorks" should leave women alone is right. It's important for a man to recognize his limitations. I suggest other losers do what I've done for the past few years—pay for sex. First, you won't have the hassle of dating. Second, by the time you've spent the money, time and effort to take out a woman who may or may not sleep with you, you've spent as much as you would in a massage parlor or with an escort. There are risks, but sex is always a gamble. You may not go on any dates, but at least you'll get laid.—T.B., Sausalito, California

It's a rare man who can survive on sex alone.

I've worked in a number of bars and I have noticed a lot of couples who I thought would never go for each other—a gorgeous redhead with a short, fat, balding guy; an overweight woman with a petite guy. I'm 6'2" and 240 pounds, and I've dated women as short as 5'1" and as tall as 6'3". In my experience, when you interact with women as you would with your friends, they respond in kind. Striking up a conversation is the hard part, because it can feel artificial. That's why you go out with a group.—M.P., Sandusky, Ohio

A reader wrote to say that no woman would go out with him because good-looking = healthy = good mate. Bullshit. When I was a teenager I broke my neck and ended up a quadriplegic. Twenty years later, I've had many lovers and am now happily married. I have little upper-body movement and no feeling below my nipples. According to this guy's flawed theory, I should be sitting home watching *Baywatch* reruns.—D.D., Winnipeg, Manitoba

It's amazing what a guy with sensitive nipples can accomplish.

A word to the wise for losers, dorks and single old guys: Writing to the Advisor about your problems with women is like a chicken asking a fox about getting on with the wolves. What you need are tips from the trenches. Take your butt offshore and leave the local beauties to feed on themselves. Even an old guy can do well in the Dominican Republic. Or try Asia. I have traveled there for years and can tell you that the nicest women in the world are waiting to welcome you into their hearts. Being a dork is not something you can do much about. Your local psychiatrist, with his eyes on your wallet, may disagree, but for now, genetics are beyond your control. Behavior patterns are formed early in life and personality disorders are largely untreatable. Stay in the game. You become a loser only if you stop playing.—N.B., St. George, Utah

You make some good points, but let's not kid ourselves about why impoverished women in Cuba, the Dominican Republic or Asia might "open their hearts" to relatively rich but dorky Americans.

I'd rather have a girlfriend
I thought I'd be alone for the rest of my life and had sort of accepted that. But on a lark I placed a personal ad online. A few months passed before I received a response—and she had replied to the wrong ad. I'm 43 and she's 21, but we chatted and then met. She said right away she didn't find me attractive, but we stayed friendly. Two weeks later she invited me over. Soon I was spending two or three nights a week at her place. One night she was busy but said, "How about my friend Amy? She's not getting any." So she called Amy, who called me, and within an hour I was fucking this 19-year-old. Then Amy told me about another friend, who's 22. Same thing happened. Now they've agreed not to share me with anyone. I don't mind, except I placed the ad to find a girlfriend. I try to meet people, but when 11 p.m. rolls around I'm knocking on one of these three doors. This is the most sex I've ever gotten, and it's high quality, but I want something more.—M.H., Chicago, Illinois

It's hard enough to give up one night a week of great sex, but seven? We couldn't do it. You could walk away and see who follows; perhaps you already have a girlfriend and neither of you realizes it. But don't expect that to happen. Instead we

suggest you restrict your booty calls to weeknights so you can devote at least weekends to your search.

I'd let her blow me

Once or twice a week my friends and I go out to lunch. Sometimes we'll see a girl and somebody will say, "I wouldn't sleep with her, but I'd let her blow me." Do women say the same sort of thing about guys? That is, do they see an attractive man and say, "I wouldn't sleep with him, but I would let him go down on me"? Please survey some women and let us know the results.—T.W., Raleigh, North Carolina

What women say is, "I wouldn't sleep with him, but I'd let him spend money on me." (Ouch.) In general, women don't differentiate between oral sex and intercourse—each is considered equally intimate—so a man judged worthy of cunnilingus is suitable for fucking by default. Marcelle Karp of Bust *magazine says the women she hangs with might announce something like, "I wish I had 15 minutes alone with that" when a beautiful guy walks by, but they rarely get more specific. Nikol Lohr of DisgruntledHousewife.com says her friends have been known to say, "I wouldn't want to hang out with him, but I'd fuck him." Hearing that, we feel objectified—and disappointed we haven't met Nikol's friends.*

Do nice guys finish last?

Nice guys finish last, as always. I went out with this girl a couple of times, and things got steamy. I sent her a letter to tell her how I felt: "We have known each other for only a little while, but already I feel like we've been together for a lifetime. When I am with you, everything feels right. I never thought that I could be so happy with someone. Do you know how special you are to me? Do you think other people notice how intense our feelings are? Do you think other people feel like we do? I thought this sort of love happened only in great fiction or the movies. I can't believe how lucky I am to have found you. Give me a call. I would love to hear your voice." When I called later she yelled that she needed some sleep and hung up on me! I understand that when a nice guy comes along many women are in a new situation and act immature. But I'm tired of being nice. I'm tired of being the shoulder to cry on. I'm tired of being the one who cares. Is this why nice guys give up and become players?—K.M., Southbury, Connecticut

Yeah, yeah, you're a martyr. We hear this complaint every month from guys who face rejection, but it's too easy. The fact of the matter is, your letter was horseshit. It's no wonder this woman needed sleep—it exhausted us, too. There's no way you can have such deep feelings for someone after a few dates, or maybe ever. Put the Hollywood ending aside and concentrate on building the friendship. That's the basis of any solid relationship.

How many women are virgins?

I am a 28-year-old Christian. When I was 15, I made a vow to save myself for my future wife. I've had the chance to lose my virginity several times and always resisted. As I get older, I'm meeting more and more women who are sexually experienced, and I'm reluctant to ask them out because I fear they will laugh at me. I wish I had never made my promise, although I know in theory that it will lead to a lasting marriage. Do you know how many women have opted to do the same for their future mates?—D.C., Dallas, Texas

Have you considered that your future wife may not want your virginity? Instead, she may prefer a guy who has thrived in and survived a few intimate relationships. We're not saying you should rush out and get laid, but you made this vow before you were emotionally or sexually mature—a true leap of faith about how your life would unfold. According to one study, 16.5 percent of men and 30 percent of women remain virgins until they marry. Other research suggests that these men and women have much lower rates of separation and divorce, but anyone who can abstain in our sexually saturated culture easily has the discipline for a long-term relationship. Don't be ashamed to explain, if necessary, why you're celibate. Your dates will either respect your convictions or become incredibly turned on, but we doubt they'll laugh. If a wily lover manages to seduce you, keep in mind that your innocence had a long life, and that you'll still have a great marriage—maybe with her.

I'll marry her, but no vows

My girlfriend of five years has been hinting that she would like to get married. I told her that sounds good to me except that I do not want to take a vow of monogamy. Although I have been faithful to this point, I certainly have been tempted. Vowing that I would never cheat would be a stretch. She says that if she can do it, I can do it. My feeling is that a vow of monogamy would be one more pressure to deal with in our relationship. I would appreciate any suggestions.—D.G., Wyndmoor, Pennsylvania

Are you kidding? Quit wasting her time.

Can you seduce a woman through hypnosis?

I've heard that you can seduce women through hypnosis. I know people stop smoking or lose weight through hypnosis, so maybe there's something to this. Are these techniques difficult to learn?—P.R., San Juan, Puerto Rico

If you have the idea that you can get a woman at a bar to look deep into your eyes, and then deep into your pants, come back to reality. Despite every man's fantasies, a woman who is hypnotized isn't going to do anything against her will, though she may show fewer inhibitions (You also can achieve this with a shoulder rub.) Your subject has to be willing and able to be hypnotized, and it takes practice to pull it off. In his guide Look Into My Eyes: How to Use Hypnosis to Bring Out the Best in Your Sex Life, *Peter Masters suggests that a couple use hypnosis as they would any sex toy. The book includes the basics of inducing a trance and supplies various sexual scripts. But Masters also presents hypnosis as a way to experiment with "erotic control." For example, he suggests that you instruct your girlfriend during a trance that she will feel aroused whenever you say, "You look sexy in that outfit." You can imagine the possibilities.*

Going to the movies

On our fifth date I took my girlfriend to dinner. During the meal I caught myself quoting Mickey Rourke's character in one of my favorite movies, *9 1/2 Weeks*. My girlfriend had never seen the movie and didn't get the reference. After dinner, we took a cab to the beach. As we fooled around in the back, I found myself quoting from the movie again. I meant no harm and it felt good to role-play. Letting her in on it would have made it feel fake. Once we hit the beach, things got heavy. I started talking filthy to her—mostly a mishmash of lines from the film—and she began to strip. We fucked like crazy. By the end of the evening I must have recited half the movie's dialogue. Yesterday she ordered a copy of *9 1/2 Weeks* on DVD. She says she wants to watch it together on my birthday because I had mentioned how sexy it was. Shit. Should I confess? I don't want her to think I'm a creep.—D.J., Indianapolis, Indiana

Your girlfriend will feel cheated when she finds out. So we worked out a plan in which you set your DVD player to French language with Spanish subtitles, then insist the disc is defective. However, some of the women in the office pointed out that this would work only if your girlfriend were a nitwit. Instead, they suggested that you give her numerous hardcore erotic experiences in which you talk filthy in your own words. She'll still recognize the dialogue when you sit down to watch the film, but she'll be more forgiving if she knows you can do it on your own. If she insists on an explanation, tell her no one had ever inspired you to talk dirty before, and you fell back on the familiar.

She touched her necklace. Does she want me?

I met a gorgeous woman at a party. As we spoke, I noticed her touching her neck in the area where her blouse button would be. Any idea what that meant?—R.T., San Diego, California

She wanted you. Or she lost her necklace. Hard to say. Men tend to overestimate women's interest, especially if they aren't getting laid. Princeton researchers asked 285 adults to interpret everyday behavior for signs of horniness. They found that "basically, if a woman goes out and stands anywhere, some men are going to think she's fairly interested in sex right now." Women, meanwhile, "just about always get the sexual intent of men right." (Well, how hard is that?) For more insight, we turned to an expert in reading body language, Mike Caro of PlanetPoker.com. Years ago he and another poker champ, Doyle Brunson, developed a system they call quick bonding. "You need to come across as somewhat mysterious in an intellectual way," Caro explains. "Don't say too much at first, but convey the impression that there might be a lot for her to peel away and discover. For example, if I were to notice a woman touching her neck, I would walk past slowly, catch her eye, smile sincerely and say confidently, 'Don't worry about it. It's fine.' There's a good chance your cryptic, caring, conspiratorial remark will connect in some way to her subconscious gesture, and you'll get credit for having perceived that connection even if you're clueless. In my experience, the woman often will track you down to investigate." As usual, it's not the cards you hold but how you play them.

I'd like to ask out a tenant

I own an apartment building. One of my renters hangs out with me while I do work on the house or around the pool, and we have a blast. I helped her assemble some furniture, and we were working way too close together. If I hadn't been her landlord I would have made a pass at her. I'm getting crazy signals, but I don't want to be stupid. A friend told me to be careful. He says that if we start dating she might stop paying rent. The rents pay my mortgage. Any guidance on this?—J.R., Chicago, Illinois

Ask her out. You can't plan your life based on worst-case scenarios.

Okay to look up her number?

I met a girl who's a friend of a friend. I know her name, so I looked up her number in the campus directory. Is it okay to call? It's one thing to know a girl's number and another for her to give it to you. I don't want to creep her out.—M.F., Potsdam, New York

There's nothing wrong with getting her number from the phone book—it's only creepy if you dial random numbers.

How young can I go?

After two years of torture I am finally divorced and starting to date again. My question is: How young can I go? I read that the formula is your age divided by two, plus three. I'm 46, so that would allow me to go out with a 26-year-old. There's a 28-year-old who wants to sleep with me, but I've been shying away because of the age difference. What do you think?—J.B., Minneapolis, Minnesota

No matter what the age difference, the challenge of any relationship that starts like this is finding something in common besides your mutual interest in fucking. But that doesn't sound like a concern for you now.

Are smart guys dumb daters?

I read an article that says intelligent guys, because they have no social skills and overanalyze dating situations, have trouble with women. True?—M.S., Fayetteville, North Carolina

Genius is a burden, but we've managed. Many guys overanalyze dating situations, as do many women, but it has more to do with insecurity than intelligence. Sometimes they hook up, and the result, for their friends, is like watching a Woody Allen movie.

He likes fast women

For some reason I keep meeting all the women I want to date at fast-food drive-throughs. There's something about hearing a sexy voice through the speaker and then looking into the woman's eyes when I pull up. Is there something wrong with me? I'm concerned that I have a fetish. I also love women with tight little bellies, and all the women at drive-throughs seem to have tight little bellies.—N.R., Madison, Wisconsin

Are you attracted to women who aren't serving you fries? That would be a sign that you don't have a fetish but simply an unusual preference. In our view you need three things: a much better diet, a girlfriend and a pair of walkie-talkies.

The worst pick-up lines

What are the worst pickup lines you can use on a woman? I would like to avoid them. —H.N., Des Moines, Iowa

We're not fans of pickup lines—desperation isn't the best first impression. "Hello" and "May I sit here?" are more natural. (Hef says his favorite line is "My name is Hugh Hefner." He also says, "The best way to get a woman interested in you is to be interested in her.") A Rolling Stone *reporter witnessed a recent example of idiot lines while trailing porn star Jenna Jameson at an event. One guy said to her, "Do you remember me from that night in New York? I spent $20,000 on you." Jenna's reply: "I would remember anyone who spent $20,000 on me." The next guy squeezed her hand and whispered, "You give me pleasure." Her response: "Ewww." Indeed.*

He's a 52-year-old virgin

When I was younger I made a decision not to have sex with anyone I didn't love. I felt sex was a spiritual matter and also feared catching a disease. As I have grown older I have refined my criteria. Perhaps I would have sex with a friend. Here's the punch line: I am a 52-year-old virgin. A co-worker considers me a trusted friend, though I don't think she finds me attractive. Should I share this with her? I wouldn't want it to affect our friendship, but I get the sense she is highly sexual, and I wonder if it would matter to her.— J.R., Oakland, California

This is more information than she needs to know. The problem is that you're falling for someone who isn't interested. Contrary to your expectations, sharing this secret won't make the relationship more intimate. And even on the remote chance your co-worker agrees to a mercy fuck, you'd still be lonely afterward— perhaps lonelier. The problem with being a virgin into your 40s or 50s is that it becomes such a distraction. Every potential relationship is approached as the "last best chance" to end the drought, and getting laid becomes a mystical, life-changing event. This leads to a vicious cycle: You can't get sex because you're needy because you can't get sex. That's why you might benefit from Intercourse 101 with a sensitive professional. It won't be the sex you imagined, but at this point it's an experience you should have, and deserve to have, and enjoy. Then you'll no longer have to think of yourself as a 52-year-old virgin—you'll be just another guy searching for love.

Can a size 16 woman find love?

Could a man ever be happy with a woman like me who has a pretty face but a size-16 body? I would like an honest answer, even if it hurts my feelings and leaves me more bitter than I already am.—J.S., Oakley, California

Most men aren't attracted to overweight women, so odds are they'll never know if they could be happy with you as a size 16. We'd like an honest answer to this: Are you attracted to strangers with potbellies and double chins or those who are slim and fit?

Your response was ridiculous. Almost every man is attracted to a woman who is confident in how she looks. That's also the case with confident men who have potbellies.—S.K., Ashland, Ohio

As a longtime reader I'm sad and angry that the writer of that letter could believe what some faceless, unimportant guy from *Playboy* thinks and would give up on the idea that someone could love her for who she is. She may so fully accept what you told her that when a man smiles at her she'll turn away, not believing he could find her attractive. What was she thinking when she wrote to a magazine that turns women into plastic fuck dolls? You had a chance to do some good, and you blew it.—R.A., Madison, Alabama

While it is true that our initial attraction or lust may be for slim people, this can fade after a short conversation. I have quickly lost interest in some very handsome men after finding that they are arrogant, conceited or stupid.—C.S., Stillman Valley, Illinois

I'm a big girl. I know the score. But life and attraction aren't that simple. The Advisor of all people should have recognized the importance of that letter. Instead you were cold and dismissive. If you can devote eight sentences to vermouth, you can at least give a few more to a reader asking a sensitive question.—V.C., Chicago, Illinois

I'm sure you've heard from a ton of angry women. As a guy, I feel for you. I just underwent gastric bypass surgery. My post-op support groups are full of ex-fat chicks who are still psycho and bitter. With my weight back to normal, women react differently to me. No one sets out to be fat, just as no one sets out to have a career in waste management. It sucks, and it's not healthy. Even though our society is composed mostly of fat people, we despise them unless they are jovial.—W.P., Toledo, Ohio

Most men don't know what they're missing. I enjoy the company of women who have curves rather than edges. In my experience larger women are more passionate.—D.C., Merrill, Wisconsin

Did a seventh-grader break into your offices and answer that question? I am a size 16 and have never lacked for companionship. I would have told her to stop giving off the "I am not worth dating because I am fat" vibe. What happened to the days when curves were sexy?—J.S., Dundas, Illinois

The reader admitted she is bitter. That's a turnoff no matter what your size. She should get a hobby. I suggest something aerobic, like belly dancing. She'll learn that even plus-sizers like us can make men cry.—S.J., Salt Lake City, Utah

In my book *Guy Logic*, single guys bluntly fess up about what they want. No one wants to be cruel, but people don't succeed until they stop living fairy tales about whom they can get. The odds are slim that a Roseanne Barr will get a Brad Pitt, so some women (and men) need to cut the crap.—Guy Sparks, New York, New York

Your reply was asinine. When all men develop perfect bodies, maybe all women will too.—M.F., Arlington, Virginia

Our response should have been more expansive. More important, we didn't answer the reader's question. So, belatedly: Yes, a man can be happy with a larger woman—as many have told us they are. But confident or not, a woman will attract the attention of far fewer men (and vice versa) if overweight. That isn't fair, but it's the honesty the reader asked for.

You took a beating for your reply to the size-16 woman who wanted to know if a cute face was enough for her to find a man. But the Advisor's honesty, brutal or otherwise, is the reason I read *Playboy*. When people ask you for the truth, they actually want you to affirm their unrealistic fantasies. Because men are confronted with the harsh realities of life and dating at an earlier age, we do not so easily find solace in fairy tales.—T.S., New York, New York

Not sure that's true—we hear from plenty of men who have unrealistic expectations.

Your critics are too harsh. The woman told you she was heavy and therefore didn't have a man and therefore was bitter. This is a common pattern. Many people gain weight to avoid intimacy, but it doesn't always work for women, because they date and marry up, while men date and marry down. That is, even a woman who is a 1 on a scale of 1 to 10 will be attractive to a guy who is a 2. You also see women who become 10s only so they can say that no man is good enough.—S.S., Chicago, Illinois

That explains why we date so many 9s.

The angry letters took up too much space, especially since you were right. Drop it!—J.R., New Orleans, Louisiana

Done. But where were you guys when we needed you?

SPIRITS

Flavors to savor.

Any value to old whiskey?

Recently I talked my father out of two bottles of Crown Royal distilled in 1957. Do these bottles have any value that should give me pause before I crack one open for a special occasion?—G.M., Lynnwood, Washington

Because it's mass-produced, even Crown Royal bottled nearly 50 years ago has mostly sentimental value. John Hansell of Malt Advocate *suggests you sip it with your father while toasting his generosity. Rather than blended Canadian whiskeys, collectors search almost exclusively for single-malt scotch produced in limited quantities by respected distilleries. (Blended whiskeys generally need to be at least 80 years old to get a second look.) A bottle of vintage Macallan from 1938, 1940 or 1950, for example, can be worth $1,000. Both Hansell and David Wainwright, who appraises whiskeys for Christie's, mentioned an elusive single-malt scotch produced by the now-defunct Ladyburn distillery. Hansell bought a bottle for $23 at a Manhattan wine-shop in the 1980s that he later sold for $2,000; a Christie's client from Scotland won hers in a raffle. Another client purchased a bottle at a shop in Spain, asked Wainwright what it might be worth, then flew back to buy the seven others.*

What is an extra-dry martini?

What exactly is an extra-dry martini? Isn't that another name for gin?—P.L., San Antonio, Texas

Some people argue that, prepared properly and served in the right glass, straight gin qualifies as an extra-dry martini. (As the story goes, Winston Churchill made martinis by glancing across the room at the vermouth.) That's ridiculous. A martini has to include some measure of vermouth, even if it's added from an eyedropper or spray bottle. The classic recipe for dry is four to eight parts gin to one part vermouth. For extra dry, swirl the vermouth in the glass to coat the sides, then dump it and add the gin. Alternatively, you can fill a pitcher with ice, add two measures of dry vermouth, stir and pour the vermouth off. When you add the gin, it will pick up the vermouth from the ice.

Eating the olive

When is the proper time to eat the olive in your martini?—M.M., Denver, Colorado

Gary Regan, co-author of The Martini Companion, *recommends waiting until you finish your drink. "Otherwise you have to stick your fingers into the martini, and you might spill some of it," he says. (Toothpicks are out, by the way.) Connoisseurs who prefer very dry martinis marinate their olives in vermouth for months, and they always add the garnish after the drink has been poured. How many olives? Regan says to go with an odd number but says three is too many (which leaves one—these martini guys love formulas). Another guide offers this rule: One is elegant, two is proper and three is a meal.*

I once read an interview with Frank Sinatra in which he said that the number of olives in a martini should always be two—one for yourself and one to share with the next beautiful woman who walks into the room.—K.M., Carmel, Indiana

God, we miss that guy.

Scotch tastings

When I was a kid, my dad used to have scotch tastings for his friends. What goes into one?—A.R., Nashville, Tennessee

First, select a sampling of single malts and blends. Use tulip-shaped glasses or brandy snifters and make sure each guest has a water glass, plenty of ice and a plate of unflavored crackers for cleansing the palate. Set out several pitchers of room-temperature, noncarbonated mineral water for adding to the scotch. Before tasting it, guests should swirl the whiskey in the glass to bring up the aroma. After sipping, they should savor the taste as it lingers in the mouth (the "finish"). When each bottle has been sampled, bring out strong-flavored foods to complement the smokiness of the scotch—one distiller suggests oysters on the half shell, caviar, smoked meats, pâtés and aged cheeses.

Blended scotch whiskey

How can you tell if you're drinking a good blended Scotch whiskey?—B.L., Oakland, California

A fine blended whiskey should taste slightly different each time you sip it. One sip could be slightly peaty, another slightly dry, another slightly peppery. In theory, blended whiskeys combine the best qualities of various malts.

Wise to pour good whiskey on ice?

As I've gotten older, I have acquired a taste for good scotch: single malt, at least 18 years old. My problem is that I drink it only on the rocks. Am I ruining $150 scotch by pouring it over ice?—N.G., Minneapolis, Minnesota

It's your scotch and your money, so you can drink it any way you want. But you're missing much of the flavor. If you were to offer us a glass, we'd take it neat. That's also how it's traditionally served in the U.K. If you need a dash of water, there are pitchers around the pub. While we're on the topic, older whiskeys don't necessarily taste better. If anything, they start to taste more like the oak barrel. You'll find more good whiskeys in their teens than older.

Who gets drunk faster?

Who becomes intoxicated faster, men or women?—B.B., Ogden, Utah

A common theory used to be that a man's body contains more water than a woman's and thereby dilutes alcohol more effectively. But researchers have found that women have less of the stomach enzyme which metabolizes liquor. As a result, more pure alcohol moves into a woman's blood, intestines and liver, making her more likely to become impaired than a man of equal weight drinking at the same rate.

What is it about champagne that makes it go straight to my head?—T.Y., Phoenix, Arizona

An experiment conducted by researchers at the University of Surrey in England confirmed that bubbly champagne gets a person drunker faster, especially when you drink from a flute. No one is sure why, but one hypothesis is that the carbon dioxide in the bubbles speeds up the absorption of the alcohol into the intestines.

The Goldeneye

Last month *Playboy* listed the "best beach drink" as the Goldeneye, available at the Jamaican resort of the same name that once was the home of James Bond creator Ian Fleming. Can you share the recipe?—M.R., Tallahassee, Florida

Happy to. Chris Blackwell, who owns the resort (he's better known for founding Island Records), and Goldeneye barman Clayton Hinds created the drink. Combine one measure lime juice, three measures clear syrup, one measure Appleton Estate Jamaica Rum (21 years old), four measures Appleton Special Rum and two measures Myers's Dark Rum. It should fill about half the blender. Add ice to fill to the top and blend at high speed until the drink is firm. Serve in a traditional cocktail glass. Garnish with a fresh flower from an orchid. If an orchid isn't available, use another small tropical flower, a wedge of pineapple or a cherry.

The half-life of Jello shots

How long can gelatin shots sit around in the fridge and still be good to eat?—M.G., San Francisco, California

If you've covered them in cling wrap, they should last for up to a week. This according to Chaz Boston Baden, the foremost authority on gelatin shots. Since 1994 he has maintained a site at boston-baden.com/hazel/Jello that offers his philosophy (shots should be served as alcoholic desserts, not as a quick way to get drunk), advice (use sugar-free gelatin for easier cleanup) and recipes, such as his world-famous margarita shot: Stir a large box of lime-flavored gelatin into 2 cups of boiling water until dissolved. Add 1 cup cold water, 1/2 cup tequila and 1/4 cup triple sec. Chill until set. Makes 8 half-cup or 16 quarter-cup servings. For a strawberry margarita use strawberry gelatin and 1/4 cup lime juice or lime schnapps. Use gin instead of tequila for a kamikaze or rum instead of tequila for a daiquiri.

Does booze have health benefits?

I've read that two or three drinks a night can have health benefits. I've also read that five or six drinks are unhealthy. I drink about half a pint of 80 proof booze, usually whiskey or rum, each night. It helps me sleep. Am I living healthily or headed to an early grave?—M.R., Scranton, Pennsylvania

You're putting away the equivalent of six shots a day, which qualifies as heavy drinking. It's also not a good sign that you can't sleep without it. The only medical value in consuming alcohol is associated with light to moderate consumption. For example, numerous studies have concluded that people who consume one to two glasses of alcohol daily have lower incidences of coronary heart disease. Apparently any type of alcohol provides the benefit, although wine drinkers seem to fare best. However, this may be because, as a group, they exercise more and eat better than the louts who drink beer or liquor. In The Science of Healthy Drinking, *published by the Wine Appreciation Guild, Gene Ford collects a variety of epidemiological studies that seem to indicate that people who consume in moderation are healthier than those who abstain—a fact he says medical and health authorities in the United States downplay because it's politically incorrect. Ford dug up studies suggesting that alcohol helps prevent or lessens the damage from upper-body pain, hardening of the arteries, blood clots, high blood pressure, cancer, heart attacks, strokes, Alzheimer's, diabetes, gastrointestinal problems, kidney stones, gallstones, osteoporosis, stress, tremors, ulcers and the common cold.*

The Hairy Buffalo

The other night a friend offered to buy me a drink called a Hairy Buffalo. He said no two are alike. I was skeptical. Have you ever heard of it?—S.O., Midwest City, Oklahoma

Some friend. A Hairy Buffalo (or Gorilla Tongue or Buffalo Sweat) is the spillage caught in the rubber mat along the edge of the bar. Not surprisingly, it's served at no charge.

Decoding cognac

What are the differences among VS, VSOP and XO cognacs?—J.S., Fresno, California

The higher the grade of cognac, the older the blend; the more flavor and color it absorbs from the oak barrel, the smoother it tastes. Although French law sets minimum standards for the aging required in each grade, the four major cognac houses raise the bar. In general, the cognacs used to create Very Special blend have been aged an average of five years, those used for Very Superior Old Pale 10 to 12 years, Napoleon 20 to 25 years, Extra Old 35 to 40 years and premium brands such as Hennessy's Paradis 55 to 60 years.

Hangover cures

The Advisor once wrote that "the best hangover treatment is to know your limits." You also mentioned one of the 50-odd products that claim to cure hangovers. As part of my medical school coursework, I read everything scientists know about hangovers and also tested products with my friends. One 2004 study intrigued me. It found that an extract from the skin of the prickly pear (*Opuntia ficus indica*) helps reduce inflammation caused by impurities in booze or mixers. With funding from the makers of an herbal pill that contains the extract, Dr. Jeffrey Wiese of Tulane University recruited 55 medical students for two experiments. Each was given the extract or a placebo five hours before drinking. Wiese found it helped reduce three of nine common morning-after symptoms (including nausea, dry mouth and loss of appetite) and that the risk of severe hangover was reduced by half.—J.R., Morgantown, West Virginia

The three main factors that contribute to hangover, Wiese tells us, are dehydration, a lack of deep sleep and mild poisoning of the body from the impurities you mentioned. So one common method to lessen the severity of a hangover is to consume a glass of water between each drink and to limit yourself to one beer, one shot or one glass of wine per hour, which is about the rate the body can absorb it. To consume fewer impurities, drink white wine instead of red, and vodka or gin instead of rum or whiskey. It helps as well to stick with better-quality liquors. Studies also have found that aspirin and ibuprofen provide only slight relief, which is probably offset by their effect on an already irritated stomach. As for the many products out there, it's safe to say that if you need a supply of hangover pills, you drink too much, too often.

What's the deal with duty free?

What's the deal with duty-free shops at airports? I've never found the booze prices enticing. Is there some other advantage to shopping at them?—N.R., Miami, Florida

A lot depends on where you are and what you're buying. If you're flying home from Portugal, for example, you won't find better values on ports. Besides savings, duty-free shops offer two advantages: (1) Distilleries use them for market tests, so you can buy products that aren't available at liquor stores (be careful—sometimes only the packaging is different); and (2) the alcohol content can be higher in duty-free booze, which may improve taste. A common misconception is that duty-free means the consumer doesn't pay tax. In fact, with some exceptions, travelers entering the U.S. are allowed to bring in only one liter of booze tax-free, no matter where it was purchased.

Is vodka only made from potatoes?

I recently saw a vodka made from grapes. I thought all vodkas were distilled from grain or potatoes. What makes vodka vodka?—K.B., Leavenworth, Kansas

Vodka is defined more by what it isn't than by what it is. Other alcohols are classified according to the ingredients used to make them and sometimes the place they were made. You need fruit to make brandy, sugarcane to make rum, barley to make scotch, corn to make bourbon and blue agave to make tequila. Scotch is from

Scotland, bourbon from Kentucky and tequila from Mexico. But vodka can be made anywhere on earth, using any distillation process, from any raw material that ferments. It has been produced using beets, potatoes, sugar, rice, rye, wheat, barley, molasses, fruit, whey, corn, flour, soy and rutabagas—each ingredient is said to produce a distinct smell, flavor, aftertaste and burn. Ciroc (ciroc.com) distills the grape vodka you saw, Vermont Spirits (vermontspirits.com) has a vodka made from maple sap and another from milk sugar, and a Russian distributor says its Cannabis brand is created with hemp seeds.

Can you bruise gin?

My understanding is that you should never shake a gin martini because you can bruise the gin. Yet all the bartenders want to shake my martini. When I ask for it to be stirred, invariably I hear, "Ah, like James Bond." But he drank vodka martinis, which need to be shaken. Am I wrong?—L.M., Austin, Texas

You can't bruise gin. The difference between shaken and stirred is that shaken will be colder and cloudier. The preferred method is whichever method you prefer, though a recent study found that shaken martinis have "superior antioxidant activity." Bond's standard was three measures of Gordon's, one of grain vodka and half a measure of Kina Lillet, shaken until ice cold, and served in a deep champagne goblet with a large, thin slice of lemon peel.

How much wine do I need?

I'm having a dinner party for eight friends. How much wine should I buy?—J.J., New Orleans, Louisiana

You should always have enough wine on hand, rather than buying on the fly before each party, so stock up. If you love wine as we do, you can never have enough vintages or bottles for your own enjoyment. You cheat yourself by not buying the best wines when they're ready for you, rather than when you're ready for them. People drink less these days, and of your eight guests, two may not partake, so open two reds and a white and go from there. As you know, the traditional service is champagne with hors d'oeuvres, dry white with fish, Bordeaux with the main course, burgundy with the cheese and port or cognac with dessert.

Is it necessary to "prime" the glass?

I was in New York with friends recently, and we ordered wine. The sommelier showed us the bottle, then stepped to the sideboard to pour a sample. He offered me the sample, I approved and then he brought the three other glasses. They each had a light residue on them, as if they were dirty. When I asked about it, he said he had primed them with a small amount of the wine, poured from one glass to the next and then thrown out, because it allows the bouquet an early start. Have you ever heard of this?—H.R., Philadelphia, Pennsylvania

We've seen it done. The explanation we got was that it ensured that whatever contaminants might have been in the glasses, such as soap residue, had been vanquished. Does it do any harm? No. Is it fun? Sure. Should you tip more for it? Forget it.

Should I smell the cork?

What are you supposed to do when a waiter hands you the cork from a bottle of wine? I've seen people sniff it, but what do they smell that prompts them to send the wine back? Until I figure this out, I'll just keep nodding and smiling as if I know what I'm doing.—K.A., Omaha, Nebraska

The smell of the cork is a good early warning if something is dramatically wrong. At its best, the cork can yield an attractive preview of the condition and quality. If the cork is dry and cracked, air may have oxidized the wine. A damaged cork may also indicate biotic problems. Before you reject a bottle by its cork, check the bouquet of the wine.

What are those white crystals?

My wife and I bought a case of Spanish wine from the Toro region, dated 1997. We found the bouquet and flavor had improved 24 hours after we uncorked it. However, white crystals formed on the wet end of each cork. What were they?—G.H., South Padre Island, Texas

The crystals, sometimes called wine diamonds, are potassium acid tartrates. Grapes grown in cooler climates are higher in tartaric acids, and during the fermentation process the acids crystallize in the vats. Because some wineries take extra steps to remove tartrates, many people take the appearance of diamonds as a sign that the wine has not been overly processed. Tartrates are tasteless and have no effect on the wine.

Foil over the cork

My opinion has always been that a lead foil over the cork gives wine a sense of quality. Over the past few years, I've seen more wineries using a plastic disc. Occasionally they are thin enough to pierce with a corkscrew, but more often they seem to be put in place by someone who caps oil wells for a living. What's the best way to remove the thicker plastic discs without chipping the rim of the bottle?—L.M., Mississauga, Ontario

Score around the edge with a lead-foil cutter or small knife. We're always glad to find a bottle that has the newer flange rim and beeswax seal introduced by the Robert Mondavi Winery. It's easy to push a corkscrew through the wax, and the bottles are elegant and appealing. Lead symbolizes tradition more than quality. Originally, lead foils kept dirt and rats away from the corks of bottles stored in cellars. These days most wines are opened within a few years of being bottled. Lead foils can contaminate wine, especially older bottles improperly stored on their sides instead of angled slightly upward. The wine makes its way around the cork to the groove at the edge of the rim, where its acids eat away at the foil. When you pour the wine into a glass, it passes over this groove and picks up traces of lead. British researchers who analyzed a bottle of red wine found that the wine itself had an acceptable level of lead (57 parts per billion). But the first glass poured over the rim had almost six times that amount (320 parts per billion). Even after the rim was wiped with a cloth, the reading was 250 parts per billion.

My wife and I went to a dinner party where the hosts served wine with screw tops. We laughed at first, but the wines were very good. Have you ever heard of this?—M.Z., Manasquan, New Jersey

Although many people can't get past the idea of a screw top on an expensive bottle, it has advantages. Of every 100 bottles, seven or eight may spoil because defective or decaying corks allow oxygen or bacteria to leak in, giving the wine a wet-cardboard smell. One culprit in the process is the chlorine used to bleach corks. Screw tops first started appearing on Australian and New Zealand wines in the late 1990s. A few European and U.S. producers are now experimenting with them, including PlumpJack, which offers its $145 Reserve cabernet sauvignon with a screw top, starting with the 1997 vintage. Some sommeliers argue that screw tops rob the art of opening wine of its romance and may not be ideal for cellared bottles. But many also expect they'll eventually be commonplace. Lisa Minucci, sommelier at the Martini House in Napa Valley, has seven white and two red screw tops on her wine list, including a 2000 zinfandel from Downing Family Vineyards in Napa, a 2001 pinot blanc from Oregon's WillaKenzie Estate *and a 2002 Riesling from Annie's Lane in Australia. She also recommends Beringer Blass's Two Tone Farm chardonnay and merlot.*

How long will opened port last?

How long will a bottle of port last once it has been opened?—P.L., Hartford, Connecticut

Generally, if you're drinking an aged tawny or a late-bottled vintage port, and it has a T-shaped bartender's cork, it will last three or four weeks. If it has a regular cork—for example, if it's a single quinta or vintage port—it will last only a few days. In the English tradition, this is rarely a problem, because ports are typically decanted into round-bottomed bottles. That way they can't be set down until the bottles are empty.

How are vintage timetables made?

I've heard about charts that indicate when you should open a specific vintage wine. Who determines the timetables and how?—R.F., Phoenix, Arizona

The charts are formulated to say: Here's what we think wines of a particular region in a particular vintage year will be like, based on general characteristics of that region's vintage as a whole. In her book Vintage Timecharts, *Jancis Robinson notes that any answer to the question of when to open a particular bottle must be "couched in conditionals—if the wine has been shipped and stored correctly, if your taste is more English than French, if you plan to drink the wine with food and at the right temperature and so on. One further frustrating aspect is that, in a sense, one never knows for sure when a wine has reached its peak until that peak is past and the wine begins to show signs of decline." Despite these caveats, Robinson provides colorful, controversial graphs that chart the evolution of classic wines over time. Her precision is the subject of heated arguments best settled over a good bottle of wine—properly aged, of course.*

Any way to tell if wine is spoiled?

Is there any way to tell if a bottle of wine is spoiled before you open it?—P.L., Denver, Colorado

Sure, if you own a nuclear magnetic resonance machine. A chemist at the University of California-Davis rigged an NMR machine, which uses the same technology as clinical MRI scans, to hold a corked bottle of wine. He tested bottles from the university's enology department for the presence of acetic acid, a.k.a. vinegar. Sample bottles from 1950, 1960 and 1968 had apparently spoiled (though their corks and seals showed no leaks), while bottles from 1956, 1970 and 1977 appeared to be drinkable. The chemist believes the technology might be useful for auction houses and wine collectors.

Prison wine

A friend who has spent time in prison told me that other inmates used to make wine using just a plastic bag, oranges and sugar. Is that possible?— K.M., Fountain Valley, California

Anything is possible when you have time on your hands. We won't give prison censors any more to do by reprinting a recipe here,* but those in the free world can find them online. Here's the basic idea: Prunes (hence the name pruno), raisins, oranges and/or other fruits are squeezed and sealed inside a plastic bag filled with water. The bag is heated under a tap, then hidden. After 48 hours, the inmate adds sugar, which can come from cubes or packets as well as from ketchup, frosting, jelly, yams, flavored gelatin, honey, hard candies—you name it. (The sugar is broken down into alcohol by yeast floating naturally in the air, or by adding bread.) The mixture is heated regularly over the next three to five days. Most batches of pruno are best consumed while holding your nose. Although many wardens prohibit inmates from taking fruit to their cells, California prison officials still seize the equivalent of 2 million pruno cocktails each year.

What is the best temperature for wine?

I received a wine thermometer as a gift. Can you tell me the optimal temperatures at which to serve reds and whites?—S.E., Bellevue, Washington

Optimal? No. It depends on the wine. General? Yes. As you know, whites are usually served chilled (but not ice-cold) and reds closer to room temperature, which is actually not the temperature of a room but a cellar, about 55 degrees. You can follow a chart. (One exercise in precision we've seen suggests serving sparkling wines at 42 to 54 degrees, roses at 48 to 54, whites at 48 to 58 and reds at 57 to 68.) But in the end you should trust your instincts. If a wine lacks flavor, it may be too cold (this often happens at restaurants, which almost always keep whites too cold and then drop them in an ice bucket for good measure). If the wine seems unfocused, it may be too warm. We tend to serve big reds or whites, such as cabernet sauvignons or California chardonnays, at cellar temp and crisp whites, such as pinot grigios and

---

* Despite our best efforts here, several inmates wrote to ask why prison officials had torn the Advisor out of their magazines.

champagnes, well chilled (three hours or more in the fridge). Lighter reds are slightly chilled, meaning for less than three hours. A thermometer can get you in range, but don't let it take the fun out of the experiment.

Tan and black

A bar in town is offering a black and tan made with Guinness and Bass. Isn't a black and tan made with Guinness and Harp? I can't imagine Guinness would want its incredibly Irish brew mixed up with an English ale. What's your take?—M.A., Tallahassee, Florida

Traditionally, a black and tan is a stout mixed with a lightly hopped ale, but there are variations, depending on where you're drinking and what's available. In the States, a black and tan is typically made with Guinness and Bass, while Guinness and Harp is considered a half-and-half. (Guinness exports both Bass and Harp to North America, so it's all one happy family.) To create a black and tan in which the Guinness floats on top—a carnival trick popular only in America—place the glass at an angle and rapidly fill it halfway with ale. Hold a spoon (inquire at your pub about one made especially for the task) horizontally and facedown over the glass just above the surface of the ale. Slowly pour the stout over the cup of the spoon. That should keep the beers separated.

Are bottles better than draft?

My friends give me a hard time because I always order bottled beer at bars. They say draft is fresher. I suppose that's true, but I've always just preferred the bottle. What do you think?—R.S., Gary, Indiana

As you like it. Michael Jackson, author of The Great Beer Guide, *says that bottled beer can be more refreshing because it has a slightly higher carbonation. But the carbonation prickle on your tongue also masks flavor. In addition, bottled beer is usually pasteurized, and that can flatten its flavor or impart a cooked taste. Draft beer is pasteurized less aggressively, and sometimes not at all, because it has a faster turnover. If "draft" appears on the bottle, the brewer may have used sterile filtration to avoid pasteurization, but that can strip some of the beer's body. So for fresh-tasting beer, a draw is the better bet. "In the U.K. and at select pubs in the U.S., casks are delivered with unfermented sugars and live yeast so they can finish developing in the cellar," Jackson says. He also points out what may be the most important attribute of a draft, which is that you rarely find yourself drinking one alone. "If anyone can find a way of putting the pub in a bottle," he says, "I might be more inclined to shop for the odd six-pack."*

What is a pint?

Last night I got into an argument with a bartender because he tried to short me on a pint of beer. This has happened before. Either they give you a big head or they pour the beer into a glass that doesn't hold 16 ounces. Have you ever noticed this, or am I sounding like a crackpot? My friends roll their eyes when I bring it up.—P.R., Omaha, Nebraska

Many if not most bars that claim to serve pints use "cheater" glasses that hold 14 ounces—and that only if filled to the brim. It's a minor scandal, and technically illegal, but don't let it distract you from enjoying your lager. They call it a pint; you know it's a large. Short measures are serious business in the U.K., where the Campaign for Real Ale estimates that 80 percent of pulls are short and where pub owners occasionally are prosecuted. "They say, 'You should have asked for a top-up,' but why the hell should we have to ask?" writes a former trading standards officer in Camra's Good Beer Guide. *The group says that pub owners who want to serve thick heads—a chief method there of shorting a draw—should buy larger glasses. A survey of British adults found that 84 percent agreed with Camra that a pint should be 100 percent liquid; the rest allowed for some froth. The trade standard is 5 percent; the government has proposed no more than three.*

Since you dragged the Brits into it, you could have noted that an imperial pint is 20 ounces, or 1.2 American pints. In answer to the question you're thinking at the moment: No, I haven't anything better to do.—S.D., Emporia, Kansas

You're right—about the pint. Have you ever had a traditional Scottish pint? It's four mutchkins, or about 3.5 American pints. So it's all relative. A short pull in London might be a full pint in New York, but we're not in New York, so serve what we ordered.

The essential bar

I always have a few bottles of essentials (whiskey, rum, gin, etc.) along with mixers for guests. The problem is that I make and drink the same thing day in and day out. Can you suggest a new type of alcohol that's somewhat exotic yet versatile and not unbelievably expensive?—M.T., New York, New York

You can use many different liquors to make cocktails that aren't American staples. First, add a bottle of Campari to your stash so you can make Campari and soda, which women love. You can also mix it with gin, sweet vermouth and an orange-peel garnish to make negronis. Both are big hits in Italy. You might also try Chartreuse, a French liqueur you can mix with tequila or fruit juices. If you value your friends, create a top shelf for them in the back of the liquor cabinet. We suggest one of Milagro's select barrel reserve tequilas, a scotch from Balvenie, Plymouth gin and Pyrat XO Reserve rum. These aren't for mixing but for drinking straight or on the rocks. They're more expensive, but you won't go through them as quickly.

SPORTS

Playing rough.

Athletic sex

What's the word on having sex the day before the big game? Good idea, or bad?—T.B., Spokane, Washington

As the philosopher Casey Stengel once said, "Being with a woman all night never hurt no professional baseball player. It's staying up all night looking for her that does you in." Some Olympic coaches have forbidden their athletes from fooling around before the big event, but research suggests that sex raises testosterone levels, making competitors more aggressive and focused. Sex also can relieve pregame anxiety. Every top athlete seems to have an opinion on the matter. Wilt Chamberlain said he had sex the day before he scored an NBA-record 100 points in a single game—although given his claim of 20,000 partners, on what night didn't he have sex? Rocky Marciano is said to have considered sex a distraction, and he avoided any distractions before each of his seven world-title fights. Some football players feel intimacy brings out emotions that make them play soft.

Brushing your table

How often should you brush a pool table if it gets at least six hours of use each day?—A.K., Nanaimo, British Columbia

Brush the playing surface every two hours, and vacuum and wipe it with a damp cloth. Be careful to remove chalk marks, especially on the cushions, as they increase friction if they accumulate. It's also wise to cover the table when it's not in use. If you're serious about your game, sharpshooter Robert Byrne suggests occasionally shaving the bed of the table and the nose of the cushions with an electric razor. Not that great for the razor, but wonderful for your angles.

Rose-colored glasses

What's up with wearing colored lenses while playing softball? Does that help, or is it just a fashion statement?—P.W., Denver, Colorado

They're a functional fashion statement. Tinted lenses can make it easier to follow the ball in the grass, or against the sky. They're usually designed to be worn

in response to weather conditions, although some are marketed to specific sports, such as golf or tennis. When it's cloudy, yellow or orange works best. If there's some sun peeking through the clouds, try a rose hue. Gray is best for full sunlight. If you're fishing or boating, use polarized lenses to cut down on glare. A mountain biker who goes in and out of shadows should consider a high-contrast amber. With any sport sunglasses, look for shatter-proof polycarbonate that provides at least 400 nanometers of UV protection. Many manufacturers, including Zeal Optics and Bollé, offer models with interchangeable lenses.

The life of running shoes

How long should I keep my running shoes before replacing them?—P.D., Lancaster, Ontario

Although there are variables, such as your weight and running schedule, Paul Carrozza, who owns Run-Tex in Austin, Texas and covers footwear for Runner's World, *suggests that casual runners replace their shoes about twice a year. More active runners may need to replace their shoes as often as every two months. (This assumes you have properly fitted shoes; if not, you could destroy them within 100 miles.) Most runners sense when they need fresh shoes because the ground starts to feel hard. But it's also a good idea to keep an eye on your midsole—if the foam there feels mushy, the shoe is dying or dead. The most durable shoes have polyurethane midsoles and carbon rubber outsoles, but the downside is that polyurethane is relatively heavy.*

Stroke of luck

What is the most popular golf bet?—K.L., Sarasota, Florida

That would be the Nassau, named for the Nassau Country Club in Glen Cove, New York, where it is said to have originated. It involves three bets. In $20 Nassau, $20 rides on the front nine, the back nine and the 18-hole total. The player or team with the best score on each hole wins a point. To make things interesting, if one side falls two points behind on the front or back, it can request a press, or a new $20 bet, on the remaining holes of the nine. One can also make side bets on who will hit the longest or straightest drive or whether a player will make par from a trap (a sandy), after hitting a tree (a barky) or without hitting the fairway (an Arnie, after Arnold Palmer). The USGA allows wagering among amateurs as long as "the amount of money involved is such that the primary purpose is the playing of the game for enjoyment." There was little enjoyment in the least popular golf bet of all time, between Sir David Moncreiffe and John Whyte-

Melville in 1870 at St. Andrews. The club didn't record the score, but the loser agreed to kill himself, and Moncreiffe apparently did.

Can a football coach get tossed?

Can a football coach get tossed out of a game for cussing at or arguing with an official? I've seen it happen in basketball and baseball but never in the NFL.—R.P., San Francisco, California

That's in part because football officials have more room to roam, which often puts them out of earshot. An NFL coach who loses his cool risks a 15-yard penalty and a fine, but he would have to punch or shove an official to be ejected. No one we talked to at the NFL could remember that ever happening, but there is a famous story about an assistant who was tossed from a game in 1957. San Francisco was trailing Chicago in the final two minutes when an official gave the 49ers a 15-yard penalty. He told quarterback Y.A. Tittle that a coach had used abusive language, and indicated offensive line coach Tiger Johnson. Tittle denied knowing Johnson. Puzzled, the official went to head coach Frankie Albert, who also denied knowing Johnson. Albert went further, claiming Johnson was a "drunk" who had been "annoying the hell out of me." Two Chicago cops escorted Johnson out, the official reversed his call and the 49ers went on to win the game.

Arm-wrestling techniques

Once in a while you hear a story about a 90-pound woman who puts down some guy twice her size in an arm wrestling match. Is there a technique involved, or is it just brute arm strength?—H.H., Indianapolis, Indiana

In general, good arm wrestlers are blessed with thick fingers and tendons of steel in their wrists and forearms. Because the typical sanctioned arm wrestling match lasts only 15 seconds (30 seconds is a barn burner), the strength of your hand, wrist and forearm is required from the get-go, and then the bicep, tricep and deltoid muscles jump in for support. For that reason, wiry guys and gals can outperform bodybuilder types. To stay on top of his game, Bob O'Leary, executive director of the American Arm Wrestling Association, does plenty of reverse curls and spends time strengthening his fingers.

Breaking in a glove

What's the best way to break in a new softball glove?—J.S., Grand Rapids, Michigan

Pour a small amount of leather conditioner or glove oil on a dry, clean cloth and work it into the pocket and back of the mitt. Allow the leather to dry for at least 24 hours. Wipe off any excess oil, then play catch for ten to 15 minutes to stretch the pocket and allow the glove to conform to your hand. Finally, position a ball in the pocket and tie or rubber-band it closed for a few days. Store your glove with a ball in the pocket, and don't oil it more than once or twice a season.

Preventing golf blisters

Three months ago I took up golf. I visit the driving range or course twice a week, but I am getting blisters on my thumbs. Am I holding the clubs too tightly? Would it help to wear gloves on both hands?—M.T., Sacramento, California

Holding your clubs with a death grip is a common beginner's mistake. Have the club pro take a look—and soon, before you ingrain any bad habits. But even if you have a perfect swing, expect blisters if you don't play every day. One study found that a golfer must pull the grip of a driver with more than 100 pounds of force during a fast swing to keep from falling forward. A slow swing requires 30 to 40 pounds. That causes some wear and tear. "When you shake hands with tour players, their hands feel like sandpaper," says Shawn Humphries, who works with many pros as director of instruction at Cowboys Golf Club near Dallas. "Yet they still fear blisters. Tiger Woods often puts medical tape on a finger or pinkie because he doesn't want his hands to split, especially in cold weather. Lee Trevino always wore a glove with tape on the outside around his thumb. If a golfer stays the course, he'll get calluses. In the meantime there's nothing wrong with using two gloves, although it may be enough just to tape your thumbs."

As I get older, I suffer more injuries

I am an outdoor-sports enthusiast who just turned 45. Lately it seems I'm constantly suffering from injuries such as torn muscles and cracked bones, even from minor falls. Am I getting too old for aggressive sports, or can I adjust my training regimen and continue to hack the occasional 20-foot cliff?—S.R., Pacific Palisades, California

You can make adjustments but also need to accept your body's limitations as you age. It helps to stretch like a madman, use proper form and make sure you have the best equipment. The most common "boomeritis" ailments that Dr. Nicholas DiNubile, an orthopedic surgeon in Philadelphia, sees among men over

40 are rotator cuff problems (typically in guys who throw around too much weight); tendinitis-related problems in the heel, under the knees and at the elbow; early arthritis in the knees and hips; and lower back stiffness and pain often caused by degenerating disks. He says it's crucial to have a balanced, year-round fitness routine. "As you get older, you can't just be a weekend warrior or a springtime softball player," he says. "You need a regular regimen that includes cardiovascular exercise, strength training and flexibility. It's the rare boomer who has all three." A trainer or physician who specializes in sports medicine can help you establish a safe zone and then design a program to expand it. When starting a new sport or returning from an injury, it's a good idea to increase your level of activity by no more than 10 percent each week.

Preventing a golf slice

What can you recommend for preventing a golf slice? I have a fair short game, but if I could get off the tee better I'd lower my score by a few strokes.—C.S., Phoenix, Arizona

Fixing a slice can be more difficult than asking your girlfriend to have a three-some. And harder to explain. The ball veers to the right because the face of your club is tilted away from you at contact. That causes sidespin, and the ball begins to curve when it reaches maximum velocity. First, you need to work on keeping the club head square to the ball. A common error is not releasing the head just before impact—that is, your right hand needs to catch up and pass through your left as the ball is struck. (Old pros will tell you to work on hooking the ball, so that everything balances out.) It's crucial that the back of your left hand remains square. If your wrist folds or cups—which happens especially if you swing the club back farther than your shoulder—your swing becomes an outside-in throwing motion. Second, check your hands. Any respectable golf book or video will include a demonstration of a proper grip (see Nick Price's guide, The Swing: Mastering the Principles of the Game.*) Third, check your stance. Your weight shouldn't shift toward your toes or lunge down the fairway during your downswing. Finally, find a place to practice where you can take your time to develop good habits. Videotape your swing, and consider taking a few lessons with the club pro.*

After a loss

I play basketball once a week in a city league. I tell myself it's just exercise, but I'm always depressed after a loss. Sometimes this mood continues to the next day. When we win, I'm a friendly guy, congratulating the other team on their play, commiserating about the officiating, probably annoying them as much as cheerful winners annoy me when we lose. Is there some biological explanation for this, or am I simply two-faced and too competitive?—P.W., Chicago, Illinois

Your reaction is natural. Your body anticipates the competition and produces more testosterone during the hours before tip-off. The surge increases your concentration, confidence and aggressiveness. If you win, your body maintains the higher level of testosterone. If you lose, the level returns to normal. The surge is most pronounced when the outcome is in doubt. "If a player is positive he's going to defeat his opponent, he won't get the rise," explains Alan Booth, a sociologist at Penn State University who has studied hormone levels in wrestlers and tennis players. The drop in testosterone isn't all bad—your body is telling you to rest and heal. The winner, meanwhile, must be ready for the next challenger (consider how tournaments are structured). Researchers have recorded these fluctuations even among men playing chess and male spectators. Testosterone doesn't completely explain your moods—some guys are just better at losing than others. In our experience, the most gracious competitors are those who don't view their time on the floor as a way to prove their manhood off the floor.

A proper rack

How do you properly rack the balls for a game of pool?—C.K., St. Louis, Missouri

In eight ball, the balls can be racked in any order as long as number eight sits at the center. Alternating stripes and solids is not required, but the shooter may ask for a re-rack if he doesn't like how things look. In nine ball (where you pocket nine balls in numerical order), rack them in a diamond shape with number one at the head, number nine in the center and the remainder in any order. For more guidance, download the American Poolplayers Association rule book at poolplayers.com. Our favorite section explains what to do if your buddy starts knocking in the wrong balls, e.g., stripes when he's playing solids: "It is permissible, though not recommended, that the sitting player allow the shooting player to continue shooting his balls in until he feels inclined to call the foul." However, if your friend gets wise and asks which balls he should be hitting, "the sitting player must tell him the truth." What kind of rule is that?

During long nights working at a pool hall in Milwaukee, I kept busy reading the rules of the Billiard Congress of America. It says that the balls should be racked with the eight ball in the center, a striped ball in one corner and a solid ball in the other corner. Every time I play, someone questions why I place opposite balls in the corners. What can I say? I like a proper rack as much as the next guy.—S.S., Portland, Oregon

We were waiting for that joke.

Healing a sprained ankle

What's the best way to treat a sprained ankle so I can get back to my running?—G.B., Toronto, Ontario

For years trainers recommended a course of treatment known as RICE—rest, ice, compression and elevation. But reformers now encourage gentle movement, or MICE. "Immobilizing an injury, unless it's fractured or shredded, shuts down the muscle," explains Jim Wharton, who runs Maximum Performance International, a New York-based sports rehab clinic. "Even the tiniest range of motion helps blood flow to the injury and repatterns the neurological firing." If you're injured, apply ice and visit a doctor immediately for X rays. To rehab, move ice over the area for 5 or 10 minutes every hour. (You also should compress and elevate the injury to reduce swelling.) Begin gentle stretching—point your toes up and down and turn the foot in and out enough that you feel discomfort but not pain. You'll see steady improvement in your range of motion. Within hours or days (depending on the severity of the sprain), add light resistance by holding the ankle with your hand as you flex. The muscle should return to form within a few weeks, but it usually takes six weeks for it to heal enough for sports.

Calculating a golf handicap

How do I get a golf handicap? I can tell people what my average score is, but I would like one to be on record from year to year for when I play in leagues or tournaments.—D.W., Cincinnati, Ohio

A handicap must be established through a golf club that operates under guidelines established by the USGA. That isn't as difficult as it sounds: A club can be any group of at least ten golfers who play together often. The system is based on peer review: Partners make sure everyone's scorecard reflects reality. (The club's handicap committee handles disputes.) To establish a handicap, you need to play at least five rounds. Once you've played more, your handicap will be calculated based on the ten best of your most recent twenty rounds and adjusted every two to four weeks during your playing season. You also adjust your handicap at each course, based on its difficulty. In addition, there are calculations to account for every kind of anomaly you might encounter while playing a round that affects your handicap, such as bad weather that postpones the final holes. And don't forget Equitable Stroke Control and slope ratings. It's a math major's delight. You'll find all the details—there are 17 chapters and six appendixes—in the USGA handicap system manual, available online at http://usga.org/handicap or by phoning 800-336-4446. The maximum handicap index for men, by the way, is 36.4, from which you can only improve.

Getting ready for softball

I play a lot of softball in the summer. Can you tell me which exercises to do or muscle groups to work so I'll be ready?—C.G., Flint, Michigan

From a sitting position, lift a full can of beer to your mouth. Repeat. Still tight? Start preparing three to four months before the season by strengthening your shoulder and upper back muscles. (See The Whartons' Strength Book *for workouts designed for softball players.) These muscles need to be in balance before you begin swinging the bat in earnest. Your cardio work should include endurance runs to get you through the season and sprints and shuffles to mimic the fast-twitch motions of a game. The goal is to prevent the soreness and injuries that cripple many players early in the season. Be creative. As part of his skills work, one guy we know swings a 34-inch section of broomstick at one-inch plastic golf balls. When the season begins, he says the softball looks as big as the pitcher's head.*

The best way to throw darts

Is there a proper way to throw darts? I just started playing, and I've received conflicting advice. Presently I throw pretty consistently—half into the board and half into the wall.—R.B., Muskogee, Oklahoma

Throw sober. That's our first rule. We asked Rick Osgood, editor of Cyber Darts *(cyberdarts.com), for more-specific pointers. "There are two fundamentals in any target sport: stance and follow-through," he says. "Stand with your feet shoulder-width apart and parallel to the line. Turn the shoulder of your throwing arm to face the board. Raise the dart to eye level. Keep it level as you fully extend your arm and 'place' the dart on the board. Don't throw the dart; guide it to the target. That will force you to follow through." A common mistake is leaning forward, which shortens the distance to the board but puts you off balance. Finally, you should never lunge. You don't need power to throw darts. Cyber Darts offers more guidance, as well as a handy list of excuses for bad throws, including "my hand hit the brim of my cap," "a fly landed on my tip," "bar noise impaired my peripheral hearing" and the classic "I was distracted by my partner's breasts."*

His hands are deadly weapons

A loudmouth at the corner bar says his hands and feet are registered as lethal weapons. He claims he's a black belt in karate and that martial artists and boxers are required to register with the police. We've been telling him he's full of it, but he insists. Can you register your hands as weapons?—P.C., Jamesville, New York

No, that's bunk. Anyone can claim his hands are lethal weapons, but no statute anywhere in North America requires registration. Unless he's been convicted of killing someone with his bare hands, which we suppose is a form of legal recognition, it's just a lame boast. Most laws specify that only an object can be considered a deadly weapon, although that could conceivably include your shoe if you were to kick someone hard enough. That's not to say body parts can't be weapons; in one case a jury convicted an HIV-positive inmate of assault with a deadly weapon for biting two guards. Legally, a person's experience as a boxer or martial artist may work against him if he seriously injures someone—the prosecutor could argue that someone with training should know when to stop.

STDs

Let's be careful out there.

Can you get an STD from panties?

Over the past year I have bought several pairs of used panties offered by women at an online auction site. The panties are vacuum sealed and shipped through UPS. Are there any health risks? I'm most concerned about the more durable diseases such as chlamydia and genital warts.—G.H., Laramie, Wyoming

It's possible you could catch a sexually transmitted disease from a pair of days old panties, but not probable. According to Dr. Peter Leone, a professor of infectious diseases at the University of North Carolina, the most likely STD to survive would be genital warts (there are concerns that warts can be passed via sex toys that aren't sterilized between users). But in this case, you would have to rub the fabric against a skin abrasion to have even a remote chance of infection. A more realistic concern would be intestinal illnesses such as E. coli, especially if you touch the panties to your lips. We suggest you microwave your purchases.

According to *The Doctor's Book of Home Remedies*, in 1989 a woman in Idaho called the fire department because of smoke in her attic. She had been zapping her nylon panties to battle a yeast infection. The book suggests instead boiling the panties, soaking them in bleach or touching them with a hot iron.—S.L., San Francisco, California

Poison ivy

My girlfriend claims that an old boyfriend once gave her poison ivy while they were having sex, before he had any symptoms. Can this really happen?—D.B., Dallas, Texas

Why not? Many men who get poison ivy inadvertently spread it to their genitals when they hold their penis to urinate, and from there it can spread just about anywhere. One physician who misdiagnosed a patient's burning, swelling lips as herpes or an allergic reaction later discovered that she'd gotten poison ivy when she gave her boyfriend a blow job after he'd been hunting. She spent the next few weeks battling a rash and blisters on her lips. His case was more severe.

Hepatitis C

I have hepatitis C. Before my fiancée and I broke up, we decided not to use condoms, and she tested negative several times. Now that I've started to date again, I'm wondering what to tell new partners. My doctor says I need to use condoms only for anal sex or sex during her period. I intend to use condoms with anyone I meet until we are monogamous, but I don't want to bring it up too early and scare women off. What do you think?—R.S., Atlanta, Georgia

You should discuss this with any woman before you sleep with her. Tell her you want her to know, even though it's extremely difficult to spread the virus during sex, particularly if you use a condom. Unlike HIV, which is present in blood, semen and other bodily fluids, hepatitis C can be shared only by blood contact. Nearly all of the 3.9 million Americans who are infected acquired the disease through transfusions or by sharing needles. The virus is scary because most people who acquire it develop chronic liver disease.

Herpes

I recently met a girl, and we hit it off. We were about to have sex for the first time when she told me she has herpes. She wasn't having an outbreak, so we used a condom and had oral and vaginal sex. I know this didn't protect me 100 percent, but I wasn't sure what else to do. I don't want to get herpes, but I like this girl. I don't want a long-term relationship, but it's fun for the moment. Is it worth the risk?—A.D., San Mateo, California

It may be riskier than you realize. Genital herpes spreads through skin-to-skin contact, but the virus can be transmitted even when no symptoms are present. A condom is essential but doesn't cover every area that can hold the virus. That's partly why genital herpes is so common—after a study of blood samples, researchers estimated that 80 percent of people with herpes worldwide don't realize they have it. The prescription drug Valtrex, used to suppress outbreaks, has been shown also to reduce by 50 percent the risk of transmitting herpes to a partner. That's something to discuss. If you have other questions, the American Social Health Association operates a herpes hotline at 919-361-8488. To her credit, your lover told you about her STD before you had sex, and let you make your own decision. That should earn many points with you.

Can you get herpes if someone who has a cold sore gives you head?—O.D., Cincinnati, Ohio

Yes. The strain of herpes that causes cold sores has also been identified as the root of 20 percent to 30 percent of genital herpes cases, suggesting these viruses were contracted through oral sex. The good news, if you can call it that, is: Research indicates that genital herpes contracted through oral sex reactivates far less often (if ever) than herpes spread through intercourse. While not every fever blister or canker sore is a sign of herpes, hold off on oral sex until it heals. Open sores or cuts in the mouth also can be a route for HIV.

Will I get AIDS?

What are the odds that a person will get HIV?—R.T., Boston, Massachusetts

We could give you numbers, but they wouldn't mean much. As one HIV expert pointed out in an online discussion group, "The risk of transmission is not like the risk of losing at the races. Because you can't recoup the loss represented by infection, you can't think of the odds in the same way." Instead, let's talk about high-risk activities. The people most at risk of acquiring HIV are those who have unprotected anal sex with an infected person, and people who share a needle with an infected person while injecting drugs. In the U.S., those two groups account for the majority of infections among men. Among American women, 75 percent of new infections are attributed to vaginal sex. Scientists believe the first row of cells in the vagina are HIV-resistant, but that the virus makes it way past them through small abrasions and cuts, which can be caused by lack of lubrication or other STDs. Since it's impossible to tell if a partner has HIV (people don't always know for months after they are infected), even if you've been together a long time (people cheat), you have to make certain uncomfortable assumptions. At the same time, no one wants to have sex with plastic for the rest of their life, and people take what they consider acceptable risks.

A recent *Scientific American* article stated that one of the reasons for the high rate of HIV infections in Africa is that the men prefer "dry" sex. Am I missing something? I have been married for 25 years, and wetter has always been better.—J.M., Newtown, Connecticut

We're sure your wife agrees. Many men in sub-Saharan Africa demand dry sex because it increases friction and because wetness is considered a sign of a woman's infidelity. The women comply because they don't have the status to refuse. They dry themselves with soap and water, detergent, toothpaste, salt, cotton, shredded newspapers, baboon urine mixed with soil or inflammatory herbs that also make the vagina tighter. Then they suffer through intercourse. Not only is dry sex painful, it causes tears or abrasions in the vaginal walls, giving HIV a route into the body.

Dry sex also does a condom no favors. These are important lessons for anyone who hopes to avoid HIV or any blood-borne disease, such as hepatitis. But in Africa, where many men believe a woman's role in sex is only to provide pleasure and/or children, ignorance is killing millions of wives, sisters and mothers. It's a sad, vicious circle: The women find sex painful and avoid it, so the men visit prostitutes and take mistresses, justifying their behavior by explaining that their wives are nonresponsive. The disease also is spreading because of low condom use, the high rates of other STDs and fallacies such as the belief that deflowering 100 virgins will rid you of HIV.

Genital warts

I'm amazed that no one has been able to find a simple, inexpensive cure for genital warts. I've tried to have them burned off at clinics. I've considered an operation, though I was told it wouldn't cure them. I've been to a dermatologist, who told me he might be able to get rid of the problem for a couple thousand bucks. I haven't had sex in three years because I'm afraid I'll infect someone. Can you help?—C.D., Cincinnati, Ohio

We can't offer a cure—there isn't one. But genital warts, which are caused by the human papillomavirus, can be managed. In many cases they don't return after treatment. In others they reappear with less severity for a few years, then disappear as your immune system gets the upper hand. The most common topical medications are a solution containing podophyllin (which must be applied by a health care provider), imiquimod cream and a podofilox solution or gel. Removing the warts doesn't eliminate the risk of infecting someone else, because the virus may remain. Condoms or other barriers help if they cover the infected area. You're not alone on this one: Researchers estimate that 75 percent of Americans who have sex have been exposed to HPV, though only about one percent develop symptoms. HPV spreads so quickly that researchers have turned their attention to treating warts rather than preventing them. The type of warts you get on other parts of your body, such as your hands, are caused by a different virus that does not appear to be transferable to or from the genitals.

I have been dating a girl for two months. Early in the relationship she told me she has HPV-16, one of the types linked to cervical cancer. We haven't had sex, and I don't know if I'm willing to get this virus just to be with her. Am I being an asshole? What are my chances of getting a vaccination?—J.J., Mobile, Alabama

How long can you hold out? Vaccines that prevent specific types of HPV, including HPV-16, are being developed, although their efficacy in men is still being tested. They're also most effective on virgins; most sexually active adults have already been infected with HPV but are unaware because they've never had warts. For most people HPV is not cause enough to abandon a relationship—if you want out for other reasons, don't blame the virus. Besides warts, which can be treated or removed, the primary risk is that HPV-16 and about a dozen other strains have been linked to cervical and penile cancer. Both are rare in North America, the latter in part because many men here are circumcised, which reduces the risk to nearly zero. But that's not true of many other places in the world, where these cancers are more prevalent. That's why a vaccine is so vital. Unbelievably, some conservative religious groups oppose the development of HPV vaccines, saying they will encourage teenagers to have sex before marriage.

You mentioned that HPV-16 has been linked to penile cancer. Can you actually get cancer in your penis?—H.M., Tampa, Florida

Unfortunately, yes. Because most tumors appear on the head or foreskin, one hypothesis is they are caused by secretions that become trapped when an uncircumcised penis is not washed regularly. Researchers are investigating the role of HPV-16 and HPV-18, which have been found in a third of all penile cancer cases. In Western countries, where circumcision is common, only about 1,000 men are diagnosed annually. But in Asia, Africa and South America, penile cancer represents 20 to 30 percent of all cancers among men. It can strike at any age but typically affects men who are 60 or older. Left untreated, it can be deadly. In one study of 1,605 men diagnosed with penile cancer, 22 percent died. What to watch for: a lesion or growth that won't heal.

STEREOS

The sound of music.

Good vibrations

I'm a car-audio installer. An instructor at a training conference told me that clitoral resonance is 33 hertz, give or take, depending on the woman's weight. This means that anything vibrating 33 times per second will cause the clitoris to resonate. Howard Stern made an example of this in *Private Parts* when he got a woman off by having her sit on a speaker, and just about any woman will respond to a bass note at that frequency if your subwoofer can play that low. Is there any truth to this?—J.B., Yuma, Arizona

Don't touch that dial. The idea that 33 Hz is the optimal resonance to get a woman off originated with an experiment performed in 1992 by car-audio consultant Todd Ramsey. While on spring break in Daytona Beach, Ramsey and his buddies spent three days asking women to sit in the front seat of a Honda Accord. The crew then swept the frequencies from high to low on an 18-inch subwoofer, powered by a 1,000-watt amp, in the trunk. The women gave the thumbs-up when the vibrations felt best. Once Ramsey had crunched the numbers for about 100 volunteers, including making adjustments for their self-reported weights, he calculated that the optimal resonance for a woman of 115 to 125 pounds is 33 Hz. Not so coincidentally, he says, that's about the same resonance as an idling Harley or a spinning washing machine. In 2001 Ramsey wrote about the CR (clitoral resonance) factor in Auto Sound & Security. *"I'm still waiting for a call from one of the big automakers," he says today. One CR disciple is Richie Warren, founder of Fuel records, which produces bass heavy music for car-audio systems. To promote Fuel at auto shows, Warren straps three models across the top of a Dodge Challenger and booms a 33 Hz tone "until they're coming all over the car." Visit the label's site at liquid injuredhearing.com, where you will find a resonator that produces tones from 30 to 110 Hz. Ask your partner to sit on your quality subwoofer, hook up your computer to your sound system and sweep through the tones to find her number (the heavier the woman, the lower the frequency). The only downside is that she may leave with your stereo.*

Thirty-three hertz also happens to be near the frequency you hear from the lowest pedal pipe on most organs. Consider that the next time you're singing hymns in church.—M.L., Brookline, New Hampshire

This could explain the fervor of many fundamentalists. A U.K. study found that many churches have organs producing not only a 32 hertz bass but also vibrations that measure below 20 hertz, which is inaudible to humans but can produce sorrow, coldness, anxiety and shivers. One researcher suggests these reactions may "lead people to have weird experiences that they attribute to God."

Speaker wire length

I've heard that speaker cables should be exactly the same length for the best sound, on the theory that you want the signal to reach each at the same time. That is, if your left speaker is connected with 10 feet of wire, the right speaker also should be connected with exactly 10 feet of wire. True?—G.F., Miami, Florida

Sure, if you have only 20 feet of wire. The signal travels at 688,498,300 feet per second, more or less. A few feet certainly won't make a difference.

Why can't I play European DVDs?

Why is it that you can buy a music CD in Europe and play it in the U.S., but you can't do the same with DVDs? It's too bad, because there are many movies released in other countries that you can't get here.—S.A., Burbank, California

Major studios have divided the world into eight markets, and they work hard to keep each one isolated to maximize profits. They do this by adding a code to each DVD that prevents it from being played anywhere but on a machine coded for the same region. (The exception is porn, which rarely has codes.) Because films are usually released in the U.S. months before their debuts overseas, the system prevents foreign consumers from buying mail-order DVDs prior to a movie's showing at their local theaters. It also prevents consumers in the U.S. from buying foreign films on DVD before their Stateside debuts. Movie buffs get around the codes by buying universal players from online retailers such as HKFlix.com. In response, a few studios experimented with a code that prevents discs from being played on zone-free machines but gave it up after about 20 titles.

Do I need a subwoofer?

I'm buying a stereo system. Do I need a subwoofer?—P.L., San Antonio, Texas

You can probably live without one unless you watch a lot of action movies. If you mostly listen to music, and your speakers can reproduce frequencies down to 40 Hz, you won't notice much improvement. Humans can hear as low as 20 Hz, but there's not a lot going on of musical interest between 20 and 40 cycles, which is the octave processed by most subwoofers. The lowest note on a rock album is typically the low E produced by an electric bass, which hits about 41 Hz. In classical music, booming orchestral drums occasionally reach the low 30s. Outside of home theater use, a subwoofer is necessary only if your speakers are not flat to 40 Hz or if your listening room is an acoustical disaster. Expect to pay at least $400, and resist buying used equipment. Subwoofers are often abused, and their quality has improved dramatically over the past decade, perhaps more than any other component. Today's models are much less boomy and sluggish and provide more flexible controls.

Speakers don't sound as good as in store

I bought a pair of speakers that sounded great in the store, but when I got them home, they didn't sound as rich. This may have to do with the layout of my room and its acoustics, but my old speakers sounded fine. Can you explain it?—B.B., New York, New York

When you buy speakers, they're displayed on "speaker walls" or in rooms full of equipment. When you test them, the other speakers vibrate as well, making your pair sound richer. Before you buy, ask to hear the merchandise in a private listening room. More important, insist on a liberal return policy.

Binaural sound

A friend who is a stereo buff lent me a CD and told me to listen to it through headphones. It sounded incredible. He said it was binaural. I've looked in record stores and haven't been able to find another disc like it. Do you have any information?—W.L., Phoenix, Arizona

Most recordings are made for playback through loudspeakers. Binaural CDs are designed to be played through headphones. They are created using a life-size model of a human head equipped with microphones where the ears would be. The recording head is placed in the audience or onstage during performances (or, in the case of nature recordings, carried into the wild) to capture sound as a listener would hear it. The rich 3D effect can be stunning. John Sunier of the Binaural Source (binaural.com) suggests starting your collection with an audio drama (Stephen King's The Mist*), nature recording (Gordon Hempton's* Earth Sounds Sampler*), jazz (Jürgen Sturm's* Tango Subversivo*) or classical music (either of two discs available on the Auracle label). For an arousing binaural experience, check out* Cyborgasm, *a collection of erotic fantasies on CD (available from good vibes.com or 800-289-8423). You'll swear the dominatrix is in the room, especially when she walks all the way around your chair.*

Beginner jazz

I have always listened to rock and some classical. Can you suggest some jazz and blues albums to add to my collection?—R.F., Minneapolis, Minnesota

Since this sort of exercise always sparks debate, we'll let our music critics stand near the fire. Neil Tesser, author of the Playboy Guide to Jazz, *suggests Miles Davis'* Kind of Blue *as a starting point, Keith Jarrett's* Köln Concert *for its classical influence, Charlie Parker's* Bird's Best Bop *on Verve and Pat Metheny's* Still Life (Talking) *for a contemporary sound. Among vocalists, you're safe with anything by Sarah Vaughan, Ella Fitzgerald or Billie Holiday. Dave Marsh, who reviews the blues, recommends the Smithsonian's* Mean Old World: The Blues From 1940 to 1994, *which begins with Ma Rainey and ends with Corey Harris, and MCA's* Blues Classics, *which covers 1927 (Furry Lewis) to 1969 (B.B. King). He also suggests* The Best of Muddy Waters, *B.B. King's* Live at the Regal *and Stevie Ray Vaughan's* In Step.

Upgrading classical

My classical CDs are by great orchestras with great conductors. But even a Karajan or a Bernstein cannot blind me to the fact that recording technology 20 years ago wasn't as good as it is now. I'd like to update my collection. The names on the cover are less important than the quality of the music. Any recommendations?—Y.K., Fort Lauderdale, Florida

The first step is to look for remastered versions of the CDs you already own. While the fidelity won't be as good as that of contemporary recordings, some performances by Karajan, George Szell and Hans Knappertsbusch are still better than anything recorded today. Gramophone (www.gramophone.co.uk) has reviews. Among current conductors, we like Simon Rattle with the Berlin Philharmonic and Nikolaus Harnoncourt with the Concentus Musicus Wien.

Cable descramblers

How can companies advertise descramblers that allow you to receive pay-per-view and premium cable channels without paying? Aren't descramblers illegal?—P.S., Boston, Massachusetts

In many states it's not illegal to sell or own a descrambler. In every state, however, it is illegal to use one without notifying your cable provider. That's the rub, and that's what you learn when you read the fine print. One mass e-mail claims you can build your own device with parts purchased at Radio Shack. A reporter for Playboy Online investigated and discovered what you'd expect: Radio Shack no longer stocks a critical part—the variable capacitor—because so many people were asking for it to build descramblers to cheat the cable company. Even if you could construct a descrambler, you'd probably be disappointed. One size doesn't fit all. Companies that sell these devices walk a thin line: A federal judge sentenced an entrepreneur who sold more than 84,000 descramblers by mail order to five years in prison. People who steal premium or pay-per-view service typically are caught and fined when a judge compels a distributor to turn over its customer list, or when a neighbor or ex-friend reports them.

Power strips

I'd like to upgrade the power strips I use with my hi-fi equipment. Can you offer guidance?—N.N., Dallas, Texas

Most people will find that a $30 to $50 strip with surge protection is sufficient. Look for the Underwriters Laboratories mark on both the box and the product, as well as the words "transient voltage." Keep in mind that many strips have only a single metaloxide varistor, which is what provides the protection, and it's a kamikaze—if there's a surge or a spike, it sacrifices itself. Once that happens, the strip may continue to work but not protect against energy bursts. Some strips have MOV indicator lights, but even those can't always be trusted. The point is, don't assume that a strip with surge protection will last forever. If you're daring, try the Wiremold L10320, which is popular among audiophiles who feel that the switches, fuses, circuit breakers and noise filters found on most strips diminish system performance. Naim, which makes high-end equipment, *recommends connecting all your components to the same strip, with the amp plugged into the outlet closest to the cord, followed by the sources. The theory is that different grounds in a house can vary a bit; on high-end audio, that may cause noise. Naim also suggests having your power and source cords flow separately and "as gracefully as possible," because "electricity does not travel efficiently around sharp corners and bends." If you just paid $5,100 for a Naim CD player, that advice is comforting.*

SWINGERS
The best of friends.

The logistics of swapping

Most of our friends know that my wife and I are into threesomes. One friend offered herself, and my wife approved. After we had set a date, our friend said to my wife, "We'll do your husband, then you can do mine." The problem is that my wife doesn't find our friend's husband sexually appealing or even moderately friendly. We are new to swinging. Is this sort of swapping considered routine? I don't want my wife to feel pressured.—S.S., San Diego, California

You ran into a swinger with a plan. Generally, those involved in the lifestyle don't attempt to swap mates, because the odds are good that at least one person among the four won't find his or her potential partner appealing. Many couples who enjoy swapping are handicapped because one partner (usually it's the woman) is more attractive than the other. So typically the woman will scout for a suitable couple and imply a threesome. If a couple shows interest, the husband suddenly appears to join the conversation. These couples soon earn a reputation, and experienced swingers avoid them. We suggest you back out of this situation gracefully.

When three's not a crowd

How many people does it take to have an orgy?—W.S., Los Angeles, California

Technically? Two is a couple, and three is a threesome. Four could be described as an orgy, but more likely it's two couples, or a threesome and a guy saying, "I thought this was an orgy." Five is more likely a threesome and a couple. Six could be two threesomes or three couples or a couple, a threesome and the same poor sap. You get the idea. It's an orgy when you lose count.

Orgy food

What food should be served at a swing party?—S.B., Rochester, New York

We've never eaten anything at a swing party that could be swallowed, but one sex gourmet tells us the smart host organizes a potluck of lighter fare. As for refreshments, experienced swingers serve coffee instead of booze. "Many people won't fulfill their fantasies unless they're in an altered state," our source says.

"That way they can say, 'It wasn't my fault.' But swingers have accepted what we're about."

Swinging softly

Among wife swappers, what is the meaning of the term *soft swinging?*—M.D., Hartford, Connecticut

Don't call them wife swappers. Swingers are actually husband swappers, because the wives control all the sexual activity. Most people understand soft swinging to include nudity, massage and some sexual touching. You start by socializing and stop wherever you feel comfortable. Other soft swingers have intercourse, but only with the person they came with. In The Lifestyle: A Look at the Erotic Rites of Swingers, *Terry Gould notes two other distinctions: Open swingers exchange partners with another couple in the same room, while closed swingers exchange partners and retire to separate rooms. Swingers never refer to themselves by these terms; they simply say "Yes" or "No, thank you."*

Swinging seems sleazy

My husband and I have been married for 17 years. We both have MBAs and high-income jobs. A year ago we decided to add more zest to our sex life by finding a couple to swap with. At the risk of sounding snobbish, we're looking for classy experiences, not quickies in a hot tub. We spent time browsing sites on the Internet, responded to personal ads in an alternative paper and researched the local swingers' scene. But the couples we've met have been crude and unappealing, and many seem desperate to save failing relationships. Frankly, it all seems sort of sleazy. Does the Advisor have any suggestions?—V.B., St. Paul, Minnesota

Don't use your local or online experiences as a barometer; the lifestyle attracts every type of person you can imagine, and there are many swingers who enjoy the socializing as much as the sex. Throw your line into a larger pond. There is a swingers' gathering every summer in Nevada that attracts 3,000 couples from around the world (for information, visit lifestyles-convention.com). If your experience is typical, you'll form a clique or a clique will find you.

That woman looks familiar

Last night when my husband and I were opening responses to our ad in a swingers' magazine, he went pale. One letter included a photo of a nude woman, and it was his sister. We had no idea she and her new husband were swingers and we don't think she knows we are (we use a pseudonym in our ads). My husband says we should return the letter and photo marked "not interested" and say nothing more. I argue that we should discuss the situation with them, because our paths are sure to cross. I'm not suggesting that we swing with them, but perhaps they could benefit from our experience. What do you think?—M.J., New York, New York

Small world, eh? Acknowledge the letter for exactly the reason you state. Rather than send a written reply, invite your sister-in-law and her husband to dinner. Don't reveal your shared lifestyle with the idea that they might benefit from your experience—who says they're beginners? Simply explain that you wanted to acknowledge the unusual situation in a comfortable, familiar setting rather than after rounding the corner at a party. Then have a good laugh. It's a great story, after all, and your husband couldn't buy a better opening line than "Say, do you know my sister?"

Games swingers play

The wives in our swinging group have agreed to participate in a game they call Who's Down There? The women will be blindfolded and receive cunnilingus from each man in turn. Each woman will try to guess which tongue belongs to her husband. The problem we're having is that no one can agree on the details. Are the women naked? Are the lights on? Are the women in a group or isolated? Is there a time limit, a referee, spectators, video equipment? Some members of the group have expressed reservations about playing unless we have formal rules. However, everyone agreed to abide by the Advisor's recommendations.—D.W., Tucson, Arizona

The women should be naked, which means the lights must be on. One room. No cameras. Three minutes on the egg timer. When the bell rings, the men rotate. Ideally, none of the men have facial hair, or they all do. No touching besides tongue to vulva. No sounds besides moans. Round one ends only after each woman has climaxed at least once. Round two begins when the men have been given the blindfolds. Rounds three and beyond you can figure out for yourself.

My girlfriend and I joined some neighbors for a swing party. We were impressed by the number of games the host couple invented to entertain everyone. After each guest had been introduced (most of us knew one another), all the men left the room. One of the men was blindfolded, as was a woman. When the group came together, we surrounded the blindfolded couple and watched as they tried to identify each other by touch alone. Next, all the women were blindfolded to see if they could recognize their partners by kiss. That progressed to oral sex. The men then wore the blindfolds, and the roles reversed. We are interested in hosting a party and wondered if you had any ideas as to how we could make it as fun and innovative as our neighbors did.—M.B., Toronto, Ontario

The downside of these type of games is that they put guests on the spot, and not everyone is comfortable performing for a group or being intimate with strangers. Typically, swingers first get to know each other in a nonsexual context. Robert McGinley, president of the North American Swing Club Association (NASCA), suggests this icebreaker for parties at which everyone is already acquainted: The women form a circle facing outward. The men form a circle around the women facing inward. Each person begins opposite his or her partner. The host instructs the women, and then the men, on how to interact with their partners. It might be as simple as running fingers softly down the person's cheek, or caressing his or her arms, or a quick shoulder rub. At the host's cue, each guest removes an item of clothing, and the women take one step to the right. The new couples interact per the host's instructions. The action can become more intimate following each rotation, but it usually doesn't progress beyond a kiss or hug. The process repeats itself until the circle has rotated 360 degrees and the women are again facing their partners. "By that point everyone is naked and probably very turned on," says McGinley. "It's nice to have your partner right in front of you, so you can act on whatever urges you're feeling."

How to start a swing club

A female friend took me to a swingers' club in Kentucky and we had a great time. The club charged $35 per couple as an entrance fee, and $50 for single guys. We filled out applications at the door to become members and to attest we weren't cops or reporters. The booze and food prices were outrageous. With at least 50 couples inside, the club must have made a fortune. I recently lost my job. What better way to get back on my feet than to start a sex club? I'm sure that wherever I set up the local authorities will fuck with me, but if I'm not breaking any laws, what can they do?—B.J., Laurelville, Ohio

If they disapprove, they'll find a way to harass you out of existence. The club you visited sounds like it's ready to be closed down—first, because it had you

join at the door, and second, because it sold booze and food. Both make it look suspiciously like a business, which invites scrutiny from zoning, health and tax authorities. That's why most owners don't open their doors to the public. Instead, they collect applications and dues at a separate office (but also may charge party fees at the door). They also have members bring their own alcohol. Sex isn't the stated reason most clubs get shut down—it's noise complaints and parking problems. It helps to have a few cops and bigwigs as active members. And you may want to host parties somewhere other than your home. One Chicago-area owner decided with her husband to move their events to local hotels. "I want my house back," she says. "People pee in our hot tub, they leave their shaving cream, razors and pubic hair everywhere, they drink too much because they're nervous and then throw up on my floor. We started with a house where we hosted fun parties and ended up living in a swing club." Even sex club owners need a hug sometimes. As for profits, you might make some money, but "it's not the road to millions," says a NASCA spokesman. He means dollars, not partners.

What should we expect?

My wife and I have decided to try swinging. What should we expect on a first meeting with another couple?—A.M., Grand Rapids, Michigan

Don't expect anything. That way, you won't be disappointed. In most cases it takes at least two dates before couples are comfortable enough with one another to have sex. In the event that either you or your wife aren't interested in a swap, work out a subtle signal to alert each other. One couple we know turns over a spoon at dinner.

My wife is a different woman when we swing

Last year my wife and I began swapping with another couple. When my wife fucks the other guy, she has more and stronger orgasms. She is also less inhibited. When we have sex, I do most of the work. My wife claims that her behavior is due to the "newness" of the situation. Now that I've seen what she's capable of, I'm thinking I should call off the swap. Is this just a common risk of swinging or is there a corrective action I can take?—S.V., Lakewood, Ohio

Many guys who have the opportunity are surprised to see how differently their wives react when they're with someone else. The best explanation: Your wife is enjoying her fantasy of being with a relative stranger, whereas the sex in a long-term

relationship tends to be more comfortable (sometimes too comfortable). Your wife also is being shown hard evidence that a stranger finds her desirable, which will perk up anyone's interest. If you're uncomfortable with the swap, suspend it. No matter what, you need to make sex as a couple less predictable. Arrange to share a few private fantasies—something out of the ordinary but perhaps as simple as a blindfold—and see what reaction you get.

Do married swingers last longer?

A female swinger who is a friend of my wife's wanted to have a gang bang. Her husband lined up four single guys, but his wife was disappointed because the fun lasted only an hour. When my wife told me this story, I said I wasn't surprised. Single guys are into pleasing themselves, which is why they're single. Married guys are into pleasing women, which is why they're married. I know this isn't always the case, but what does the Advisor think?—W.B., College Station, Texas

That's not a bad setup to get yourself invited. The reason four married guys would last longer is that they'd each be thinking, I better take this slow, because it's never going to happen again.

Obstacle course

My wife and I are friends with a couple who are swingers. One night while drinking and playing cards we all engaged in masturbation and oral stimulation. As we played, my wife pushed my hand or head away several times to clear a path for the others. Should I be concerned that she doesn't find me attractive or satisfying?—J.B., Allentown, Pennsylvania

Let her know how you feel, but don't jump to conclusions. Your wife saw an opportunity to enjoy the sensation of unfamiliar fingers and tongues. She was less interested in having sex with you while others watched. Whatever her motivations, this wasn't a good move on her part. There's a difference between swinging with your partner and leaving your partner swinging. That's why it's smart to discuss these situations before they occur, to avoid surprises and hurt feelings in flagrante delicto.

A single guy in swinging

How does a single guy get into the swinging scene?—R.T., Santa Barbara, California

The few clubs that welcome single men (and their entrance fees) typically do so only on certain nights, so you end up with a crowd of mostly guys. Fun! Traditionally, single women have been admitted for free to balance the ratio, but gender-discrimination laws are putting an end to that. (In fact, the North American Swing Club Association had to revise its own guidelines to specify that it admits only male-female partners to its events after a gay male couple that was refused entry threatened to sue for $1 million.) NASCA president Robert McGinley says allowing too many single men drives couples away. "You always get single guys who argue that couples love having spare men around," he says, "but even at couples-only parties there are lots of guys who will happily fill that role." He also says the presence of single men can irritate swingers who value the honesty of the lifestyle. They assume the guys are alone because they're cheating on their partners. If you do attend as a lone wolf, don't be too grabby. A breathy play-by-play or shouting "Move over, Rover, let Jimi take over!" is not the best way to introduce yourself.

A free pass

For her 10th wedding anniversary my wife's best friend got a pass from her husband to do anything or anyone she wanted for a week, as long as it happened far away from home and he didn't learn any details. She immediately booked a beach trip and called my wife to invite her along. That was fine with me. As long as my wife returns with videos and photos, I will forgive her anything. The idea turned me on even more after my wife mentioned that a 40-year-old woman will do things to a 20-year-old guy that a 20-year-old girl can't imagine. How can two husbands who would allow such adventures be so different? When I mentioned to him that the most erotic thing I had ever seen was my wife having sex with another guy, he looked as if he might cry.—M.E., Philadelphia, Pennsylvania

He's making a sacrifice, and you're making an investment. We'd bet this wasn't his idea, which makes us wary of endorsing it. Guys who get off watching their wife get fucked usually have a lot of confidence about whom she'll end up with at the end of the night or the week. You benefit twofold here because both women will want to share details, and you'll be the only one listening.

THREESOMES

When four is a crowd.

What we learned

How can I persuade my wife to have a threesome? And if I do, how should I arrange it?—B.F., Atlanta, Georgia

After reading through the hundreds of e-mails we solicited from readers, asking them to describe real-life threesomes and how they came about, here's what we gleaned:

(1) Don't beg. You don't want your partner to do this as a favor, because that breeds resentment. It should come up as part of a discussion about fantasies. If she's curious about being with another woman, encourage her. If she isn't, back off. You may have planted a seed. Or it may not be in the cards. As Hef notes in his Little Black Book, *"It's foolish to squander the tomorrows that exist in a relationship for a momentary adventure. It's not a smart way to live your life."*

(2) Don't bring this up unless you have a strong relationship. Threesomes have been known to cause serious damage. That's why it's crucial, if your wife agrees to it, to establish ground rules. Can you kiss the other woman? Can you have intercourse with her? Does your wife want to have sex with the other woman? Will you use a condom? How about a dental dam? It isn't prudent to negotiate during the encounter. Regardless, your wife should command your full attention, particularly during the first experience.

(3) Many threesomes develop when a guy finds himself alone with two horny, intoxicated women (the women must kiss before anything else happens). Most threesomes begin tentatively as the participants grow comfortable with the extra body in the room. If you blurt out something like "I can't believe this is happening" or "Yeah, baby!," you risk making the women feel that they have been cast in your personal porn movie. It also implies that you'll be blabbing about it to your buddies for the rest of your life. Play it cool and make the experience about their pleasure. As one reader pointed out, "You have to be in the right place at the right time with the right women."

(4) There are two kinds of women you can approach: known and unknown. For the former, your wife should invite an open-minded friend for dinner and

drinks. Once everyone is cozy, either (a) invite the friend to your bedroom straight-out ("We'd like you to stay") or (b) bring up the topic more casually by recalling past adventures, how men and women have different approaches to sex, why guys are turned on by women kissing, etc. Your wife will need to make the first move, usually by massaging her friend's shoulders or otherwise getting touchy-feely. There is a risk that the friend will react badly. That's why it may be better to recruit a stranger, preferably an escort, who doesn't expect anything but an envelope of cash on the dresser. You should budget $500 or more an hour. Some couples compromise by making fast friends in the swinger community, which has no shortage of bisexual women.

I'd like to do my date—and his brother

I have been on a few dates with a guy and think we'll have sex soon. I'm also interested in his brother, and I'd like to do both of them at once. How do I ask if they'd be interested in a threesome?—J.K., Columbia, South Carolina

This may sound prudish, but we usually wait until we've slept with a woman at least once before asking if we can invite her sister (twice before we ask about her mom). Don't package your fantasy as a threesome with his brother. A threesome involves a guy and two women, always. You're thinking of a gang bang. After you've been together a few times, gauge your boyfriend's reaction by presenting it as your curiosity about having two men at once. If he's agreeable, ask him who he would suggest for the third. Then grab for the ring: "Okay, this is completely wild—and maybe too wild—but what about your brother? I'm not sure I would feel comfortable with any of those others." Don't be surprised if he says no—men generally don't invite family to their fantasies. Then again, he may one-up you and reveal he has two brothers.

You wrote that a threesome always involves a man and two women, and that a woman and two men is a gang bang. That's ridiculous. My husband and I have had threesomes with another man. Why is it that two women and a man gets the wholesome tag of "threesome," while a woman and two men deserve the crude "gang bang"? Your answer reeks of sexism.—M.Z., Cincinnati, Ohio

We like your idea of wholesome. If anything, our answer reeks of heterosexism. When you and your husband arrange a threesome, do the men have sex with each other? Probably not. That makes it a gang bang—i.e., one person having sex with

two or more partners simultaneously. Technically, a three-way could involve two men and a woman, three men or three women. We just don't fantasize about those scenarios—except for that last one, and it always ends up as a gang bang.

Does my fiancée want two guys at once?

My fiancée always sucks my thumb during sex. Does that mean she wants to have sex with two men at once?—S.S., Fort Lauderdale, Florida

Hard to say. When a woman sucks your finger it's usually a preview of what she plans to do with your cock. If your fiancée is curious about having two men, we suggest you shop together for a dildo. It's an extra penis that doesn't require an invitation.

My husband got angry when I kissed a woman

My husband and I went to a bar one night, and a female friend of ours hit on me. Later, my husband wanted to know why I hadn't let her continue so he could watch. A few months later we ran into the woman at a party. This time, I had enough wine in me to let her kiss me. I glanced over and my husband looked shocked. Suddenly I felt dirty, like a pervert. My husband said he was upset because of all the people there who might have seen us. I thought I was fulfilling a fantasy for him. Can you explain?—T.B., Youngstown, Ohio

Your husband prefers to keep his fantasies behind closed doors, or at least in the relative anonymity of a bar. He likes to watch, but he doesn't want to be watched while he's watching. If he hopes to see you with another woman, he didn't play his hand well.

The mother-daughter duo

I'm a bodybuilder, age 23, who makes ends meet as a personal trainer. My two favorite clients are a drop-dead gorgeous mother-and-daughter exotic dance duo. I train them together at their home. Both women are voluptuous and muscular. They act more like sisters. We had always flirted, but for professional reasons I never acted on it. One day I joked that it would be fun to shower together. To my amazement, they agreed. I found myself pressed between mother and daughter as they soaped my body. They did things with their hands and mouths that were beyond belief. After the shower, they led me into the bedroom. The daughter rode my cock while her mother kissed my mouth, nipples and stomach. Then I fucked the mother doggy style, with the daughter hugging me from behind. While this wasn't the first time I'd been with two women, the fact that they were mother and daughter enhanced the eroticism. Now I'm dating both. How common are mother-daughter threesomes?—C.A., Houston, Texas

They're common—as fantasies. The "exotic dance duo" is a nice touch in yours.

My wife only lets me watch

My wife and I have threesomes with a friend of hers, but I am only allowed to watch. The friend has told me she wants me, but when I ask my wife, she says no way. Is this fair? The frustration of having to remain on the sidelines leaves me not only wanting her friend all the more but yearning to have sex with other women as well. I've tried the "gentle approach" but get no game.— J.T., Dallas, Texas

That's rough. You need to attack from a flank. Your wife's friend should bring up the idea privately with your wife, who will certainly suspect you encouraged the idea. But she may be more receptive to rounding up from two and a half to three if it's presented as a favor to a friend rather than an indulgence for her husband. You also could attempt to ease yourself into the situation. Volunteer to hold the vibrator. Or wait on the women as their slave (candles, wine, whatever they need). Or perhaps your wife would like her breasts kissed and fondled while she's receiving oral sex. If she says no to any or all of that, well, you're out of luck. Having sex with the friend or anyone else without her okay is trouble. One more bit of advice: Don't complain too loudly to your buddies about how you only get to watch.

You ignored the inherent unfairness of the situation: The wife is allowed to have sex with another person, but the husband isn't permitted the same courtesy. Let's say J.T. had written: "My wife and I have threesomes with a friend, but I only allow my wife to watch. Am I being unfair?" We both know your answer would have been different. For starters, you would have ridiculed him for his male privilege.—J.K., Chicago, Illinois

It's not a courtesy, it's a contract. If J.T. felt the terms were unfair, he was free not to accept them. If his wife then had sex without his consent, it would be cheating and a problem for the marriage. That works both ways.

... And then he began to sob

Last weekend I went out with a friend and his girlfriend. They've been together for five years. We had a lot to drink and ended up back at my place at 4 AM. I suggested they sleep over, and we crawled into my bed. After a few minutes, my friend's girlfriend said, "I know what you guys are hinting at, so let's do it." The next thing I knew we were all going at it. She and I hit it off, and I think he noticed the sparks. He climbed out of bed, sat in a chair and began to sob. After a little fussing, she managed to calm him down and they left. I have spoken with her only once since that night, and she assured me everything was cool. Do I have a chance to get back into her pants, and how should I go about it?—J.M., New York, New York

Threesomes would be much simpler if they didn't involve so many people. Your friend had probably daydreamed about countless threesomes, but none involved watching you fuck his all-too-eager girlfriend. When the fantasy hit the fan, he wasn't prepared. You can ask this woman to return alone, but don't be surprised if she declines, at least for now. You were all drunk, she loves her boyfriend, it was a misunderstanding, etc. Chalk it up as one of life's little tragedies.

My friend wants me in the room

A friend of mine is a virgin. I suggested to another friend that she take care of him, and she's up for it. He said he'd do it but only if I were in the room and did whatever he did. I told him that was sort of weird, but he says he's just nervous. Should I go along?—S.D., Weehawken, New Jersey

Are you going to hold his hand during the train? Set these two lovebirds up on a date and let nature take its course. She can explain what to do as easily as you can. You've also overlooked the fact that while your friend may be up for deflowering a virgin, she may not be so enthusiastic about a threesome with a virgin and his handler.

My husband wants to go down with me

My husband has a fantasy that turns me off. He wants the two of us to perform fellatio on another man at the same time. The thought of my dear husband going down on another guy is too much for me. We tried fantasizing about it during sex, but it shuts me down. How can he enjoy this without my doing it or hearing about it?—A.T., Sudbury, Ontario

We find it interesting, first, that your husband, knowing the reaction most women would have, had the confidence to tell you this fantasy and, second, that you didn't ask if we think he's gay. We don't necessarily—many people aren't so easily labeled. But both observations tell us you have a relationship that is stronger than most. So we suggest this: Let your husband go down on you—while you're wearing a harness and a dildo. That way he's not sucking another guy's dick, he's sucking yours. The idea is to make this fantasy less about what your husband does and more about you playing the man. That may help you past the initial shock. Or it may just be beyond you. That's okay, too. At the least you may pick up some new techniques.

Years ago my wife and I were using a dildo when she told me to lick and kiss it. When she saw how much it turned me on, she bought a strap-on. We did 69s, and now she sometimes demands that I fall to my knees and service her. She also gives me an ass pounding two or three times a month. I imagine these two letters will open a lot of eyes. —R.S., Lewisburg, Pennsylvania

You bet. One couple with experience in this scenario, M. and B. in Chicago, wrote to say that our suggestion that the reader use a dildo to fulfill her husband's fantasy missed the mark. In their view, he found the idea of giving a blow job exciting simply because it involved his wife having sex with another guy. "He wants to share the pleasure she feels," they wrote, "and also feel the other man's pleasure as his wife sucks him. His wife, not the guy, is the focus of his desire. If he just wanted to suck a cock or receive anal sex, he could do that without her." Which is a good point.

A birthday surprise

My wife turns 40 next year and I want to do something special, so I told her I would take her to Las Vegas. She loves Vegas but gave me a look that said, What's so special about that? Then I told her I want to watch her pick up a stranger at a bar and screw him. I don't think I could stand watching, but if she wanted me to join in I'd be willing. How can I convince her? She hasn't said no, but I could tell from the look on her face that she is less interested in the idea than I am. Do women who've been with only one guy all their life get curious once they hit their 40s? My wife says no, but I disagree.—B.V., Los Angeles, California

It doesn't matter if other women get curious in their 40s; your wife may not be. Besides the fact that she would be doing all the work, these things are messy, especially when you involve a random barfly. We suggest you ask your wife what she wants for her birthday.

THREESOME STORIES

Because so many readers write the Advisor to ask how to arrange threesomes, we wanted to find out how they come about, for better or worse. So we asked readers to submit their real-life threesome stories. Below are a few of the hundreds of responses.

I was talking to two women when one said, "Friends who play together stay together." We started making out while her friend slid her hand down my pants. When we got to my place, they asked what I wanted to see. I told them to fight over me. So they gave me head while bickering over whose turn it was. It was fantastic.—M.F., San Francisco, California

The last time I had anything close to a threesome was two years ago. My wife and I watched *Eyes Wide Shut* while her friend blew me. Now I have blue balls because my wife says those days are over. She says she has grown up and that I should too. —D.P., Kansas City, Missouri

I was hosting a frat party when I noticed two girls flirting with each other. I told each girl that the other had asked to meet her upstairs in my room. I waited a while, then went up to see how they were doing.—M.C., Parsippany, New Jersey

It's happened three times, all with my current girlfriend: (1) We invited a waitress back to our hotel. The next morning, as we were checking out, the manager kept saying, "You had two girls!" (2) We were on a cruise. A blonde asked if I was single. I told her I could be single if she wanted and took her to meet my girlfriend. (3) We were playing golf. A woman playing alone caught up with us. I asked, "Do you ever get hit on by other golfers?" She said, "All the time." So I asked, "Do you ever get hit on by couples?" We've had other prospects, but it usually happens when we least expect it. —R.W., Phoenix, Arizona

This chick at a party asked if she could sit on the arm of my chair. Some guy bumped her and she fell into my lap. We talked and started making out. Five minutes later I opened my eyes and 30 people were watching us. Another chick said, "This shit is making me horny." Everyone cheered as the girls led me away. I always thought a threesome would be confusing, but I didn't have to do much.—P.L., St. Louis, Missouri

My date pushed me against a wall, crouched down and unbuttoned my jeans. That's when I saw her roommate. It turned into an up-and-down swap. The key is to let the women be in control.—G.C., San Diego, California

My fiancé introduced me to his ex. I suspected he wanted to sleep with her one last time, so I organized a threesome. I had two ground rules: He couldn't kiss her, and he had to give me most of his attention. But they tried to slip in a kiss, and he fucked her four times and me only once.—A.T., Provo, Utah

My wife and I had three-ways with her friend. Things were great until I decided to fix up the friend with a co-worker. He told her he would love to swing with her. She was pissed. I had no idea he'd go for the gold within 15 minutes of meeting her. I learned the hard way not to screw and tell.—W.W., Chicago, Illinois

My girlfriend and I did it doggy style while her friend stood over her back and pretended she was riding a mechanical bull. No matter how much you fantasize about a threesome, you're never ready for it.—B.T., Milwaukee, Wisconsin

My buddy and I met this adorable girl at a club. We all went back to his place. He asked her, "What do you dream about?" She said, "I don't know." He said, "Close your eyes." She closed them, and he asked, "Do you dream about this?" and kissed her. Two hours into the lovemaking, she asked, "Can I open my eyes now?"—J.K., Limbazi, Latvia

The best part of my threesome was watching the women get dressed together in the morning. I wished all my guy cousins and dead ancestors and all the male friends I ever had were there to witness it.—M.O., Los Angeles, California

I stepped outside a bar for some fresh air and spotted two women making out in a car. The car door swung open, and a co-worker called to me. She asked me not to say anything to her husband. Then another co-worker poked her head out and said, "When was the last time you had two women suck your cock?"—M.L., Philadelphia, Pennsylvania

My girlfriend and I double-dated with two cops. We went back to my date's place, and he and I started kissing. My friend started to pout, so her date joined us. Four cop hands and two cop mouths all over my body! The real fun began when they used parts of their uniforms. Batons, cuffs—oh, man! My suggestion for a threesome is to double-date with two cops and a flop.—S.B., Dallas, Texas

Our newly divorced neighbor came to dinner and kept saying she wanted an alternative relationship. When she began rubbing my wife's shoulders I moved the massage in an alternative direction.—J.K., St. Louis, Missouri

My wife's sister, who was renting our upstairs apartment, wanted an air conditioner put in. After I installed it she sat on my lap and wiggled until I got hard. Then there was a knock on the door. It was a friend of hers who needed a place to stay. My sister-in-law said it was up to her landlord. Her friend said to me, "I'll give you whatever she's giving you." I am divorced now, and sadly enough the only thing I miss about my marriage is my sister-in-law.—A.L., Tampa, Florida

My girlfriend asked me if I thought one of her friends was cute. I said, "Sure." She said, "Great. She's your birthday present." I tried to play it cool later at the hotel, but my girlfriend got impatient and said, "Get over here and fuck us."—J.T., Milwaukee, Wisconsin

I live a few blocks away from a club, so my girlfriend and her friend decided to use my bathroom rather than wait in line. I found the two of them on my

couch. "Don't be mad," my girlfriend said. I still call it my holy weekend.—
J.T., Los Angeles, California

While thumbing through a magazine I came across an article on threesomes.
Two days later, I found the magazine on our coffee table, opened to the
article. I asked my girlfriend what was up, and she said she and our new
(female) roommate had read the article together. The next morning I woke
up to a kitchen full of sex toys, champagne, whip cream, cherries, a kiddie
pool filled with hot water and bubbles—and two horny women. Never
underestimate what your girl will do for you.—M.T., Phoenix, Arizona

When I was in college, I dated a radiology technician who I met while having
a barium enema—no kidding. He asked me what I wanted for Valentine's
Day. I told him I'd always wanted to make out with the girl next door. We
visited her. My boyfriend told me to leave for a few minutes. When I came
back, he had her shirt off. I enjoyed the experience but prefer to give a
partner my full attention.—A.L., San Antonio, Texas

On my 40th birthday my wife strapped me to our bed and blindfolded me.
The doorbell rang. When she returned, I felt two sets of hands caressing me.
The women kissed and pinched and sucked everywhere except my cock.
They shaved my chest and pubic hair, then rubbed oil over me. When they
reached my thighs I started climaxing—they had made me come without
touching my erection. They took turns fucking me until I had come three
more times. My wife says my 50th will be even better. Time goes by so
slowly.—M.T., Las Vegas, Nevada

At 5 AM I went to shower for work and found my wife with her face in her
best friend's crotch. I asked if I should leave, and my wife said, "Only if you're
a fool." We had a few threesomes, but it turned out that the friend wanted to
steal me away. She did for a while. I've since remarried. My new wife brought
up the idea of a threesome, but I took a pass.—C.H., Seattle, Washington

We spent the weekend with another couple and on the drive home, the two
women sat in the backseat and read aloud from a dirty magazine. The other

couple broke up soon after, but the woman came over to share photos from the trip. She and my wife talked about how aroused they had been during the drive. The drinks flowed and it got late. We invited our friend to stay in the guest room. My wife and I went to our room to fuck. We could hear our friend moaning. That was too much for my wife. She asked if I would mind if she went to our friend's room and masturbated with her. I just about shot my load. I heard her knock on the door and say, "Can I come in?" A few minutes later they yelled through the wall that they needed a man.—B.S., New Orleans, Louisiana

I was hanging out with two girls during my junior year of high school. We climbed into the backseat of my Camaro but there wasn't enough room to do anything but make out.—C.K., Chicago, Illinois

Two women I met while drinking asked me if I had money for a room. At the hotel one woman cuffed me to the bed. They both sucked my cock. When I told them I was close, they stood up, took my wallet and clothes and left. The maid who found me in the morning didn't speak English, so soon the room was filled with the manager, two cops and two EMTs. At least I can say I've had a threesome.—R.K., Houston, Texas

TIPS AND TRICKS

You never stop learning.

The big tease

Quick, I need a new sex trick. Can you help?—J.N., Aspen, Colorado

At times like these, we're glad to have friends like Laura Corn, author of 101 Nights of Great Sex. She shared two tricks with us. The first she calls Popping Her Clutch. "You'll need a vibrator with a cord and a separate on-off switch, such as a remote-control egg, positioned on her clitoris," she says. "Your partner needs to tell you when she's about to come. As she's having her first contraction, turn it off. She'll look at you funny, so turn it back on. Then turn it off for a second or two. Then turn it on. You get the idea. The anticipation will drive her wild. This was by far the most popular trick among the couples who tried it for my book. Back for More also got a great response. With the woman on all fours, her partner alternates licking her labia from behind, pressing a vibrator or tongue against them and inserting his erection for a few thrusts. Because it's at the opposite end from the clitoris, the back of the labia usually doesn't get much attention, so the sensations will surprise her." We need to call Laura more often.

Pearls on penis

My husband loves it when I wrap a strand of costume pearls around his erection and slowly unravel it. The only thing we can think of for him to do with me is to slowly pull the strand out of my vagina. It feels good, but I prefer something more subtle. Any suggestions?—C.H., Elkhart, Indiana

More subtle than pearls in your pussy? That's a tough one. Your husband could place a section of the strand over his tongue and go down on you; you may enjoy the pearls against your clit and vulva. (Gather and grip the other end of the strand and you have a nice bridle.) He could roll the pearls under his palms as he massages you, including running them over your nipples and across the soles of your feet or lightly spanking your vulva and bottom. He could lay the pearls across your clit and vulva, hold them firmly in place and touch a vibrator to them, experimenting with speed and pressure. When it's your turn again, Laura Corn suggests this: "Grasp one end of the strand in each hand. Slide it left, then right, over his erection, spinning the pearls high and low and fast and slow, so it feels like a hundred fingers." Add your warm lips to the head of his cock and he'll be a puppet on a string.

Finger-point control

Many people who write to the Advisor about sex seem to expect their partners to know what they like in bed without being told. I've discovered an effective form of nonverbal communication that might be helpful. The other night, as my wife was giving me head, she reached up and put her fingers in my mouth. I asked her to mimic what I was doing to her index finger, and she agreed. When I licked the side of her finger, she licked the side of my erection. When I opened my mouth and blew gently on the tip of her finger, she opened her mouth and blew gently on the tip of my erection. You get the idea. It was absorbing because my wife had to focus on what she was doing to stay in sync with me, and I was in control of my pleasure. She says she has learned a lot about what makes me feel good, and we didn't have to exchange a word. The next time we'll change places and see how good I am at following directions.—J.S., Torrance, California

That's a great technique. When it's your turn to go down on her, extend your hand and make a victory sign.

Ideas for a hand job

My boyfriend loves hand jobs, but I've run out of ideas on how to make them more exciting. Do you have any suggestions?—W.J., Amarillo, Texas

Are you using both hands? You may be able to double his pleasure. Lou Paget of the Sexuality Seminars has written a sex manual for women, How to Be a Great Lover, *that diagrams 21 techniques for giving good hand. To start things off, she suggests having your boyfriend pour lube into your cupped palms. "By rubbing your hands together seductively, you'll not only warm the lube, you'll also let him know how good it feels to you and how good you are soon going to make him feel." A favorite technique is called the Ode to Bryan: (1) Hands out, thumbs down. Wrap one hand around his penis so that your wrist is flexed and your thumb rests against his pubic hair. (2) Stroke up the shaft. When you reach the head, twist your hand slightly as if you were opening a jar. (3) Rotate your entire palm over the head as if you were sculpting it. (4) Come over the top and down the shaft firmly until your pinkie touches his pubic hair. Immediately move your other hand into position on top of your "finishing" hand and begin the next cycle. You'll quickly establish a rhythm—the goal is continuous motion and sensation. How well do this and other techniques described in Paget's book work? Just reading the instructions turned us on, and one wife offered this testimonial: "The only audible words in my husband's reaction were, 'Oh Jesus, Mary and Joseph.' And he's Jewish."*

Shooting great nudes

I finally got my wife to let me take nude photos of her with our digital camera. Can you offer any tips for lighting and poses?—N.P., Fort Smith, Arkansas

You've come to the right place. First, discuss with your wife the poses you would like to try. Scan Playboy's *pictorials with her for ideas, and ask her to choose the lingerie or bikini she would like to start with. Put on some of her favorite music and ask her to strip. This will help make the shoot more fun, get her involved and keep her from looking stiff. Be sure to move in close enough that your subject fills the frame. Arny Freytag, who has shot more than 150 Centerfolds, says to "find the nicest environment you can and hide it with the girl." Don't obscure her face with an elaborate hairstyle or exaggerated makeup. Try baby lotion to give her skin more sheen. The most challenging part of the exercise will be the lighting. Freytag prefers shooting outside in sunlight either early in the morning or during the last moments of a cloudless day when the setting sun throws an orange light. "Keep the sun over your shoulder, directly on her," he says. If you're shooting inside, use two lamps, one over the camera and one under, evenly balanced, to kill shadows. Or light her from the side by posing her next to a window. Even if you don't produce* Playboy-caliber *images, there's still a great chance you'll get laid.*

How to give a lap dance

My boyfriend wants me to give him a lap dance, but I've never done anything like that before. How can I make it good for him?—S.K., Atlanta, Georgia

Sometimes this job can be a real grind. To research your question, we were forced to spend several afternoons ordering lap dances and observing the dancers' techniques at Crazy Horse Too in Chicago. Our favorite, Kennedy, provided this advice free of charge: "Dim the lights, put on some Sade or Enigma and make him sit on his hands. There will be no touching, except what you initiate. As you dance and tease him, imagine you're a cat. Purr if it helps you get in the mood. Start on the opposite side of the room and walk slowly toward him, so he can take you in. You can dress in lingerie or as a librarian or businesswoman or maid and strip as you dance; whatever turns him on. Just don't give it up during the first song. Take your time; the longer he has to wait, the crazier he'll get. Blow in his ear and whisper to him. Taunt him a little. 'You like what you see?' Show him your ass. Rub your hands up and down your body. Cup your breasts. Wet your nipples. Place your breasts close to his face. Lick your lips. Look yourself over as if it were the first time you'd ever seen yourself nude. I call it the Playboy *gaze, because the Centerfolds often have it. When you've teased him plenty, sit on his lap facing away from him and lean your head back. That gives him a nice view of your tits. We can't touch the men who visit our club, but you have more freedom. If you feel generous, let him put his hands on your hips as you grind. If he tries to move them anywhere else, whisper in his ear, 'No touching.' One last thing: Always remember to get your money." Kennedy accepts only cash, but how your boyfriend pays for his dance is negotiable.*

The love glove

When my girlfriend and I are in the heavy, panting, slippery phase of love-making, I will frequently spread my fingers like a fan and place my little finger in her anus, two fingers in her vagina and my index finger on her clitoris. If she's in the doggie position, it's reversed, with my index finger in her ass. I then stroke in and out. I'm always struck by the classic beauty of this move, which I call "the peacock tail" because my fingers are spread out. I'm wondering if there is some other name in the sexual archives that better describes it.—J.W., Boise, Idaho

We've heard it called the love glove, the trident or the double trigger. Typically the thumb is placed on the clit and the fingers advance from there, but you can arrange your digits in whatever manner your partner prefers. Make sure she is well lubricated and that your fingernails are trimmed.

How to give a foot massage

I've heard that women go nuts over foot massages. Can something like that get me laid? Any secret techniques I should know?—T.H., Nashville, Tennessee

A foot massage is always a step in the right direction, in part because lovers typically overlook and underestimate its sensual power. Use lotion instead of oil (too slippery) and warm it first in your hands. Alternate a firm stroke on the soles with a light touch on the top of the feet. To begin, massage the edges of her foot, working from heel to toe. Next, make small, circular movements on her sole with your thumb. Place both thumbs at her heel, then stroke toward her toes, making a T. You also can use your knuckles on the ball of her foot. Squeeze and roll each toe between your thumb and index finger, then give each a gentle tug. Press the flesh between. A good massage should last at least 10 minutes on each foot. Move on to the ankles, legs, etc., until she demands sex.

You should have let a foot fetishist answer the question. Don't bother with oil or lotion. Instead, use a hot towel. This will help if the woman is concerned about odor. When the towel has cooled, set it aside and continue the massage with your hands but finish with your mouth and tongue. Light nibbling and licking on the soles and between her toes will drive her crazy. Take three, four or five toes in your mouth and lick between and around rapidly. This technique will help any guy get laid.—H.G., Greenville, South Carolina

Sure, if she can get you to stop.

Brushes with greatness

One of the things I love to do with my girlfriend is to use paintbrushes on her back, neck, legs and genitals. I use a variety of sizes—small for delicate areas and larger ones on her back. Last spring I bought a vibrator. I was doing my routine with the brushes and decided to hold them against the vibrator, using both to massage her. The result was a long night with a very aroused girlfriend. Have you heard of this combination?—J.W., Auburn, Alabama

It's new to us. You couldn't have chosen a better canvas.

The art of sex

I am working on a class project on sex as art. The women I've interviewed have shown incredible interest, and one suggested we paint our bodies different colors, then have sex on a giant sheet of paper to display with the assignment. I thought this was an excellent idea, especially because she's gorgeous. Where can I find paints that dry slowly and that won't irritate tender body parts? We've chosen the colors already: purple and yellow.— M.B., Indianapolis, Indiana

We are curious—yellow? That may not be bright enough to reflect the meditative luminosity of the figurative curve. Purple we like. We don't have much experience touching up anything in the bedroom besides the trim, so we asked Rob

Blaine of MessyFun.com for his input. Blaine, who dumps buckets of paint and other liquids on naked women for fetish videos, says: "I use standard latex (water-based) indoor house paint which I cut with dishwashing detergent to help with cleanup. Eight gallons on three women doesn't get a chance to dry, and the time the girls are covered is kept to a minimum. I wouldn't recommend sex in latex paint; instead I would use nontoxic finger paints. You can buy them by the case through a school supply or art supply house." We'd love to see a copy of your work when it's finished—sign it with whatever's handy.

How to write a dirty story

My wife is reading Susie Bright's *Best American Erotica* and I thought it would be fun to surprise her with a personal story. I'm not much of a writer. I know a few friends who could help, but I don't want to share secrets about what turns my wife on. Can I hire someone to write a sexy story that contains personal details?—S.C., Boulder, Colorado

Don't be too quick to discount the do-it-yourself approach. You know your wife better than anyone. She'll be touched, if not turned on, and she won't correct your grammar. If you'd rather go pro, Custom Erotica Source offers one-page quickies for $25 each that might be fun. You fill out a questionnaire to provide the names of characters, a setting, information about the reader, specific turn-ons he or she might have and how explicit you'd like the language and activity. A writer then crafts a fantasy that you can preview and approve before it's mailed or e-mailed to your wife. You also can order a six-page story for $125 or a 12-page story for $250, put the fantasy on tape for an additional $30, add an illustration for $75 and up, or order custom stories by writers whose work has appeared in Best American Erotica *and other series. Visit Customeroticasource.com or phone 415-664-6602 for details.*

Short strokes, or long?

During intercourse, do women prefer short strokes or long ones? I try to vary my technique, but sometimes my partner says I'm not pushing deep enough, or that I'm pushing too deep. Which way should I go?—H.D., Akron, Ohio

Go the way your partner tells you to go. If there are no verbal signals, pay attention to the nonverbal ones. Don't make a plan—sometimes shallow is good, sometimes you need to go deep. One Taoist technique calls for the man to repeat a sequence of nine shallow thrusts and one deep. Our advice: Don't count out loud.

Hankie panky

On a cozy Sunday afternoon a few weekends ago, a girlfriend and I fumbled onto a wonderful sexual technique. I took a hankie and folded it into a triangle. Holding a corner in each hand I slipped the hankie under my scrotum, pulled up the ends and tied them in a knot. The knot was tight enough to cause my testes to jut forward and my penis to become engorged. I tied the loose hankie ends into four more knots. The knots went up toward my belly button. After I slid on top of her, my girlfriend went nuts. The combination of my testes on her anus and the knots rubbing her clitoris gave her an earth-shaking orgasm. I too benefited from the experience. Have you heard of this? If so, what's it called?—H.C., Arlington, Virginia

Ingenuity, man. Ingenuity.

Perfecting the touch

When I finger my girlfriend, she says that I'm too rough. My exes never complained about my touch. When I lighten it, she says it tickles. What can I do?—S.C., Toronto, Ontario

Ask your girlfriend to masturbate for you. Place your hand over hers to get an idea of the pressure she applies and where. She shouldn't be shy about giving you specific instructions about what turns her on.

Reader suggestions

I invented a way to please myself and my wife at the end of a long day when one or both of us isn't in the mood to make love. My wife lies on her stomach and I position myself so I can cradle my erection between her butt cheeks, pointed toward her head. As I grind myself to orgasm, I massage her back. We call it back-rub sex. Have you ever heard of this? Does it have an official name?—B.C., Duluth, Minnesota

An official name? Like, from a committee? The scientific name is probably related to coitus interfermoris, *which is the act of rubbing yourself to orgasm between a woman's thighs or against her perineum. It also could be related to* coitus à mammilla *(having sex with her breasts),* axillism *(armpit) or* genuphallation *(between the knees) with a dash of* pygophilia *(arousal from fondling, kissing or licking the ass). Like an astronomer who discovers a new star, this position may be yours to christen. May we suggest* coitus à gluteus?

My girlfriend and I enjoy something similar. She lies on me facing the ceiling. With a good sweat going, we don't need lubrication, just sliding and grinding. It puts me in a great position to fondle her breasts, ass and clit.—S.C., Dallas, Texas

A reader from Philadelphia tells us the position is known as slip-dogging.

I've developed a wonderful new massage technique. I have my girlfriend lie on her back with her knees bent. I slowly slide my right index and middle fingers into her pussy and make a come-hither motion to stimulate her G-spot. I then place the heel of my left hand on her mons and stroke her clitoris. My girlfriend likes to raise and lower her knees while I do this. What do you think?—D.S., Los Angeles, California

Sounds like fun. Isn't that how they used to churn butter?

I want to share a technique I use to give my lovers intense orgasms. While she is on top and I am inside her, I ask her to move her hips in a circular motion. Then I press my open hand or fist on the area three to four inches above her clitoris. By doing this, the head of my penis makes direct contact with her G-spot, which has given many of my lovers their first ejaculatory climaxes.—M.W., Silver Spring, Maryland

Fixing a squeaky bed

My girlfriend moved into a furnished apartment that has a metal bed. It makes more noise than we do. Do you know how to silence a squeaky bed?—D.E., Des Moines, Iowa

Have your girlfriend finger each nut while you add lube. Then do the same to fix the bed.

Mood lighting

My wife has suggested that we liven things up with new lightbulbs in the bedroom. What color do you suggest?—P.W., Memphis, Tennessee

We're happy just to have the lights on. In The Great Sex Weekend, *Pepper Schwartz and Janet Lever tackle this question with Marsha Hunt, a writer and producer for Playboy Home Video. "We always use blue light in our bedroom scenes," Hunt says. "It creates a mysterious and sensual atmosphere. It gives sufficient light to see, but it's dim enough to cover flaws. Pink bulbs provide light that is soft, romantic and flattering—it makes most people look much younger—but stick to a 40-watt bulb. Stay away from green—that's monster movie lighting—and yellow, which makes skin look sallow." Schwartz and Lever don't recommend red bulbs because "they make your bedroom look like a brothel." Considering the wild sex that can go on in whorehouses, red may not be such a bad choice. You'll find colored bulbs at well-stocked hardware stores.*

Riding the dome

Have you ever heard of a "dome ride"? If you have shaved your head, you must give your girlfriend or wife this experience. To prepare, don't shave your dome for a day or two. If you're someone like me who suffers from male-pattern bullshit, there will soon be a spot on your crown where you have smooth skin surrounded by slightly rough hair growth. Slide your head between her legs, let her find her spot, tell her to clamp down and start the ride. Not only is this great foreplay, but with a quick turn, your mouth is right where it should be. Finding the best position for the ride might take a few minutes, but that can be hot (and humorous) in itself. As a man who loves to satisfy his woman, it's incredible to feel her come all over my dome.—G.W., San Francisco, California

You just helped several million balding guys get laid.

LETTERS THAT DIDN'T MAKE THE CUT*

* but not for lack of trying

---

(1) "Fleas are ruining my life . . ."

(2) "I've had several nervous breakdowns. Obviously I can't be an astronaut or an airline pilot. But could I be a lawyer?"

(3) "Can a human catch any animal venereal diseases? I own a large dog, and I was on my knees and elbows, naked, searching for a CD, when . . ."

(4) "Do you know of any movies in which love is portrayed as the main theme but with lots of penis-in-vagina shots?"

(5) "Do you think my gallbladder problems are related to my coffee enemas?"

(6) "Our mother-son relationship has gone to the next level, and now I'm pregnant. How do I tell my husband?"

(7) From a prisoner: "Can you tell me who sells the book *Escape and Evasion*? I'd also like information about GPS systems."

(8) "You missed the boat with the reader concerned about his wife's pale areolae. Why not have her areolae tattooed dark brown? Dear Abby would have thought of that."

(9) "The ghosts of my parents often visit our house. We're planning to move. Are there any religious procedures that will get them to come to our new house?"

(10) "Although I'm a Christian, here is a list of things I would do if Marie Osmond were here with me . . ."

(11) "Whenever I cover the head of my penis with purple nail polish, I glue the hole shut so none will go in. I've enclosed four photos. Please write back if you would like to know more."

(12) "I have found the perfect toothbrush. If I buy 200 of them to last me the next 40 years, can you provide storage instructions?"

CONTACTING THE PLAYBOY ADVISOR

All reasonable questions—from fashion, food and drink, stereo and sports cars to dating dilemmas, taste and etiquette—will be personally answered if the writer includes a self-addressed, stamped envelope. The most interesting, pertinent questions will be presented in the column each month. Write The Playboy Advisor, 730 Fifth Avenue, New York, New York 10019, or send e-mail by visiting our website at playboyadvisor.com.